An Officer and a Lady

Studies in Canadian Military History

The Canadian War Museum, Canada's national museum of military history, has a threefold mandate: to remember, to preserve, and to educate. It does so through an interlocking and mutually supporting combination of exhibitions, public programs, and electronic outreach. Military history, military historical scholarship, and the ways in which Canadians see and understand themselves have always been closely intertwined. Studies in Canadian Military History builds on a record of success in forging those links by regular and innovative contributions based on the best contemporary scholarship. Published by UBC Press in association with the Museum, the series especially encourages the work of new generations of scholars and the investigation of important gaps in the existing historiography, pursuits not always well served by traditional sources of academic support. The results produced feed immediately into future exhibitions, programs, and outreach efforts by the Canadian War Museum. It is a modest goal that they feed into a deeper understanding of our nation's common past as well.

Cynthia Toman

An Officer and a Lady
Canadian Military Nursing and
the Second World War

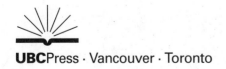
UBCPress · Vancouver · Toronto

16 15 14 13 12 11 10 09 08 07   5 4 3 2 1

Printed in Canada on ancient-forest-free paper (100% post-consumer recycled) that is processed chlorine- and acid-free, with vegetable-based inks.

Library and Archives Canada Cataloguing in Publication

Toman, Cynthia, 1948-
     An officer and a lady : Canadian military nursing and the Second World War / Cynthia Toman.

(Studies in Canadian military history, 1499-6251)
   Includes bibliographical references and index.
   ISBN 978-0-7748-1447-8 (bound); 978-0-7748-1448-5 (pbk)

        1. Canada – Armed Forces – Nurses – History – 20th century. 2. Military nursing – Canada
     – History – 20th century. 3. World War, 1939-1945 – Canada – Participation, Female. 4. World War,
     1939-1945 – Women – Canada. 5. Canada – Armed Forces – Women – History – 20th century.
     6. Women and war – Canada – History – 20th century. 7. World War, 1939-1945 – Medical care
     – Canada. 8. Nurses – Canada – History – 20th century. I. Title. II. Series.

D807.C2T64 2007   940.54'7571082   C2007-903461-6

Canadä

UBC Press gratefully acknowledges the financial support for our publishing program of the Government of Canada through the Book Publishing Industry Development Program (BPIDP), and of the Canada Council for the Arts, and the British Columbia Arts Council.

This book has been published with the help of a grant from the Canadian Federation for the Humanities and Social Sciences, through the Aid to Scholarly Publications Programme, using funds provided by the Social Sciences and Humanities Research Council of Canada.

Publication of this book has been financially supported by the Canadian War Museum. The author and publisher also acknowledge the financial assistance of the Faculty of Health Sciences, University of Ottawa.

Printed and bound in Canada
Set in Fairfield by Blakeley
Copy editor: Barbara Tessman
Proofreader: Gail Copeland
Indexer: Patricia Buchanan

UBC Press
The University of British Columbia
2029 West Mall
Vancouver, BC V6T 1Z2
604.822.5959 / Fax 604.822.6083
www.ubcpress.ca

Contents

Illustrations and Tables

Illustrations

Acknowledgments

There has been increasing interest in the Second World War Canadian nursing sisters since the early 1990s, resulting in several television documentaries and news articles, especially during the annual November Remembrance Week commemorations. Like other veterans, there are fewer nursing sisters every year and fewer opportunities to learn from their first-hand accounts about war as nurses' work. But, unlike the men who served during the war, these military nurses are marginalized within the official histories and seldom visible within official documents and archival collections.

I am deeply indebted, then, to the twenty-five nursing sisters – well into their eighties and even nineties at the time – who participated in oral history interviews. I extend a personal thanks to each one, for they are the main actors of this history, and it has truly been a pleasure and a privilege to work with them. Lt.-Col. (retired) Harriet J.T. Sloan patiently introduced me to military contexts, fielding a multitude of inquiries and providing introductions to military nurses across Canada, and graciously read developing manuscripts. She is a remarkable friend who served during the Second World War and later, became the matron-in-chief of the combined Canadian Forces Medical Services (1964-68). I dedicate *An Officer and a Lady* to the Second World War Canadian nursing sisters, with the hope that they might recognize themselves and their experiences within its pages.

A number of organizations and archives provided important and timely assistance and encouragement. In particular, I thank colleagues from the Canadian Association for the History of Nursing, the British Columbia History of Nursing Professional Practice Group, the College and Association of Registered Nurses of Alberta Museum and Archives, and the Margaret M. Allemang Centre for the History of Nursing. They helped to identify significant material relevant to the research, as well as potential nursing sisters from across Canada for the interviews. Judith Young facilitated the transcription of Margaret Allemang's oral history interviews, which included an additional fourteen Second World War nursing sisters, and pointed out other sources held by the centre. The late Edith Landells shared generously from her experiences of publishing a collection of letters solicited from military nurses who served with various armed forces and periods. Anne Crossin, archivist at the Winnipeg General Hospital and Health Sciences Nurses' Alumnae Archives, and Lorraine Mychajlunow, archivist at the College and Association of Registered Nurses of Alberta Museum and Archives, facilitated access to the collections held by their respective organizations. Dr. Charles Roland, Hannah Chair for the History of Medicine at McMaster University, generously gave me a transcript of his interview with Nursing Sister Kay Christie shortly before her death in 1994. In addition, there were innumerable research assistants at Library and Archives Canada, the Canadian War Museum, and the Department of National Defence Directorate of History and Heritage who helped me with the mysteries of military records, photographs, documentary art, audiovisual collections, and even musical scores related to nursing sisters.

I was extremely fortunate to work with two excellent supervisors at the University of Ottawa during doctoral studies there. Dr. Ruby Heap guided me through the intricacies of history and women's studies while Dr. Meryn Stuart introduced me to nursing history as a field and mentored me along the paths of scholarship and academia. The Social Sciences and Humanities Research Council generously supported my studies and research through a doctoral fellowship.

Emily Andrew, senior editor for UBC Press, offered her enthusiasm and support for a book on the nursing sisters – even before I was ready to take that step. Dean Oliver, general editor of the Studies in Canadian Military History series at UBC Press, and the Canadian War Museum have generously supported this book as part of the series. Many thanks are due to the anonymous manuscript reviewers for their time, insights, and suggestions. The University of Ottawa Press and the Canadian Museum of Civilization, Sumach Press, and *Histoire sociale/Social History* kindly permitted the use of overlapping material from my previously published articles with them.

Families inevitably share in the process of "making history" through their many accommodations to the author's research and writing activities. A very special thanks to each member of my family for their sustaining support, even as they eagerly tracked my progress towards the finish line.

Abbreviations

CAMC	Canadian Army Medical Corps
CCS	casualty clearing station
CEF	Canadian Expeditionary Force
CGH	Canadian General Hospital
CHC	Canadian Hospital Council
CMA	Canadian Medical Association
CNA	Canadian Nurses Association
DVA	Department of Veterans Affairs
FDS	field dressing station
FSU	field surgical unit, also called a field surgical centre
FTU	field transfusion unit
ICN	International Council of Nurses
MO	medical officer
NS	nursing sister
NSAC	Nursing Sisters' Association of Canada
POW	prisoner of war
QAIMNS	Queen Alexandra's Imperial Military Nursing Service
RCAF	Royal Canadian Air Force
RCAMC	Royal Canadian Army Medical Corps
RCN	Royal Canadian Navy
RNAO	Registered Nurses Association of Ontario
SAMNS	South African Military Nursing Service
SEC	Special Employment Company
SIW	self-inflicted wound
USANC	United States Army Nurse Corps
VAD	voluntary aid detachment
WD	Women's Division

An Officer and a Lady

Introduction

From the late 1800s through the Second World War, Western societies significantly changed their perceptions of medical and nursing care for sick and wounded soldiers. These shifts escalated during the First World War, coming to the fore in Canada with the political activism of veterans who engaged in a prolonged struggle for medical and social rehabilitation during the postwar period. They came to view care increasingly as a right, or a type of "social wage" that societies "owed" soldiers for services on behalf of their country or nation.[1] These changing social perceptions precipitated debates about who should provide such care and where it should be given, how military medical units should be organized and administered, and how civilian and military needs for medical personnel should be balanced during times of war when the demands for care increased dramatically. The role of nurses and skilled nursing care became increasingly important in these debates, which were conducted in the context of gendered constructions of femininity and masculinity – particularly within the military – as well as of nurses' own personal and professional agenda for an emerging field of paid women's work.

This book focuses on Canadian military nurses and their work during the Second World War (1939-45). It examines how gender intersected with class, ethnicity, and, to a lesser degree, race in transforming at least 4,079 civilian nurses into military nurses. Although race is not a primary focus in this analysis, it was a critical tool for the selection of the 'right kind of nurses' for the armed forces during this era – that is, white nurses. An exploration of white privilege in this context can inform understanding of broader issues of race. We are very limited in what we can and cannot know about the workings of race within this context, however, because non-white women are conspicuously absent from the rank and from the records.

I also seek a nuanced understanding of the complex issues of who became nursing sisters, why they enlisted, and the legacies of military nursing for postwar civilian practices. Through the study of a specific cohort of military nurses, this book explores the incongruities and ambivalence associated with nurses and war work. It analyses how nursing skills and knowledge regarding medical technologies enabled civilian nurses to create female spaces within the male-dominated military world and illuminates ways by which nurses facilitated the expansion of medical technologies and nursing care within the armed forces.

The military – including its medical services – was a masculine environment throughout the nineteenth century. Physicians, surgeons, stretcher bearers, and orderlies selected from the ranks of enlisted men served with military medical services, staffing regimental aid posts and field ambulances as needed. During the Crimean War (1853-56), women such as Florence Nightingale exerted considerable social and political pressure for medical and sanitary reform within the British army. They were successful in introducing a small number of women volunteers, some of whom had formal training as nurses, to care for soldiers but these women served in an auxiliary capacity and not within the military itself.[2] By the time of the First World War, diverse groups of women in many countries sought ways to become involved in the care of soldiers as one way for women to participate in the war effort. Efforts varied from privately funding and operating their own women's hospitals located near battle zones to joining Voluntary Aid Detachment units or enrolling with auxiliary nursing services such as Red Cross hospitals. This range of trained, semi-trained, and untrained women precipitated a great deal of controversy both within and outside of the allied armed forces. Some of the controversies developed because volunteer nurses were not under military control; other controversies arose because they often lacked necessary skills, training, and discipline for military environments.[3]

With the formation of the first permanent nursing service as part of the Canadian Army Medical Corps (CAMC) in 1904, civilian nurses were fully integrated into the Canadian armed forces as soldiers; they enlisted as lieutenants with the specially created officer's rank and title of Nursing Sister (NS).[4] Graduation from a recognized school of nursing had become one of the basic requirements for enlistment with the CAMC by 1914, effectively excluding untrained and semi-trained women from the Canadian forces. Civilian nurses readily filled every available position with the CAMC during the First World War, thereby assuring an adequate supply of military nurses as well as a standardized set of nursing skills based on civilian training and credentials. They constituted the first generation of Canadian Nursing Sisters.

Trained Canadian civilian nurses volunteered again during the Second World War in numbers so large that the military placed a moratorium on their enlistment only ten days after the call to mobilize medical units, contradicting military historian C.P. Stacey's pronouncement of Canada as a very "unmilitary community."[5] They eagerly filled all nursing positions with the Royal Canadian Army Medical Corps (RCAMC) and, later, with the Royal Canadian Air Force (RCAF) and the Royal Canadian Navy (RCN) when separate nursing service branches formed in 1940 and 1941. Thousands more added their names to a waiting list that grew longer each year; still others, tired of waiting, joined the allied American, British, and South African nursing services. This enthusiasm for enlistment contrasted sharply with the conscription of Canadian men beginning in 1940 and the contentious American campaign to conscript nurses in order to fill national quotas between 1943 and 1945 for the United States armed forces.[6]

This second generation of Canadian nursing sisters benefited from the legacy of their foremothers during the First World War, inheriting officers' status, privileges, and pay as well as work opportunities, travel, adventure, and access to the frontlines, where large numbers of men spent the war. Although nurses enlisted under the protection of the Geneva Convention, which classified medical personnel as non-combatant and neutral, Canadian nursing sisters increasingly perceived themselves as soldiers; they called themselves soldiers and they understood their work as "winning the war" through the salvage of damaged men.[7] They actively sought opportunities to move closer to the frontlines, readily accepting increased risk and danger as part of the job. The armed forces highly valued their knowledge and skills, reluctantly moving them forward as they demonstrated better outcomes for the soldiers under their care than less well-trained personnel could achieve. The military was adamant, however, that nurses were temporary; they were intended to serve only "for the duration" of the war, regardless of what the nurses wanted or needed.

These ordinary military nurses and the everyday work that they performed are the subjects of this book. Through social history and feminist approaches, I shift the analysis away from stereotypical portrayals as angels and heroines (images with which the nurses themselves are uncomfortable) to examine how gender, war, and medical technology intersected to legitimate their participation in a predominantly masculine military domain. Nursing sisters were witnesses to everyday events in hospital wards, tents, operating rooms, and casualty clearing stations as they cared for civilians and refugees as well as soldiers throughout the war. Their accounts offer alternative perspectives to irresolvable debates about the causes, politics, and strategies of war. As Erich Maria Remarque, author of the 1928 novel *All Quiet on the Western Front,* suggested, "A hospital alone shows what war is."[8]

The association of nurses with the armed forces, war, and killing is unsettling, partially because these contexts have been constructed as masculine domains and therefore antithetical to nursing, which is often seen as the epitome of femininity and pacifism. Our uneasiness and ambivalence regarding nurses as soldiers, however, has obscured their presence as well as the work that they performed on and behind the frontlines. They are women "out of place" or "dis-placed" from the more familiar civilian practice environments of the 1930s and 1940s such as hospitals and private duty settings.

Although positioned at the intersection of multiple fields of historical inquiry, military nurses remain all but invisible within national histories, military histories, women's histories, and nursing histories. For the most part, historians have treated them as a homogeneous category regardless of the very different historical contexts in which they served or the diversity among them. Nursing sisters contributed to their own invisibility through self-censorship and a reticence about sharing their war experiences, thus compounding the usual challenges of studying women's history through official records and documents. Jan Bassett, referring to the historiography on Australian military nurses, concluded that historians have generally ignored or sanctified military nurses while feminists have overlooked them as ideologically unsound, and that most military nursing histories consist primarily of anecdotes and chronologies.[9] A small body of international literature permits limited comparison of military nursing contexts and experiences, although little attention has been given to nurses' actual work or what it meant to larger war endeavours.

Canadian literature on the Second World War includes official histories, political and social histories, organizational histories, and popular histories that establish the chronology and document the larger contexts of the war, enabling us to situate the Canadian nursing sisters in relation to other men and women as well as major military campaigns that shaped their work.[10] The military medical services subsumed nursing sisters within their records and, similarly, within their histories while focusing on physicians (medical officers) and portraying nurses mostly as ancillary personnel.[11] One can catch glimpses of nurses' work hidden between the lines of these accounts describing infections, illnesses, trauma, medical technology, and medical and surgical procedures used during the war. When the Nursing Sisters' Association of Canada commissioned its organizational history in the 1970s, that volume became the first publication to focus specifically on military nurses.[12] It has remained the most commonly referenced account of Canadian military nursing, contributing importantly to documentation on the formation of various units, chronologies, and nursing leaders – a daunting task given the mobility of hospital units following the troops in battle. Veteran nurses frequently comment, however, that it is difficult to see rank-and-file nurses or their work reflected in this account. Jean Bruce referred to a "great historical silence" surrounding Canadian women and war service in 1979, when she documented women's activities on the home front and with military and paramilitary organizations. She described her book as a montage of personal stories, statements, and visual images. Her chapter on military nurses, like three other collections and an art book about women who served in the Canadian armed forces, relies heavily on the organizational history of the Nursing Sisters' Association of Canada.[13]

Most of the research related to women and war focuses on the First World

War period and tends to dismiss nurses as women whose gendered involvement in war neither threatened nor altered the status quo. This literature
seldom distinguishes between trained professionals and semi-trained or
untrained volunteers, however, treating "nurse" as a universal category. For
example, Susan Grayzel, Angela Smith, and Margaret Higonnet have each
studied women's participation in the First World War and contributed significantly to the field. Grayzel compared the porous boundaries between "war
fronts" and "home fronts" in Britain and France, considering both informal
and formal nursing as one type of wartime involvement and concluding that
war continued, rather than shattered, the reconstruction of gender relations
and identities.[14] Smith, who examined private testimonies and published
accounts by three trained and semi-trained women who did nursing work
in French hospitals during the First World War, used post-modern discourse
analysis to uncover links between warfare and literary development.[15] She
refers to military hospitals as a "second battlefield," challenges the angel
metaphor, and suggests that women's power over hospitalized male bodies inverted the usual roles and expectations related to gender, class, and
sexuality. Higonnet examined writings by two of the same women as Smith
did, a trained nurse and a novelist/hospital volunteer, but from the perspective of literary criticism of their self-representation and portrayals of their
soldier patients.[16] The strong dependence in this literature on a small body
of women's writings limits what we can know, especially regarding everyday
military nurses and their work.

Cynthia Enloe was one of the earliest scholars to include military nurses
in her analysis of the militarization of women's lives. She argued that war
and military discourse depend on women's support for the recruitment and
re-enlistment of men, for sanitary and caring tasks required to keep troops
healthy, and for replacement labour that released men for war.[17] Revisiting
the topic fifteen years later, Enloe examined the insidious and pervasive ways
in which both civilian and enlisted women become militarized. She analysed
ways in which individuals and whole societies "come to imagine military
needs and militaristic presumptions to be not only valuable but also normal,"
defining militarization as a "process by which a person or a thing gradually
comes to be controlled by the military *or* comes to depend for its well-being
on militaristic ideas." In this study, I build on significant questions raised by
Enloe concerning what is gained and lost when nurses become integral to
military systems.[18]

During the late 1980s and early 1990s, important work emerged on war as a
"gendering activity." Both Joan Scott and Ruth Roach Pierson synthesized this
body of literature, identifying key debates within it. Scott suggests there is
one basic theme, which frames war as either a positive or negative "watershed"
experience for women. The theme has four variations: new opportunities that
did or did not open up for women during war; new political rights such as

suffrage that were based on women's wartime participation; women's antipathy to war and their consequent leadership of pacifist movements; and the long- and short-term impact of war on women.[19] For example, some authors challenge the construction of war as stereotypically male while others suggest that power, economics, and status among men and women tend to remain unchanged even in the armed forces. This argument is best represented by Margaret Higonnet's "double helix" concept that allows for variation while maintaining the same relative positions of power between military women and men.[20] According to Scott, these debates are irresolvable and problematic. She calls for more attention to state policies related to women and to metaphoric uses of gender representations. Pierson suggests that the women and war literature perpetuates two stereotypical, dichotomous metaphors that portray women as "beautiful souls" and men as "just warriors."[21] Jean Elshtain is a notable exception with her study of gendered discourses that contradict these images and portray both women and men as potential beautiful souls or just warriors. Elshtain refers to nurses as "battle zone witnesses to the spectacle of war," suggesting that nursing "allowed women to get close to that action of which they are not an active part."[22]

Recent circumstances have converged to facilitate historical research on Second World War nursing sisters. Although time was running out due to advancing age and declining health, many of these women were still available for interview during this study, offering unique opportunities to document their first-hand accounts. Families of deceased nursing sisters are also discovering letters, photographs, and diaries created during the war and are beginning to make them accessible to researchers. In addition, many recent fiftieth- and sixtieth-anniversary commemorations of war-related events, along with the creation of a new war museum in Ottawa and an increased urgency among aging veterans to share their experiences with Canadian youth, have generated renewed interest in the Second World War period. Now in their late eighties to mid-nineties, nursing sisters were ready to recall what it was like to make the transition from civilian to military life and back again, to care for both soldiers and civilian casualties in a wide range of settings and circumstances, and to work with other medical personnel under less than ideal conditions.

Twenty-five remarkable nursing sisters shared their first-hand accounts with me in audiotaped oral history interviews conducted during 2001.[23] We share a professional status as nurses, although I am an outsider to the military community, and when they occasionally chose not to share particular experiences, I respected the boundaries they set. I refer to these nursing sisters by their birth surnames (the names by which they were known on enlistment), and identify them directly within the text. I reference each individual's interview only when used for the first time in a chapter and thereafter, refer to that nursing sister simply by name. The appendix contains a brief biographical profile for each. In addition to their interviews, I selected another thirty interviews from various collections in national, provincial, and private archives across Canada, to represent a broad range of wartime settings and contexts. I document the source for these additional interviews with both footnotes and names within the text. This combined set of oral history interviews is supplemented by memoirs, letters, diaries, scrapbooks, artifacts, and personal photographs of additional nursing sisters as well as material published in nursing and medical journals during and after the war.

To complement the interviews, oral histories and published materials, I generated a database based on demographic variables extracted from 1,145 individual Second World War nursing sister personnel files of the Department of National Defence (creating a 26 percent sample).[24] The resulting aggregated data provide new insights related to places of origin, residence, parentage, training, previous experience, average age, marital status, religious affiliation, languages spoken, postings, and postwar plans. In addition, these data include nurses who were dead or who were unavailable for interviews because of their location, health status, or memory loss. The data thus broaden our understanding of the cohort as a whole. The department's records were created during the war and originally intended to document the government's postwar obligation to veterans. Like other sources, they are limited according to who created each file, the modification of forms during the war, methods of transferring them between settings, and conditions of preservation.[25]

Official military documents and records were helpful in establishing the various contexts in which nurses served, although they revealed surprisingly little of these women's actual nursing practice. According to historian Tim Cook, the Army Historical Section produced a mass of documentary evidence on the Second World War: 200,000 Canadian Military Headquarters subject files, 20 million sheets of paper, and 132,000 war diaries. Cook concludes that "Clio's soldiers were not simple scribes or passive archivists ... They actively sought out the war record, influencing ... how the war would be captured and ultimately codified in print."[26] He points out how army historian C.P. Stacey directed the production of war records in the field during active campaigns as well as after the war and how he circulated accounts for revision and censored other information.[27] There are over five hundred individual war diaries pertaining to different types of medical units such as general hospital units, casualty clearing stations, field surgical units, field dressing stations, and transfusion units. A sampling of these diaries demonstrates their focus on organizational aspects and accounting rather than reflection of medical or nursing work. Depending on who was assigned recording duty, the records obscure as much or more than they reveal, especially about nursing sisters, who seldom appear except as personnel who transferred into and out of medical units.

Several theoretical perspectives inform my analysis of military nurses and their work. Building on historian Kathryn McPherson's argument that the mastery of nursing techniques provided civilian nurses with marketable skills and expertise that differentiated them from non-professional caregivers, I analyse military nurses' work through the lens of medical technology associated with the Second World War.[28] Following social construction of technology approaches, I have adopted a broad conceptualization of technologies as large technological systems that are historically situated within specific socio-political and economic contexts.[29] Such systems are both socially constructed and society shaping. They include all the components and actors considered necessary in order to achieve a common system goal, such as physical artifacts; organizational structures such as manufacturing, transportation, and banking; scientific components such as books, articles, university teaching, and research programs; legislative and regulatory policies; and natural resources.[30] Within this framework, the artifacts may be physical or non-physical, and all components are interrelated, meaning that changes in one aspect effect changes in the rest of the system. Technological systems are constructed by system builders who hold the balance of power by controlling as much of the system as possible, for as long as possible.

Military medical technology, as understood within this framework, consists of more than instruments, equipment, and pharmaceutical products. It includes the skilled application of these tools, the associated knowledge to innovate and improvise under wartime conditions, and the therapeutic use of self when technology reached its limits. It includes the participation of medical personnel in research on drugs and surgical procedures as well as policies and regulations governing decisions about patient care. Technology includes training programs, transportation components in the chain of evacuation, physical and psychological screening tools that held power to determine who was a casualty, and systems for sorting patients and documenting their care – to name only some of the elements that constituted the Second World War military-medical-technological system.

By conceptualizing military nursing through this lens, it becomes possible to explore the complexity of nurses' work as well as the multiple variables that shaped it. Nurses mobilized their skills for the war effort, capitalizing on their expertise to secure decently paid work that also relocated them closer to the centre of wartime events. In the process, they also facilitated the use of increased medical technology ever closer to the frontlines, significantly increasing the number of casualties who were able to return to active duty as well as reducing the time involved for recovery. As a result, the provision of adequate nursing care became an important part of strategic planning for battles and campaigns such as the Invasion of Italy in 1943 and the Invasion of Northwestern Europe in 1944.

Focused primarily on system builders, however, the social construction of technology approaches may deny or minimize agency for other actors within the systems. Such approaches also have limited explanatory ability regarding how social shaping takes place, how power is distributed and contested, and how variables of difference such as class, race, ethnicity, and gender work within such systems – questions that call for gender as an analytical concept. Gender analysis exposes the multiple ways in which power is unequally distributed within military medical systems, as well as "fundamental differences that divide gendered subjects" and the "historically specific processes that unite people into a shared gendered consciousness."[31]

War, gender, and medical technology intersected to transform civilian nurses into military nurses "only for the duration" of war, but many nursing sisters constructed an enduring identity as military nurses based on shared experiences. Yet most of them worked and socialized within the relatively confined environments of their immediate medical units during the war. How then did such a strong military identity develop? What purposes did this collective identity serve? And how has it contributed to shaping both a personal and social memory based on this period of their lives?[32] The concept of "symbolic community" has guided this part of the analysis. Although much of the original scholarship on symbolic community focused on nation building, sociologists and historians have expanded the concept well beyond spatial structures and regional boundaries to encompass social structures and relationships.[33] A.P. Cohen identified more than ninety definitions of community within the social sciences literature, for example, arguing on behalf of community as a mental construct distinguished through the constructed meanings shared by those who claim membership. He directs us to examine important questions such as how a community creates particular symbols, how it constructs a public face, how it remembers the past, and how it uses the past for present integrity.[34]

This book begins by situating Second World War nursing sisters in relation not only to nurses who served with the Canadian armed forces prior to 1939 but also to the socio-economic contexts of the 1930s. Most of these women were born or grew up during the First World War and either trained or searched for work as nurses during the Great Depression. The professional, technological, and military contexts of the interwar years made military nursing service a very attractive alternative. When Great Britain declared war on Germany in August 1939, civilian nurses were once again ready to enlist.

The armed forces considered nurses, once they were enlisted, to be an expandable and expendable workforce – one that it could readily transform into military nurses for the duration of the war. Civilian nurse leaders and hospitals resisted the flood of nurse resignations to enlist, lobbying the armed forces in efforts to balance the need for nurses in both practice settings. The military carefully controlled the public perceptions and media portrayals related to nursing sisters, particularly reinforcing messages about their safety and femininity. Nurses, in turn, negotiated significant social and professional space within this traditionally male domain, although gender shaped all decisions about what they could do, and where and when they could do it.

The admission of women to the ranks generated a great deal of anxiety, especially in relation to their continuous close proximity to men in social and work settings as well as the potential for various types of danger. According to prevailing discourse of the time, women needed the protection of men, and wartime service threatened their femininity.[35] Therefore, the armed forces developed specific gender- and class-based regulations and policies that ensured that nursing sisters comported themselves as "officers" and "ladies" at all times. Although nurses contested these expectations to different degrees, the nurses' success was contingent on geographical distance from Canada and changing conditions during the war itself, which permitted increased flexibility.

Nurses were able to capitalize on their skills and knowledge as actors within a large military-medical-technological system dedicated to the care of military personnel. Innovations in medicine, surgery, and drugs brought opportunities to move closer to the frontlines of war and the frontiers of medical technology, where they learned new skills and challenged the established boundaries between physicians' work and nurses' work. The technological and military contexts in which they practised shaped the nursing care of soldiers, reconfiguring some aspects while maintaining others. But for the most part, those changes failed to transform postwar and non-military settings to any significant degree.

At the end of the war, there was no longer any need for a large military nurse contingent. The armed forces demobilized them as rapidly as possible, downsizing the number to a total of eighty nurses within all three service branches. Although a nursing shortage began to emerge in civilian settings during the 1940s, most nursing sisters married, left the profession, or sought non-traditional practice settings. Many of them maintained contact with one another through local and national nursing sister associations that met regularly over the following sixty years, developing an enduring symbolic community based on gender, shared experiences, and identities as military nurses. With time, this community solidified around certain portrayals of military nursing, adopting a set of rituals and symbols and forging a collective social memory. They actively promoted military nursing to younger generations of nurses while seeking to reconcile nursing ideologies with military objectives.

"Ready, Aye Ready": Enlisting Nurses

Nursing became respectable paid work for Canadian women, gradually more acceptable from the 1870s through the 1930s, due to a number of changes in both the medical and nursing fields. With medical technology on the rise in hospitals, nurses increasingly shifted their emphasis from domestic duties to technological skills, and such skills became the basis of nurses' claims to scientific legitimacy and professional recognition.[1] The standardization of nurses' training, improvement of their working conditions, and pressure for adequate pay became important issues that prompted the Canadian Medical Association and the Canadian Nurses Association to commission a study of nursing in Canada in 1929. The *Survey of Nursing Education in Canada*, published in 1932 and known popularly as the Weir Report, provides an excellent portrait of the state of civilian nursing and working conditions at the beginning of the decade prior to the Second World War.[2] One can safely infer that these conditions only worsened as economic depression deepened in Canada.

Like many Canadians, nurses struggled with varying levels of deprivation and uncertainty during the Great Depression. Nursing was often a second or even third occupational change for many single women in search of economic security. Historian Kathryn McPherson has described training programs as analogous to "riding the rails" for men of the same period, arguing that "while their brothers rode the rails looking for work and handouts, rural women went to nursing school."[3] Student nurses were able to trade their labour for room, board, and skilled training for at least three years, but this survival strategy could only be temporary. On graduation, these new nurses worsened the employment situation as the profession struggled with oversupply and underemployment in relation to the public's ability to pay for private nursing care in the days before universal public medical insurance. The vast majority of working nurses were single women practising in private duty, as hospitals did not typically employ nurses after graduation from training programs. Without the support of male relatives as breadwinners (thereby reducing the burden on their families) and without hospitals as a significant source for employment, nurses experienced the Depression in particular gendered ways because government efforts to combat the economic crisis focused primarily on relief measures for jobless men.[4] Moreover, graduate nurses frequently found themselves with additional social and financial obligations that included needy family members. Attractive as it might have seemed during the Depression, joining the military medical services was not an option: the Canadian military system languished during the interwar years under the economic constraints, policies, and isolationism of the Mackenzie King government. With only a small reserve and an even smaller permanent nursing force, the military relied on the civilian profession to fill the ranks should the need arise.

This was the situation in August 1939. Combined social, professional, technological, and military contexts had shaped a large, readily available, feminine workforce in need of employment. Nurses were able to capitalize on their technical skills and extra post-training courses in operating room technique, teaching, supervision, administration, and mental nursing to enhance their qualifications to become nursing sisters. They exerted personal, family, and political influence wherever possible to get a coveted position in the armed forces. Military nursing provided work while permitting women to fulfill family obligations and enjoy perks associated with wartime service. One physician referred to military nurses in 1940 as "Happy Warriors" whose "training has taught ... [them] to go in company with pain and fear and blood-shed – a strange privilege."[5] While nurses saved the military by supplying an essential workforce for the duration of the war, the military also saved nurses by providing them with much-needed work, and more.

Civilian Workplaces during the Great Depression

Hospitals grew in size and acceptance over the first half of the twentieth century, meeting the need for a cheap, dependable workforce by relying heavily on the labour of student nurses in their training schools. Hospitals typically hired only a small number of graduate nurses to serve as supervisors, educators, and "specials" for privately paying patients or patients needing more complex care than students could manage. At one large hospital, for example, student nurses constituted 70-80 percent of the nursing staff between 1924 and 1944.[6] For the most part, graduate nurses such as Gertrude LeRoy Miller, who was a Red Cross Outpost nurse during the 1930s, had to seek employment outside of hospitals. Miller valued the hardiness and autonomy of her remote practice setting, but she also described the working and living conditions as characterized by isolation, loneliness, dependence on the community, poverty, and improvisation.[7]

Most graduate nurses worked in private homes, depending on referrals from physicians or a local nursing registry and paid by the patient or patient's family.

Between 35 and 43 percent of all employed nurses during the early 1930s were private duty nurses, and according to the Weir Report, approximately 60 percent of these were either "intermittently" or "almost continuously unemployed," illustrating the dire circumstances of private duty nursing during this period.[8] Even when they found paid work, there was such a discrepancy between their wages and living expenses that they could not meet the basic costs of living during the 1930s.[9]

More than half (51.7 percent) of the 1,052 military nurses included in this study were private duty nurses before enlistment. Nursing Sister (NS) Eva Wannop, who worked to pay for a public health nursing course at the University of Toronto, earning $5 for a regular twelve-hour shift, noted that "if you had an alcoholic patient, it was $10. So it was more lucrative to get an alcoholic patient so that the money would accumulate [faster]."[10] Private duty nurses often reported waiting from two to four weeks between cases and sometimes working only five days in a month. Nursing registries tried to distribute work equitably among several nurses by regulating the number of working days each one could be assigned to a case. NS Muriel McArthur, however, "didn't get called for many patients" because she had trained in Toronto, and the local hospital near her home in Barrie, Ontario, "gave preference to their own graduates."[11]

Some hospitals experimented with reduced hours per shift for any graduate nurses that they did hire, and with hourly or "group nursing" fees, wherein a privately paying patient could hire a nurse by the hour rather than for the whole shift or a group of patients could share the costs of a private duty nurse, as ways to distribute available work among more nurses. Meanwhile, nursing schools reduced enrolments to stem the rising number of unemployed graduate nurses.[12] Graduate nurses who did find work in hospitals reported wages of $25 to $65 a month plus room and board. Some nurses crossed the border to the United States in search of work. NS Lois Bayly worked in Albany, New York, for example, while Betty Riddell travelled across the river daily from her home near the border to work in Detroit, Michigan. Many other nurses joined the ranks of the unemployed or took jobs as waitresses or sales clerks. NS Dorothy Grainger combined construction work with nursing, finding that laying steel reinforcements for concrete and reading blueprints was easy, and the wages were higher than in nursing jobs.[13]

At least 1.5 million Canadians were on relief by 1933 (an unemployment rate of 30 percent). Unemployment and welfare programs stretched dwindling resources that were inadequate at the best of times. Family members, including women, were considered responsible for the financial support of parents and siblings regardless of their own marital status or their ability to be self-sufficient, and welfare entitlements were adjusted accordingly.[14] Nurses bore social and legal responsibilities for parents and siblings, even when it was difficult to find enough work for their own support. As all soldiers enlisting during the Second World War did, nursing sisters completed a form indicating the number of dependants and the amount of financial support they had provided to each one prior to enlistment. This information determined their eligibility for an additional "Dependent's Allowance" benefit, intended to compensate dependants while soldiers were on active duty. One nursing sister claimed poignantly that although she was her mother's only relative and would have liked to support her, she had not been able to do so "because [her] nursing salary was not big enough."

Within hospitals, student nurses found working conditions increasingly intolerable. Indigent patients crowded public wards, taxing both human and material resources and sometimes provoking drastic attempts to create change, such as the 1939 nurses' strike at St. Joseph's Hospital in Comox, British Columbia.[15] Changes in medical technology increased the workload for novice nurses, as hospitals became repositories for technology that had become either too expensive or too seldom used for individual physicians to own and operate, or too difficult to transport to private homes for either diagnosis or treatments. Physicians relied increasingly on nurses' constant presence at the bedside and their growing familiarity with medical technology such as X-rays, hydrotherapy, electrical therapy, specimen collection, and thermometry.[16]

Prior to the 1940s nursing techniques focused on preparing the equipment and the patients for procedures, assisting physicians during procedures, and cleaning up afterwards. Nurses perfected and routinized techniques such as the administration of counter-irritants, medications, enemas, douches, catheters, lavages, poultices, packs, stupes, and foments, creating parameters of safety around patient care and claiming scientific status related to the acquisition of these skills. They sterilized equipment and supplies, followed elaborate instructions for isolating infectious patients, and developed strategies for "feeding patients, assisting them with ablutions, and maintaining the cleanliness of bed and patient alike."[17] Graduate nurses worried about losing their skills in private duty, perceiving hospitals as easier places to maintain or update skills. They were continually taking certificate courses and acquiring additional skills in areas such as operating room technique, X-ray technique, tuberculosis nursing, teaching, supervision, and administration. These extra courses also enhanced their credentials for military service whenever positions did become available.

Military Workplaces between the Wars

Vacancies in permanent military nursing positions seldom occurred during the interwar years. When the First World War medical units demobilized in 1920, nursing sisters found themselves in a situation different from that of medical officers who had been assigned positions with various regiments, sanitary stations, and field ambulances − units that continued to function after the war but on a smaller scale. Physicians could combine their reduced military responsibilities with a return to their private practices, but nursing sisters had been assigned to field hospitals that ceased to exist once the postwar care of soldiers came under the mandate of the Department of Pensions and National Health civilian rehabilitation hospitals. Some nurses worked in these hospitals initially, but as soldiers returned to civilian lives, this work tapered off.[18]

The postwar permanent force medical services, known as the Royal Canadian Army Medical Corps (RCAMC) after 1919, planned for twenty-five nursing sisters. Several reorganizations and economic recessions during the interwar period reduced military staffing and funding overall and authorized only twelve nursing positions throughout the period, with two exceptions where the transition of personnel overlapped briefly. The 1930 reorganization, for example, called for the small core of permanent force nursing sisters to be supplemented by a non-permanent reserve force of 1,110 nurses, but this plan was never implemented. Analysis of personnel records and annual reports of the Department of Militia and Defence for the Dominion of Canada demonstrates that the number of permanent nursing sisters ranged from eleven in 1920 to fourteen in 1931, with an average of twelve nurses and a reserve list that ranged from 127 nurses in 1923 to 399 nurses in 1925 – far short of the plans on paper.[19]

Only the permanent force nursing sisters had the stability of full-time paid work and military pensions at retirement. They served primarily as supervisors and administrators during the interwar period. They also trained "other ranks," or enlisted men, as medical assistants and stretcher bearers. Among other topics, nursing sisters taught first aid, certifying more than 50 percent of the "other ranks" and consequently keeping the requirement for nurses during peace time at a minimum level.[20] Reserve nurses were expected to be available for emergencies, epidemics, and occasionally for summer training-camp duty. This limited involvement left them economically dependent on private duty cases or a very flexible employer who could grant them time to fulfill their military assignments. For example, five reserve nursing sisters were "called out" to care for soldiers at the Royal Military College at Kingston, Ontario, during an influenza outbreak in 1924.

R.B. Bennett, prime minister from 1930 to 1935, developed a scheme to deal with massive civilian unemployment and labour unrest during the Depression by converting military camps into labour camps. The military benefited through the construction of airfields and fortification repairs at Halifax and Quebec, but medical services related to these projects were handled mostly through reserve nurses and local civilian hospitals. NS Elizabeth Pense, one of the reserve nurses, described the ratio between military patients and unemployed men in these relief camps as 5:50 with "lots of pneumonia" among the unemployed.[21]

As the decade progressed, it became increasingly clear that another war was imminent. Yet only one summer camp included military field training opportunities for medical units during this period, the one held at Camp Borden in 1938. No equipment had been added to the medical units or updated since the First World War. Policies indicated that units were to use British supplies if, and when, Canada entered another war. The RCAMC continued to rely on the civilian nursing profession to "fill the ranks," beginning with nursing sisters in the permanent and reserve forces. Nurses, like the physicians with whom they worked, were well qualified professionally but almost completely inexperienced with regards to wartime conditions. Physicians formed a special Military Section within the Canadian Medical Association in 1930, anticipating the need to plan for military and civilian needs during wartime as well as responses to bacteriological and chemical warfare.

The Canadian Nurses Association and the Canadian Red Cross shared a concern over civilian shortages if nurses enlisted in large numbers.[22] Beginning in 1926 they jointly created and maintained a "Reserve List" of nurses who had agreed to be available for emergencies, either within or outside of Canada. The officer commanding for each military district was supposed to have an updated list for his district. The "list" became problematic, however: nurses moved around in search of private duty cases or married and left nursing, making it difficult to keep the list current or to locate the nurses on it.[23]

The interwar permanent force nursing service consisted initially of eleven First World War nursing sisters who transferred directly from active service to the postwar permanent RCAMC in July 1920. Nine of them were over thirty-five years old at the time and remained in the military until retirement with pensions after serving between sixteen and twenty-eight years. The twelve nurses who eventually replaced them ranged in age from twenty-six to forty-six on enlistment. With the exception of six nurses who trained in the United States, the majority of the interwar nursing sisters trained in Ontario or Quebec, graduating between 1898 and 1915.[24] In 1939 they welcomed into their ranks the second generation of nursing sisters, to whom they passed the torch of military nursing in Canada.

American political scientist Cynthia Enloe has pointed out that the generation of Americans who grew up during the interwar period became a valuable pool of potential recruits for the military based on their experiences as children of the First World War and their socialization towards ideological expectations that made war a foregone conclusion.[25] In Canada, the severe working conditions of the 1930s combined with a legacy of military nursing that bestowed officer status, military benefits, and overwhelming social approval in addition to similar ideological expectations. Military nursing was consequently attractive to the large, valuable, and underemployed pool of trained civilian nurses. Indeed, Jean Wilson, writing on behalf of the Canadian Nurses Association, assured the Canadian government in August

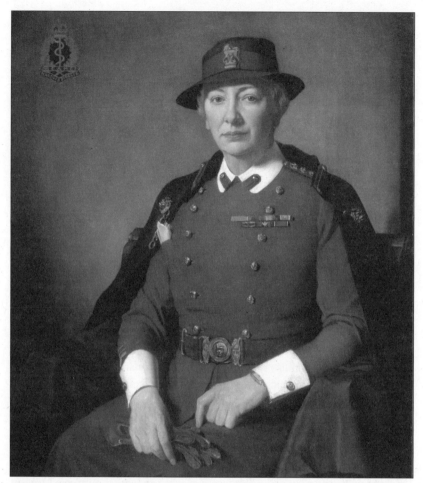

Miss Smellie, as she was popularly known, began her military nursing career as a nursing sister during the First World War and rose through the ranks to assistant matron in the postwar CAMC nursing service. She retired from the CAMC to take public health courses, teach at the McGill University School for Graduate Nurses, work for Victorian Order of Nurses, and then assume leadership of the VON. The RCAMC seconded her at the outbreak of the Second World War to become the matron-in-chief of its nursing service. She often referred to herself as the "most retired" nurse in Canada due to her diverse roles in both the civilian and military nursing fields. *Kenneth Forbes, Colonel Elizabeth Laurie Smellie C.B.E., R.R.C., L.L.D. AN 20000105-054, Beaverbrook Collection of War Art, © Canadian War Museum*

1939 that, should the need arise again, "there would be an immediate rush by nurses to answer 'The Call' for their professional services." She claimed that civilian nurses would be ready to answer, "'Ready, aye Ready' to any emergency call."[26] And they did respond enthusiastically when the call came. The issues then became which nurses would serve and how to select the right ones from such a large number of applicants.

The "Right" Kind of Nurse

One might expect the demographic composition of national military forces to reflect that of the larger population, but many factors skew enlistment in favour of the privileged classes while exploiting persons disadvantaged by education, race, or gender. Some of these factors include prevailing socio-economic conditions, whether enlistment is voluntary or conscripted, who is deemed to be exempt from military service, specific eligibility criteria, and strategies used to either avoid or achieve enlistment. Conscription had threatened Canadian unity during the First World War, bringing down the governing Liberals and creating a crisis within the new Conservative administration, which narrowly averted dissolution through the formation of a coalition Union government.[27] The government enacted two special pieces of legislation that ultimately permitted the conscription of men in 1917. The Military Voters Act (1917), popularly known as the "Soldiers Vote," extended the suffrage to all serving soldiers, including nursing sisters, while the Wartime Elections Act (1917) enfranchised mothers and wives of soldiers. These groups of women thereby became the first Canadian women eligible to vote in national elections, a year before other women received the same legal status.

William Lyon Mackenzie King, prime minister during the Second World War, had been a member of the Liberal government at the beginning of the First World War, and he understood first-hand the dangers associated with conscription. He also understood Canada's position within the British Empire and the inevitable requests for an increasing number of Canadian troops in Europe. Prior to the war, King had been well known for his politics of diplomatic appeasement and for fiscal decisions related to armed forces budget reductions despite the threat of impending conflict. He wanted to avoid not only Canadian involvement in distant wars but also the conscription issue, which had caused so much political and social turmoil during the First World War. King had promised as late as the 1940 election not to implement conscription but, when events during the war forced him to alter his stance, he called for a plebiscite in 1942 to release him from that promise. King's government then brought in the conscription of men in stages, initially for home defence only, but later for overseas duty as well.[28]

Canadian nurses were exempt from conscription for at least two reasons other than gender: they volunteered far in excess of the numbers required, and the previous "oversupply" of nurses during the 1930s had turned into a national nursing "shortage" by 1942. While the conscription of nurses was never necessary in Canada, however, the United States struggled to meet its nursing quotas in spite of special training programs such as the Cadet Nurse Corps established in 1943, raising the age limit to permit older nurses to enlist, eliminating the marriage bar, increasing nurses' pay, and improving their status within the armed forces. A protracted struggle took place between Congress, the American Nurses Association, and American military institutions over the conscription of nurses. A bill calling for their conscription passed the House of Representatives in March 1945 and narrowly missed Senate approval in April. Meanwhile a massive recruitment effort mounted by the army, Red Cross, and American Nurses Association proved successful, and by May, the War Department withdrew its second request for a draft of nurses, just days prior to the end of the war in Europe.[29]

Multiple factors influenced which nurses ultimately became nursing sisters. The civilian nursing profession controlled the training school admission criteria, curriculum, and examination process that credentialed a pool of the "right kind" of nurses for recruitment. The *King's Regulations and Orders for the Canadian Militia, 1939* included specific sections that established the basic eligibility requirements for nursing sisters related to citizenship, gender, age, marital status, and graduation from an approved school of nursing. The *Regulations* also required nursing sisters to be physically fit, less than forty-five years of age on enlistment, and either single or widowed without children.[30] Applicants were not accepted until the military verified their registration number and good standing with the relevant provincial professional nursing association. Thus, the demographic profile of military nurses closely reflected the civilian nursing workforce except for the relatively low number of French-Canadian nurses, which can only partially be explained in relation to prevailing French-Canadian perceptions of the war as a British endeavour.

The requirement to be graduates of approved training programs also meant that nursing sisters reflected and reinforced entrance criteria established by schools of nursing that were based on class, race, gender, age, and marital status. At the time, training programs systematically excluded black, First Nation, and Asian women as well as most men – with a few exceptions.[31] For example, a small number of Jewish women gained admission to the School of Nursing at Montreal's Women's General Hospital, while a small number of men trained as nurses at mental hospitals in Ontario and Alberta, as well as at the Victoria General Hospital in Halifax, Nova Scotia.[32] Although gender was not specifically mentioned by the *King's Regulations and Orders,* the military accepted only women as nursing sisters. According to prevailing social constructions of masculinity and femininity, men were combatants, not nurses. Men could go where women could not go, and by filling all nursing positions with women, the armed forces effectively reserved men who were fully qualified as nurses for the battlefield.[33]

The military required nursing applicants to submit references from an employer and from their clergy. A rigorous interview with the district commanding officer and a physical fitness test came next. The Royal Canadian Air Force (RCAF) went so far as to investigate the applicant's family background and home setting by sending investigators into the neighbourhood. Once a candidate was accepted, moreover, the armed forces used an initial training period of several months to screen out women perceived as being difficult to manage. Reports on nurses discharged within the first six months (1.5 percent of my sample) typically described them as either "not suited" to the military or "unable to adjust to discipline," or commented that they "didn't fit in."[34]

The nursing profession itself exerted yet another influence on the composition of military nursing services by continuing to resist the use of volunteer nurses and voluntary aid detachments (VADs).[35] No VADs worked in Canadian military medical units overseas, and while a very few worked in military hospitals within Canada, that change occurred only towards the end of the war, when civilian hospitals grew anxious regarding an emerging nursing shortage. With the volunteer question resolved, the nursing profession turned its attention towards an equitable process for selecting and enlisting civilian nurses.

The Canadian Nurses Association (CNA), in conjunction with the Canadian Red Cross and the RCAMC, began to negotiate the recruitment process at the beginning of 1939 based on common concerns to balance civilian and military nursing needs in the event of war. Their "Plan for National Enrolment of Nurses for Emergency Service" used the responses of registered nurses to a survey administered through their respective provincial associations. The survey asked nurses to categorize their availability according to four options: Class A for both war and disaster; Class B for war only; Class C for disaster only; and Class D (nurses over age forty-five) as a reserve for the first three classes. Classes A, B, and C had a minimum quota set at 3,000 nurses each.[36] The lists were forwarded from the provincial nursing associations to each military district within that province for the purpose of calling up only nurses who were on the lists and had applied in that district. The *Canadian Nurse* journal reported in October 1939 that more than 3,000 nurses had already enrolled and were "now ready to be called upon for service in an orderly manner and without delay."[37] NS Fran Oakes was one of them. She had completed extra courses at both the Montreal and Toronto General Hospitals in operating room technique and supervision and had over ten years' experience when she became one of the first two nurses in the newly organized RCAF nursing service. Oakes said:

> We didn't know we were the first nurses ... You see we were [enrolled for both] war and disaster at home or abroad ... When we first graduated as nurses, you were given this piece of paper. Were you willing to serve at home or abroad, in war or in disaster ... ? They contacted you; they gave you a post card. And I went to London and a little colonel, who wasn't as tall as I was, told me they had 999 well-qualified, experienced Army nurses. And they didn't need me. So I went back and minded my own business. And then, I got called in for the Air Force because when we signed up for war and disaster, it wasn't for any [particular] service.[38]

During the First World War, the medical and nursing staff of large teaching hospitals had mobilized together and formed complete medical units that moved overseas together. This practice depleted major Canadian hospitals such as Toronto General and Montreal General of a great proportion of their staff – especially experienced teachers and supervisors. The CNA was determined not to repeat this pattern. Each provincial association received an initial quota in proportion to the number of nurses registered in their province. By 1940 all provinces except Quebec and New Brunswick had exceeded their quota, and 4,080 nurses had volunteered for various categories of war service. Of these, only 150 nurses were actually on active duty.[39] The Association of Registered Nurses of the Province of Quebec issued a rebuttal to reports that Quebec had not met its quota, reporting a total of 4,064 members in good standing, with 1,040 names (25 percent) on their enrolment list and 900 nurses willing to serve in the military.[40]

In spite of these strategies to ensure that military enlistment would be proportionally distributed across the provinces and hospitals, the list soon fell into disuse – partially due to difficulties of maintaining its accuracy, and partially due to the penchant of commanding officers for independent decisions.[41] In September 1940 Col. Potter, director general of Medical Services, told the CNA he could not ensure the use of the list because applicants were screened and selected in the local districts.[42] As was often the case, district medical officers requested nurses whom they knew and had worked with in civilian hospitals. Surgeons in particular developed preferences for specific operating room nurses who were familiar with their techniques and equipment preferences. NS Helen Morton recalled that one Toronto General Hospital physician went through the building over the Labour Day weekend immediately following the call to mobilize units in 1939, personally recruiting Agnes Neill as matron and forty staff nurses for duty with No. 15 Canadian General Hospital (CGH).[43] NS Betty Nicolson moved directly from the operating room at Winnipeg General Hospital to Fort Osborne Barracks because, as she said, "the surgeon was one of our doctors from Winnipeg General and he wanted a scrub nurse from his hospital, of course. So I was taken on strength immediately."[44] The RCAMC called up NS Doris Carter shortly after she met a surgeon from Montreal's Royal Victoria Hospital who assured her, "I've got your name on my hospital [staff list] and I'm going to be chief surgeon."[45] Although military medical units preferred nurses with at least two years' experience beyond training, NS Beatrice Cole received a phone call within two months of graduation from the Regina General Hospital in 1944, asking her if she wanted to enlist. Because she had not applied and was therefore surprised to get an interview, she asked the recruiter if they were calling all the new graduates. Told that they had been advised to phone her, she didn't find out until after the war that one of her patients, a First World War nursing sister, had recommended her.[46]

Nurses themselves circumvented the list in various ways. They submitted multiple applications, either to the same service or to different service branches in order to increase the selection odds. One nurse applied to and was accepted by the RCAMC three times, according to her personnel file.[47] Nurses applied in several military districts in search of unfilled personnel quotas. NS Hallie Sloan applied to the navy, air force, army, and South African nursing services, for example. When each service replied that they had plenty of people "waiting in line," Sloan returned to her home community of Regina, where she found a vacancy with the RCAMC.[48] NS Lois Bayly gave up work in New York and returned to Canada in order to enlist.[49] As NS Mary Bower summarized, "We all were trying to get into the Army or Air Force or anything. We tried to go to Africa! Anything to get in the armed forces."[50]

An unknown number of Canadian nurses decided the waiting list was too long. They enlisted with Queen Alexandra's Imperial Military Nursing Service (QAIMNS) in England, or the United States Army Nurse Corps (USANC). Crossing the river to work in Detroit, Betty Riddell saw a billboard message every day: "Uncle Sam needs you!" She decided to inquire one day "if they would take Canadians. I almost didn't get back [to Canada]. They wanted to hold me." Other nurses, such as Isabel Morrison, served with the South African Military Nursing Service (SAMNS) as part of a special South African draft of Canadian nurses in 1942. After serving one year there, she remustered to the RCAMC.[51] Not all SAMNS nursing sisters were accepted into the RCAMC, however. Matron-in-chief of the RCAMC Nursing Service, Elizabeth Smellie, made it clear in a letter to the Department of National Defence that "many [nurses] were on the Reserve list with no immediate prospect of being called, and were glad to go to South Africa. They should not be considered before those who have been waiting a long time, with no opportunity to serve as yet."[52]

Other nurses took civilian positions at military hospitals, hoping that proximity and work record would favour their selection by commanding officers. Air Commodore J.W. Tice, director of Medical Services for the RCAF, expressed concerned over this practice, noting that some nurses were not "suitable" for appointment and that civilian positions on RCAF bases should be "without any undertaking as to subsequent appointments."[53] After 1941, a few nurses enlisted with the newly formed Women's Divisions to work as hospital assistants while hoping to remuster as nursing sisters. The military refused to allow changes in status, however, as this practice undermined plans to balance supply and demand with the civilian workforce. As well, nursing sisters belonged to the medical corps and were completely separate from Women's Divisions, with different rank, pay, and administration.[54] Nurses also used personal and familial influences such as mutual acquaintances or letters to members of Parliament requesting military appointments. They capitalized on relationships to fathers or brothers who were already serving in the forces, as illustrated by the files of underage and inexperienced nurses in the records.

By 1941, *Canadian Nurse* editorials reveal that professional concerns for meeting military nursing needs had shifted to concerns for meeting civilian nursing needs. Medical and nursing leaders took measures to prevent the enlistment of nurses who were already employed in civilian settings, to prevent nurses from leaving the country for employment elsewhere, and to increase the number of students in training. They interfered directly when specific skills or experience were required to maintain civilian practice. In October 1942, for example, Associate Minister of National Defence C.G. Power received a request to avoid enlisting public health nurses from a certain province since there was a "greater danger of epidemics in certain provinces where there are very large numbers of men in small areas."[55] The letter further explained that there was a crucial need for public health nurses to follow up with venereal disease cases among soldiers mobilizing in port areas. Public health nurses already required an official release from provincial ministers of health in order to enlist, but, as this letter complained, nurses were generally "dissatisfied" if denied permission and therefore it would be easier if the military didn't even offer them positions.

Thus, both nurses and their civilian employers influenced military enlistment, using a variety of strategies that altered the composition of military nursing services regardless of careful plans to be representative and provide equal opportunities for selection. As I will illustrate later, additional factors emerged during the war, such as the need for particular skills or knowledge, that enabled still other nurses to circumvent waiting lists and quotas.

Too Many or Too Few Nurses?

Provincial and national associations were anxious to meet the dual obligations to support the war effort and stabilize civilian nursing services.[56] With the military quota of nurses more than adequately met, Ethel Johns as editor of *Canadian Nurse*, challenged civilian nurses to consider home service as being as much a sacrifice as "spectacular" service overseas. Marion Lindeburgh, president of the CNA from 1942 to 1944, referred to nurses as soldiers "whether serving overseas or on the home front. The professional nurse ... displays the marks of the good soldier. She will not desert the ranks at a time of crisis, nor will she seek shelter, leaving others to face the hardships and the struggle." Even public health nurses adopted the language of "soldiering" on the home front, as is evident, for example, in a poem on the civilian Air Raid Precautions program.[57] Wary of a return to the employment conditions that characterized the Depression, the profession was reluctant to increase the number of students in training, and ultimately the number of graduate nurses. The professional associations preferred to make full use of existing nursing resources, limit the number of military nurses, and continue the employment restrictions on civilian nurses for the duration of the war.

The total number of graduate nurses available for work in Canada during the war remains ambiguous. On one hand, the CNA reported an increasing membership of 16,758 in 1940, 18,266 in 1942, and 19,137 in 1943. On the other hand, the 1941 census reported 27,114 active graduate nurses and 11,907 student nurses, for a total of 39,021 nurses, and data from the National Health Survey conducted during March 1943 suggest there were almost 55,000 "active" nurses (Table 1.1).[58]

Because it was not mandatory for a nurse to be a member of the CNA, the organization's records do not reflect the full number of Canadian nurses. At the same time, while many, if not most, nurses belonged to their provincial association, some belonged to more than one association in order to be able to work in several provinces. Because the 1941 census took place after nurse-recruitment campaigns, it potentially over-reports the number of actively practising nurses: retired and married nurses may have identified themselves in this category given the emergency plan focus on both active and inactive nurses. While these issues pose limitations on the interpretation of statistical analyses, the data reveal significant new demographic information and raise important questions about the nursing workforce and nursing shortages during this period.

The Royal Canadian Army Medical Corps (RCAMC) initially supplied medical and nursing services for the Royal Canadian Navy (RCN) and the Royal Canadian Air Force (RCAF) as well as for the army itself. All nursing sisters enlisted with the RCAMC until the RCN and RCAF organized their own respective services in 1941 and 1942, with small groups of nurses remustering to these nursing services. Because the Canadian troops overseas were initially stationed only in England, the RCAMC built up its nursing service slowly, minimizing effects on the civilian profession yet bringing some welcome relief to the employment crisis of the 1930s. By the time of the ill-fated assault on Dieppe in mid-1942, the number of nursing sisters had increased 110 percent, and the civilian profession began to worry about a shortage of nurses.

Before embarking on a general recruitment campaign for more nurses to enter training and the workforce, however, the CNA decided to obtain updated, accurate information about the nursing workforce through at least two endeavours. In January 1942, the organization appointed Kathleen Ellis as the CNA emergency nursing adviser, responsible for surveying nursing needs in each province and making recommendations at the annual general meetings. Suzanne Giroux was her French associate.[59] By December of the same year, CNA president Marion Lindeburgh warned nurses that if the profession did not ensure adequate nursing services throughout Canada, the federal government would do so by way of the National Selective Service of the Department of Labour and its Canadian Medical Procurement and Assignment Board.[60] The CNA also sent representatives to this board and participated with the board in the National Health Survey conducted during March 1943, the nursing alternative to the National Selective Service registration of all Canadian women under twenty-five years of age for the war

Table 1.1

Active Canadian nurses by province and enlistment status, March 1943

Province	Number of civilian nurses	Number of military nurses	Total	Percent enlisted
Prince Edward Island	391	43	434	9.9
Nova Scotia	939	151	3,090	4.9
New Brunswick	2,002	111	2,113	5.3
Quebec	7,834	317	8,151	3.9
Ontario	23,884	735	24,619	3.0
Manitoba	2,963	179	3,142	5.7
Saskatchewan	2,901	138	3,039	4.5
Alberta	3,600	110	3,710	3.0
British Columbia	5,937	224	6,161	3.6
Yukon/Northwest Territories	33	0	33	0
Canada	52,483	2,008	54,491	3.7

Source: Based on Canada, *Report of the National Health Survey,* part 8, *Nurses,* (Ottawa: King's Printer, 1945) 219.

effort.[61] This survey of graduate nurses, however, included everyone under the age of sixty-six, active or inactive, married or single, inquiring about their availability for emergency nursing service in Canada and their intentions regarding military nursing service.[62]

The CNA and the Canadian Hospital Council had access to both sets of data (from the emergency nursing adviser and the National Health Survey), as well as information about the number of nursing sister appointments forwarded from the armed forces branches. They combined these sources to analyze the nursing situation in Canada, make decisions about nursing education, and impose limits on civilian nurses' mobility.[63] The data generated by these surveys provide significant information regarding the availability and intentions of civilian nurses to enlist (Table 1.2), their pattern of application to the armed forces (Table 1.3), the number of nurses enlisted as of March 1943 (Table 1.1), and the number of military nursing sister appointments over the course of the war (Table 1.4).

As of March 1943, according to the National Health Survey, there were 52,483 civilian nurses in Canada. Of these, 47.5 percent indicated that they were unavailable for military service and another 29.6 percent did not indicate their availability (a total of 77 percent). Another 7.1 percent had already applied to the military and 15.8 percent were willing to apply. The armed forces reported only 2,008 nursing sisters on active duty at this time, a mere 3.7 percent of the combined total of 54,491 civilian and military nurses. Meanwhile, the number of applications had increased considerably (to 3,741) and exceeded the actual number of appointments, perhaps due to the National Survey query about willingness to apply (Tables 1.2 and 1.3). Some

20.5 percent of those who had already applied to the armed forces applied to more than one branch, and 4.4 percent applied to all three branches. With another 8,300 nurses willing to apply for military service, there would be no difficulty in recruiting military nurses in Canada. Based on these data, with nursing sisters constituting a mere 3.7 percent of active registered nurses – a much smaller proportion than the 37 percent reported for the First World War – the impact on the civilian nursing workforce should have been manageable.[64] Although the number of nursing sister appointments increased again in preparation for the 1943 Italian campaign and the 1944 European invasion, the armed forces can scarcely be blamed for creating a shortage, given the relatively low proportion of military nurses overall.

It is therefore highly doubtful that the perceived development of a nursing shortage was due to military enlistment. Rather, as the interim report of Emergency Nursing Adviser Ellis identified, there were multiple problems with the maldistribution of nurses. Based on information from the provincial registered nurses organizations, for example, 950 nurses were practising outside of the province in which they were registered, with an additional 625 nurses working in the United States. In addition, there had been a 10.9 percent increase in the actual number of hospital beds along with a 21.6 percent increase in overall bed-utilization. Lesser-skilled workers had replaced the experienced personnel lost to enlistment. Certain health care sectors such as mental hospitals, sanatoria, and rural areas were inadequately staffed. Hours and salaries varied by region and health care setting, and nurses often sought work in the better-remunerated areas. Moreover, discrimination against married nurses contributed to the perceived shortages.[65] These issues combined to create a nursing shortage perception that was out of proportion to the data, whereas other causes may have had more to do with the distribution of nursing services across regions and practice settings. Ellis' final report revealed a large gap between the total number of registered Canadian nurses and the number of nurses engaged in active practice (22,136) or potentially available for practice (16,818). At least 27,044 nurses reported that they were "employed other than as nurses," of which 93 percent stated they were housewives and mothers.[66] When comparing the proportion of nursing sisters to Ellis' total of 38,954 available or potentially available nurses then, military nurses still constituted only 5.2 percent of the active nursing population in 1943.

Nonetheless, the CNA called for constraints on nurses' mobility and employment options out of fear that the situation would worsen. A special appeal was made to Matron-in-Chief Elizabeth Smellie not to deplete hospital training schools of their experienced instructors and supervisors. In conjunction with the National Selective Service, the CNA was involved in decisions on all labour exit permits requested by Canadian nurses after May 1943. There were four categories of applicants, and "it was felt that only in very special circumstances could requests for permits from nurses in group

Table 1.2

Availability of Canadian nurses for enlistment, March 1943

Province	Available for military service (Not yet applied)	Available for military service (Applied)	Unavailable for military service	Not indicated	Total
Prince Edward Island	62	28	244	56	390
Nova Scotia	466	253	1,210	1,010	2,939
New Brunswick	318	125	1,057	502	2,002
Quebec	890	568	3,815	2,561	7,834
Ontario	3,845	1,555	11,335	7,149	23,884
Manitoba	611	236	1,194	922	2,963
Saskatchewan	506	214	1,483	698	2,901
Alberta	619	299	1,544	1,138	3,600
British Columbia	982	462	3,015	1,478	5,937
Yukon/Northwest Territories	7	1	12	13	33
Canada	8,306	3,741	24,909	15,527	52,483

Source: Based on Canada, *Report of the National Health Survey,* part 8, *Nurses,* (Ottawa: King's Printer, 1945), 218.

one [defined as registered nurses actively engaged in nursing in Canada] be given consideration; this would include nurses asking permission to go to the United States for post-graduate study during the duration [of the war]."[67] The CNA referred problems associated with the other three categories – "potential" student nurses applying to schools of nursing in the United States, married nurses who claimed they could not find work in Canada, and appeals from industries in other countries for Canadian nurses – to the individual provincial associations. Exceptions to the moratorium on labour exit permits were made for nurses over fifty-five years of age, nurses with "indifferent health," and student applicants "of special religious faiths and coloured students who cannot be placed in Canada."[68]

Changing Needs for Nurses during the War

Socio-economic conditions of the 1930s had shaped the context in which nursing sisters trained and entered the workforce, while leaders of the profession influenced the selection process, but events during the war itself constituted a third influence on the number and selection of military nurses.[69] In contrast to the First World War, the Canadian forces (and their medical units) entered this war as Allies with full responsibility for meeting the medical needs of Canadian troops rather than as "British soldiers recruited abroad." Defence Scheme No. 3 formed the basis of prewar planning, providing for an overseas field force. An official War Book contained details for organizing such a force but little else. The King government, aiming to strengthen national identity while distributing burdens and opportunities

Table 1.3

Applications to the armed forces submitted by Canadian nurses, March 1943

Province	Army	Navy	Air Force	Service Navy Army	Navy Air Force	Army Air Force	Navy Army Air Force	Total
Prince Edward Island	18	3	2	1	4	0	0	28
Nova Scotia	137	59	21	14	5	8	9	253
New Brunswick	72	22	11	7	1	9	3	125
Quebec	283	89	79	42	16	34	25	568
Ontario	801	255	186	105	34	106	68	1,555
Manitoba	n/a	n/a	n/a	n/a	n/a	n/a	n/a	236
Saskatchewan	93	28	34	11	5	26	17	214
Alberta	n/a	n/a	n/a	n/a	n/a	n/a	n/a	299
British Columbia	230	73	64	27	14	33	21	462
Yukon/Northwest Territories	1	0	0	0	0	0	0	1
Canada	1,635+	529+	397+	207+	79+	216+	143+	3,741

Note: For Manitoba and Alberta, only the total number of applications was reported. Thus the Canadian total for each service was greater than the figure given in each case. The total for all services nationwide is accurate, since it includes the Manitoba and Alberta figures.

Sources: Based on *Report of the National Health Survey*, part 8, *Nurses* (Ottawa: King's Printer, 1945), 219.

(depending on one's perspective) equitably throughout different geographic regions, sought proportional representation for the armed forces.[70]

The initial commitment called for two military divisions (consisting of 50,000-60,000 all ranks) in support of the British army, as well as extensive involvement in the British Commonwealth Air Training Plan, with forty-eight air training centres scattered across Canada.[71] By the summer of 1940 a rapid German expansion into Belgium, the Netherlands, and France resulted in the formation of two more divisions, enactment of the National Resources Mobilization Act (NRMA), and a transition from "phony [sic] war" to "total war." The NRMA required all persons, services, and property to be available "as deemed necessary or expedient for securing the public safety, the defence of Canada ..., efficient prosecution of the war, or for maintaining supplies or services essential to the life of the community."[72] The main medical needs during this first phase of the war involved screening recruits, administering immunizations, and managing communicable illnesses that occurred as large numbers of young men were transported across Canada, living together in large communal settings. A relatively small number of medical units in Canada and England, with limited nursing staff, were sufficient for these needs.

Between the summers of 1940 and 1943, a second phase of the war brought devastating air strikes during the Battle of Britain, the defeat of British forces in Hong Kong, and the failed Dieppe raid. There were five Canadian divisions (100,000-125,000 all ranks) overseas. With the exception of two battalions (1,975 soldiers) whose remnants became prisoners of war in Hong Kong after December 1941, Canadian troops were posted primarily for the defence of England and in preparation for the invasion of northwestern Europe.[73] Medical units increased correspondingly, particularly in preparation for casualties from Dieppe. Hospital units remained in England during this phase, and medical plans focused on evacuation of the wounded by trains and ships from the continent to military hospitals on the English coast. A small medical team, including two nursing sisters, accompanied the Canadian contingent sent to Hong Kong, working within British hospital units. They were there only three weeks when the Japanese attacked Pearl Harbor and overran Hong Kong in December 1941. The two Canadian nursing sisters were taken as prisoners of war, spending the next twenty-one months in a Japanese prison camp and a civilian internment camp.[74]

From the perspective of medical units, the second phase of the war involved treating more trauma, an increase in surgical care, and more experience in working under war conditions. This phase exposed various problems to be resolved prior to major campaigns and provided training opportunities, also known as "schemes," in northern England and Scotland.

The third phase of the war involved Canadian participation in two major campaigns: in Sicily and Italy beginning in July 1943, and the Allied invasion of

Table 1.4

RCAMC, RCAF, and RCN new nursing service appointments, 1939-45

Year	RCAMC	RCAF	RCN	SAMNS	Total	Cumulative
1939	151	0	0	0	151	151
1940	369	4	0	0	373	524
1941	380	237*	7	80	467	991+
1942	659	–	100	221	980	1,971+
1943	687	–	114	0	1,038	3,009**
1944	1,140	148	82	0	1,370	4,379
1945	270	23	38	0	331	4,710
Total	3,656	412	341	301	4,710	

* Total for 1941-43.
+ Total plus RCAF appointments.
** Includes previous RCAF appointments.
Note: Table reflects only the total number of appointments made per year without adjusting for attrition or repeat appointments. It also includes non-nurses in the appointment statistics. The RCN and RCAF had no appointments initially because they had no nursing services. The SAMNS cohort was a one-time limited recruitment.
Sources: Based on data from "Appointment Statistics – Nursing Sisters, Physiotherapy Aides, Occupational Therapists, Dieticians and Home Sisters," 000.8(D93), Department of Defence Directorate of History and Heritage and RCAF memos of 2 December 1940, 23 October 1944, 30 January 1945, and a 1943 nominal list in files 400-1-1 and 400-2-1, RG24, E-1-b, v. 3365, LAC.

northwestern Europe beginning in June 1944. Involvement in these campaigns brought the medical units to peak strength and moved nursing sisters forward to the frontlines as they followed the troops in rapid advances across long distances. This phase introduced new settings in the Mediterranean and Europe (North Africa, Sicily, Italy, France, the Netherlands, Belgium, and Germany), different working conditions (frequently under canvas and requiring great mobility), and treatment innovations (increased use of blood transfusions and the introduction of penicillin). As well, the number of experienced nursing sisters in the field by this time permitted, and even favoured, the recruitment of younger nurses with less work experience as reinforcements to the rank.

The fourth and final phase was quite short in duration. By May 1945, 1,412 nursing sisters had volunteered for the Pacific campaign as the war in Europe drew to a close.[75] They had returned from overseas early to join others serving in Canada, in preparation for embarkation to the South Pacific, when Japan surrendered after atomic bombs were dropped on Hiroshima (6 August) and Nagasaki (9 August). For the military medical units, this last phase involved closing down hospital units and moving patients, first to England and then to Canada. For many patients and many nurses, there still remained long months and years of surgeries, recovery, and rehabilitation.

After they enlisted, almost all nursing sisters received an initial six-month posting in Canada. Some remained in Canada for their entire service, either by choice or because there were no overseas vacancies. RCAF nurses served at most of the air training centres across Canada, often in small, relatively isolated units with only a few beds and little backup support. They also served at large training camps such as the one in St. Thomas, Ontario. Several small groups served in England at East Grinstead in Sussex, which specialized in the care of burn patients (typically pilots wounded during bombing assignments flown out of Britain), or with No. 6 Bomber Command in southern England at Odiham and Bournemouth. Two RCAF nursing sisters with No. 52 RCAF Mobile Field Hospital were the first Canadian nurses to arrive in Normandy, just thirteen days after D-Day on 6 June 1944.[76] RCN nursing sisters also served primarily in Canada, with the exceptions of those posted to RCNH *Avalon* in Newfoundland and HMCS *Niobe* in Scotland – land-based naval hospitals. A group of 301 nurses responded to the call for volunteers in South Africa.[77] They carried the same title and wore the same uniform as RCAMC nurses but once they left Canada, SAMNS nursing sisters served under the South African military authority with postings primarily in South Africa, although nurses who extended the original one-year contracts were posted to the Middle East, North Africa, and Italy as well.

Many facets contributed to the social construction of military nursing and nursing sisters. Medical units became an important part of strategic planning for major military campaigns – to manage human resources efficiently and minimize war "wastage." Whenever there was an increased need for nursing skills on the frontlines, eligibility criteria and military policies could be altered to enlist more nursing sisters.

Profile of Second World War Nursing Sisters

There is considerable variance in the literature regarding the number of Second World War nursing sisters, with an unknown number of non-nurses typically included in these reports and members of the RCN, RCAF, and SAMNS typically excluded from them.[78] After adjusting for multiple enlistments by the same persons, remustering of personnel when new nursing services formed, and non-nurses enlisted to the rank, I compared archival documents to reports from the secondary literature and estimated the total number of Second World War Canadian military nurses alone as 4,047 without the South African cohort or 4,348 with the South African cohort, compared to the 3,600 to 4,800 range found within the literature.[79]

I planned originally to review at least a thousand individual personnel records to increase the representativeness of my sample. On preliminary analysis, however, it became clear that non-nurses accounted for at least 8.2 percent of the records, that there were redundancies for some individuals, and that a few records contained insufficient data. The RCAMC was the only service to clearly document occupational categories other than nursing, and its figures of 64 dieticians, 64 occupational therapists, 58 home sisters, and 104 physiotherapist aides in its postwar statistical summary confirm the proportion

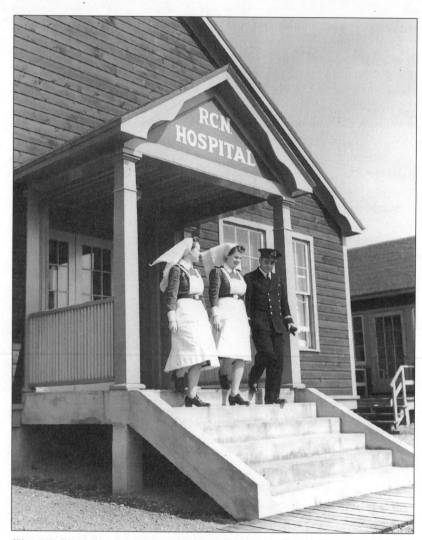

Although land-based hospitals, RCN medical units such as this one retained full naval traditions and language. Here unidentified nursing sisters and Surgeon Lieutenant Riddell leave the hospital at St. John's, Newfoundland, on 27 July 1942. *LAC/DND fonds/PA-137827*

of occupational categories within the rank that emerged in my analysis.[80] I therefore oversampled to ensure a final data set of at least a thousand nurses' records after adjusting for these factors. I sampled RCN, RCAF, and SAMNS records proportionately to the RCAMC records, resulting in a data set of 1,145 individual records: 1,052 nurses, 22 dieticians, 34 physiotherapist aides, 15 occupational therapists, and 22 home sisters (the last were responsible for the care and household management of the living quarters). Analysis indicates that, as nurses constituted 91.8 percent of the sample and non-nurses 8.2 percent, my

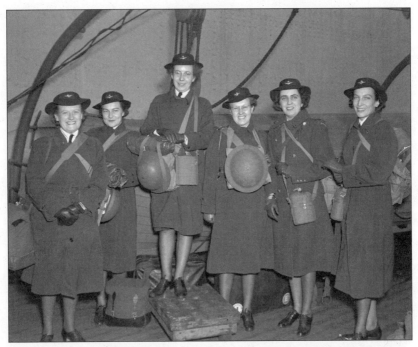

RCAF Nursing Sisters Jessie Young, Edna Millman, Elaine Matheson, Vera Soper, Jean Steinhoff, and Jackie Vanier arrived in England in September 1943, part of the newly formed No. 52 Mobile Field Hospital. They trained on the coast, receiving and evacuating patients to prepare for the D-Day invasion. Although an advanced team landed in Normandy only two days after D-Day, the full unit (including nurses) arrived on 19 June 1944. *Canadian Forces Joint Imagery Centre, PL-19964*

final sample represents 26 percent of the estimated 4,047 nurses who served through the Canadian armed forces during the war. This, then, is the sample for the demographic analyses that follow, compared to and supplemented by existing archival reports and records.

There were no legal restrictions on the title of nursing sister, and since gender superseded occupational classification, all women enlisted in the Canadian forces as nursing sisters prior to 1941. The Canadian Women's Army Corps (CWACs) and other Women's Divisions were formed between 1941 and 1942; in fact, RCAMC Matron Smellie was responsible for organizing the CWACs initially. When RCAF Matron Jean Porteous inquired if occupational therapists and physiotherapy aides could be called nursing sisters, for example, CNA General Secretary Kathleen Ellis replied that there was no objection because it was not a civilian title and "it only concerned the military."[81] Given that at least 8.2 percent of the nursing sister rank consisted of professionals other than nurses, it is important to clarify exactly who is included in particular demographic analyses and to differentiate between nurses and non-nurses.

The Canadian Army Medical Corps (CAMC) had established a precedent of including non-nurses in the rank, based on the very few women involved during the First World War. A small number of CAMC nursing sisters (nurses and non-nurses) served as physiotherapists, for example, but following the war, physiotherapy emerged as a distinct profession. The CAMC also included at least three dieticians and two women physicians as nursing sisters. During the Second World War, the different service branches made their own decisions regarding occupational categories included within the nursing sister rank. While physiotherapy aides and dieticians enlisted with the RCAMC and RCN as nursing sisters, the RCAF employed civilian physiotherapists in their units and delayed their enlistment until 1944, whereupon they assigned them to the Women's Division rather than include them in the rank. RCAF dieticians were also members of the Women's Division.[82] RCAMC and RCN occupational therapists enlisted as nursing sisters, but the RCN was the only service to include female laboratory technicians as well.[83] Home sisters were always members of the RCAMC and RCN nursing sister rank. They came from various backgrounds and occupational experiences, chosen for their "adaptability, resourcefulness, and diplomacy, ... good educational background, pleasing personality, knowledge and experience in household management, and ability to direct as well as work with others."[84]

This practice of including non-nurses in the nursing sister rank proved problematic at times – for example, when immediate emergency nursing assistance was required during British air raids but the general public was unable to distinguish which nursing sisters were actually nurses. At the RCN land-based hospital in Scotland, the HMCS *Niobe*, policy required all nursing sisters to take turns being "on call" for night emergencies. As NS Elizabeth Dean, a dietician, recalled, "So I was put on call, too. I said, 'Well, that's fine. I can go down and make a cup of coffee or do something like that.' And the first time I was on call, a couple of Navy ratings ... had had a real fight in a bar. And one of them was shot. So my kitchen became a morgue, and the others had to be surgically looked after, and the Matron decided, 'Well, I don't think Elizabeth should go on call because she is not much use.' Well, my kitchen was used!"[85]

Besides including non-nurses in the rank, the literature on distribution of nurses according to nursing service branches overestimates the total number of Second World War nurses. Without close critical examination of the data across the whole of the armed forces, it is easy to miss the impact of multiple enlistments and remustering when relying on enlistment figures tallied from monthly or annual official reports. My analysis, for example, reveals that at least 2.9 percent of the nurses served in more than one Canadian forces branch, while 22.8 percent of the Canadian nurses who initially served with the SAMNS served with a Canadian branch later (Table 1.5).[86]

The type and number of personnel required varied from service to service.

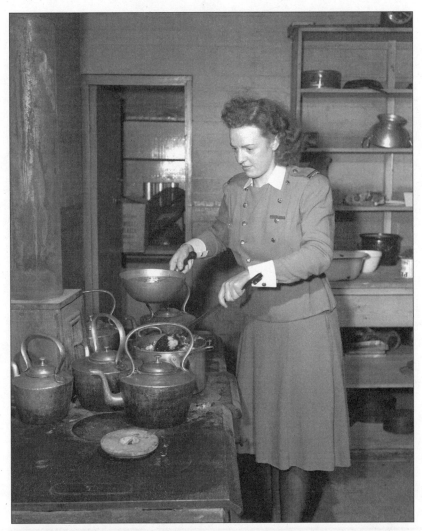

RCAF Nursing Sister Lynn Johnston, with one of several small Bomber Groups posted to southern England, may well have been one of the RCAF dieticians serving in the nursing sister rank. According to one caption for this photograph, she spent "many a long hour in the hospital kitchen trying to make British war rations please patients' palates." The RCAF was particularly interested in the nutrition of pilots as it related to peak performance on long bombing missions and excellence of night vision for air raids. *Canadian Forces Joint Imagery Centre, PL-33084*

The RCAF, for example, required fewer non-nurses because its medical units remained mostly within Canada, where civilian employees were readily available to work on local military bases. And because nurses contested RCAF attempts to alter their rank and status, the authorities seemed increasingly determined to keep other women workers out of the military. In contrast, the RCAMC operated at least 117 hospitals within Canada, 25 hospitals

Table 1.5

Distribution of sampled nurses within Canadian Armed Forces nursing services, 1939-45							
	RCAMC	RCAMC and SAMNS	SAMNS	RCN	RCAF	RCAF and SAMNS	RCAMC and RCAF
Number	964	27	19	21	18	1	2
Percentage	91.6	2.6	1.8	2.0	1.7	0.1	0.2

Source: Based on data extracted from Department of National Defence personnel files for 1,052 Second World War Canadian military nurses, Library and Archives Canada.

of various sizes overseas, 2 hospital transport ships, several hospital trains, a small number of air ambulances operating between the continent and England, and a variety of mobile medical units deployed in several theatres of war.[87] With such a large organization and the need for flexibility in staffing them, it was essential for the RCAMC to have full control over all their personnel, both nurses and non-nurses.

Initial eligibility criteria required nursing sisters of all branches to be between twenty-five and forty-five years of age, although the minimum was lowered to twenty-three in May 1942, and to twenty-one by September 1943, while the upper limit increased to fifty-five years as the military prepared for two major campaigns.[88] With an abundance of applicants, the armed forces could be selective, and they were particularly interested in the more experienced nurses who had teaching and supervisory abilities, skills often missing in new graduates. NS Pauline Lamont recalled enlisting on her twenty-third birthday. NS Ella Beardmore applied every time she went to Toronto but always received the same response, that she was too young, until she finally got her acceptance.[89] Once there were sufficient experienced nurses in place, younger nurses could be safely accepted as reinforcements into established units where they could be mentored and monitored. As a result, the average age of nursing sisters decreased after 1943. Prior to 1943, only 0.9 percent of the nurses were between twenty-one and twenty-two years old at enlistment; after 1943, however, 3.6 percent were in that age bracket. Prior to 1943, 9 percent of the nurses were over thirty-five, and 3.2 percent of these were over forty. Nurses in their late forties and early fifties brought years of experience, including previous war experience, as was the case for the two oldest women in this sample, who were fifty-two and fifty-four years old on enlistment and had served during the First World War. Diversity of practice settings and roles accommodated this wide range of ages.

The nurses tended to be older, on average, than dieticians, physiotherapist aides, and occupational therapists, but younger than home sisters (Table 1.6). This can be explained partially by different training requirements. Nursing schools required applicants to be at least eighteen or nineteen years

Table 1.6

Canadian nursing sisters by occupation and age on enlistment

Occupation	Number in sample	Average age	Minimum age	Maximum age
Registered nurses	1,052	28.03	21	54
Physiotherapist aides	34	26.08	20	42
Dieticians	22	26.95	22	36
Home sisters	22	33.04	25	45
Occupational therapists	15	23.26	19	32

Source: Based on data extracted from Department of National Defence personnel files for 1,052 Second World War Canadian Nursing Sisters, Library and Archives Canada.

old, with junior matriculation as the minimum educational requirement for admission, and the training programs extended over three full years. The military preferred a minimum of two years' experience after graduation and often gave higher priority to more-experienced nurses. In addition, in a bid to enhance their credentials for application, many nurses took extra courses of six to twelve months' duration after graduation from training programs. While the youngest age for a nurse with full nursing credentials was twenty-one to twenty-two years, those with post graduate courses and required experience were typically twenty-three to twenty-five years old. Additional experience raised the average age higher still. In contrast, physiotherapist aides and occupational therapists were not only eligible for university programs at a younger age than nursing students but they had no experience requirements prior to enlistment. Some even completed the internship component of their training as part of their military service.

Many of the nurses (40.8 percent) were born during the First World War, trained during the Depression (between 1933 and 1937), and graduated into the nursing workforce during one of the worst employment periods. Like other children of their generation, many had lost one or both parents to the war or the global influenza epidemic of 1918-19: more than 30 percent of them reported the death of one or both parents. These nurses needed to work, not simply "to fill time" between school leaving and marriage, but for personal survival and family obligations: 8.4 percent indicated that they supported dependent relatives – parents, siblings, or relatives who had raised them in lieu of parents. The range of such support, which varied from $5 to $90 per month with an average of $30 per month, needs to be understood in comparison to average civilian nursing salaries during the 1930s. In spite of recommendations from the Weir Report and the CNA, the Depression had continued to exert downward pressure on nurses' salaries. The support of dependants was a significant commitment for nurses – one that a regular military salary of $150 per month plus food, lodging, clothing, and medical care made much easier.

As noted earlier, there were quotas for each military district in an attempt to equalize nursing losses to civilian hospitals. These quotas were proportioned according to provincial population and nursing needs but failed to take into account the large numbers of nurses who trained outside of their home provinces or their practice of registering both where they trained and in their home communities. Nurses could, therefore, apply to the military in more than one district. More nurses enlisted in British Columbia, Ontario, and Quebec because they trained at the large, well-known training schools in Vancouver, Toronto, and Montreal. Nurses frequently wrote their registration exams in the province where they trained and, because registration in a provincial association was required for enlistment, they could then apply to the military in that province.

By far the greatest proportion of military nurses in my sample were born in Ontario (31 percent); those born in Quebec (11 percent) and Saskatchewan (10.4 percent) constituted the second- and third-largest groups in the service. The largest number of enlistments also occurred in Ontario (35.6 percent), with enlistments in Quebec a distant second (16.7 percent). The Maritimes and the Prairie region, with the exception of Alberta, had substantially higher percentages of nurses enlisted compared to their civilian nurse population overall (4.5 to 9.9 percent), partially reflecting regional economic disparities. A small number of nurses enlisted in England, for a variety of reasons that will become apparent later.

Although the armed forces initially required at least two years' experience, some nurses evaded this restriction either by personal influence or because the military needed a particular set of skills. Nurses enlisted with an average of 4.7 years of experience, although 13.6 percent had ten or more years of experience. In reality, these averages meant that experience ranged from none, for those few nurses who enrolled as reinforcements at the end of the war, to twenty-nine years of teaching, supervision, and hospital administration.

At least 80.4 percent of the nurses in this study reported having had experience either in general duty nursing, private duty nursing, or some combination of both. Other nurses combined general duty nursing with a range of practice settings or even non-nursing work experience. Although they preferred private practice, they needed to take cases in hospitals as well, where they "specialed" patients too complex or unstable for student nurses to manage and wealthy patients who could afford a private nurse for hospital care. Other types of experience listed by the nurses included: public health (6.4 percent), operating room nursing (14.1 percent), psychiatric or mental nursing (1.7 percent), teaching (3.0 percent), supervising (19 percent), X-ray (1.6 percent), and military nursing experience either from the First World War or a term with the SAMNS (1.6 percent).

Nurses, in general, used a variety of educational paths to climb career ladders and the profession benefited from a trend of more girls completing high school during the 1930s. As nursing programs increased the minimum age for entry to training, young women used this interim period between leaving high school and the start of nurses' training to develop a variety of other work skills that ultimately proved to be assets in their nursing roles.[90] A small number of Canadian nurses (1.1 percent), for example, were among other university students who "quietly endured a Depression economy, hoping to use their education as an instrument of survival" and armed themselves with "credentials expected to pay rewarding dividends at some point."[91] Other nurses took advantage of a variety of business courses marketed to young women of this period. Such courses were important for working- and middle-class women during the 1920s and 1930s, offering them ready access to overwhelmingly female courses such as typing, shorthand, stenography, and bookkeeping.[92] For many nurses, these secretarial courses had paved the way for earning teaching certificates, which, in turn, had covered the expenses associated with nurse-training programs such as uniforms, shoes, and textbooks. As well, during the Depression both clerical and teaching jobs were increasingly reserved for men but nursing was a "safe" and socially acceptable field of employment for women – one with little competition from men. Successful completion of prior educational programs was considered an asset when applying to a school of nursing. Business courses and teaching certificates provided good backgrounds for myriad educational, supervisory, and administrative roles that became part of graduate nurses' responsibilities. A surprising number of nursing sisters (6.2 percent) had earned teaching certificates and teaching experience before entering nursing programs, and at least 7.7 percent had completed business courses.

It was also a common practice for nurses to take so-called postgraduate courses after completing their basic training, in order to gain additional skills and consolidate recently acquired ones. Courses in operating room technique, obstetrics, pediatrics, tuberculosis nursing, industrial nursing, mental nursing, and dietetics supplemented basic training and created a more flexible, more experienced workforce. Larger teaching hospitals, such as the Montreal General, the Toronto General, and the Montreal Neurological Institute for mental nursing, typically offered these courses, which consisted of three to twelve months of specialized training. Teaching, supervision, and public health nursing were typical postgraduate programs, earning a certificate (for a one-year course) or a diploma (for a two-year course) at the University of Toronto, McGill University, or the University of British Columbia. At least 22.6 percent of the military nurses reported the completion of one or more of these courses prior to enlistment.

One conspicuous, although not surprising, characteristic of the nursing sister population was its exclusively feminine construction. In Canada, nursing had been stereotyped as women's work since at least the 1880s, and hospital schools of nursing reinforced this perception by admitting only women to their programs, with a few exceptions such as the Victoria General Hospital in Halifax, and psychiatric hospitals in Alberta and Ontario.[93] As one CNA recruitment brochure promised, "You will not, as in other professions or business, be handicappéd by having to compete with men for top positions – nursing is a woman's profession, and women hold top positions."[94]

Few men challenged that convention during the 1920s and 1930s, and although the Canadian census for 1941 reported 153 male nurses and 73 male student nurses, military policy continued to prohibit men from serving as professional nurses until 1967.[95] Hospital training schools typically required student nurses, and even graduate nurses hired as hospital employees, to live in residence – providing a ready argument for the exclusion of men based on prohibitive costs for separate facilities. As early as 1940, however, the Ontario Hospital at Hamilton, part of the provincial mental hospital system, accepted men into nurse-training programs that included an affiliation period at the Toronto General Hospital. Other Ontario Hospital sites followed suit, enrolling at least forty men on four sites.[96] Even when men gained access to training programs and could register in some provinces such as Alberta and Ontario, other provinces denied them registration, as the Association of Nurses of the Province of Quebec did until December 1969.[97] Without eligibility for provincial registration, these men could not join the armed forces as nurses. NS Estelle Tritt recalled working with a male ward master at No. 7 CGH who was a trained nurse and had been denied rank.[98] A few male nurses enlisted with the RCN and served as sick berth attendants on ships. But this was not the equivalent of serving as a professional nurse, nor did it carry the rank and status granted to nursing sisters. The RCN Nursing Service was for women only, just as the other armed forces nursing services were.

The marriage bar was another issue that caused a great deal of consternation between 1939 and 1943. Initially, as set out in *King's Regulations and Orders*, nursing sisters had to be unmarried or widowed without children. A candidate signed an "undertaking" on enrolment, not to request permission to marry within her first year of service and promising that if she did marry while overseas, she would "relinquish all claims" that she might have "to be returned to Canada at the public expense, and undertake to make no claim for transportation pertaining to such return." After the first year, nurses still required permission to marry from the commanding officer and had to resign their commissions.[99] Since schools of nursing admitted only unmarried and widowed women, and civilian graduate nurses who married had to resign their positions as well, the armed forces' policies were consistent with social expectations.

With an abundance of nurses waiting to enlist, there was little incentive to alter the marriage policy during the first years of the war. As the need for nurses increased and the war continued, however, obligatory resignation upon marriage became both unenforceable and problematic. One nurse who signed the undertaking in June 1942 requested permission to marry only four months later. When denied permission, she married anyway and informed her commanding officer two days after the wedding. Marriage without permission carried the possibility of court martial, as well as the loss of benefits such as medals, war gratuities, and educational credits. It required the intervention of Matron-in-Chief Smellie to prevent such serious consequences in this particular case.[100] By January 1943, Matron-in-Chief Smellie informed nurses that "appointments of Nursing Sisters are not now automatically relinquished on marriage and the Nursing Sister would have to request her discharge if desired."[101]

According to RCAMC statistics, marriage was the primary reason for nursing resignations: two in 1939, twenty-five in 1940, fifty in 1941, and seventy-four in 1942. Discharges for 1943 dropped to sixty-two as more married nurses chose to remain in the service once that option became available. Three specific examples from the records illustrate how changes to marriage policy affected nurses. One nurse married in 1922, divorced, remarried, and then became a widow – making her eligible for enlistment. Another nurse married in 1942 but had to resign based on the current policy. She re-enlisted after becoming a widow and subsequently remarried in 1944 without having to resign. A third nurse married after the policy change and chose to remain in the service; she later became a widow and married again in the military.

RCAMC statistical reports support the analysis of marital status in my sample that 83.3 percent of nursing sisters remained single throughout their term of service; 0.8 percent were widowed on enlistment; 0.2 percent were divorced; 0.3 percent were married; and 15.3 percent married while in the military.[102] Married nurses presented problems, however, because of their repeated requests for postings near spouses and their pregnancies, which required them to be "boarded out" of the service. The director of Medical Services (Air) summed up his opinions in a 1943 memo: "Nursing Sisters rarely give as wholehearted service to the RCAF following marriage for the reason that their interests have changed and they naturally would prefer to live with their husbands." He even went so far as to document the changes in attrition rates after marriage with statistics.[103]

The military was losing experienced nurses to marriage just as plans were developing for the two major offensives of 1943 and 1944. At a matrons' conference during May 1943, Matron-in-Chief Smellie confirmed that married nurses would not be admitted to the armed forces but, if they married after enlistment, they could remain on duty as long as they were "medically fit" (i.e., not pregnant) or they could retire "on compassionate grounds."[104] A Department of National Defence memorandum justified the change, noting that "if nurses coming into the service feel that they must refrain from marriage during their service, very few nurses of the proper age could be induced to enter the Army, and one year 'undertaking not to marry' was all

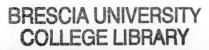

that [could be] demanded of them."[105] Additional policies shaped marriage as a career-limiting move, however: married nurses were not permitted to serve in active theatres overseas. As a result, nurses typically delayed marriage until the end of the war, when they had little to lose in terms of nursing opportunities. Although only 0.6 percent of them had married prior to 1943, 2.9 percent married during 1943, and 9.4 percent between 1944 and 1946.

Canadian nursing sisters were a relatively homogeneous group in terms of race, ethnicity, origin, religion, and language, raising the question why. Scholars now examine race and ethnicity as socially constructed and historically situated concepts that require careful analysis of supposedly objective data such as census information, attestation papers (the official personnel information forms filled out on enlistment) and even one's self-identification, given what was at stake in claiming certain racial or ethnic origins.[106] Identities held different meanings that worked both for and against individuals. Decisions to disclose or hide ethnic origin or linguistic ability could ensure social acceptance that hinged on an individual's "sameness" with the dominant group. Conversely, identification with a non-dominant ethnic or language group could be perceived as a potentially valuable asset for overseas postings where soldier patients spoke a variety of languages. Some nurses who indicated that they spoke German or Ukrainian claimed these respective ethnic origins on the forms, for example, but others did not. Birthplace offers another potential indicator of ethnicity, as in the 1921 Canadian census, in which the population was assigned to one of two main categories: Canadian- and British-born persons, and those "Born in Other Foreign Countries."[107]

In order to examine race and ethnicity in relation to military nurses, I used multiple sources of information from the attestation papers regarding place of birth, citizenship, language, and religion, because no one type of information was adequate. All nursing sisters claimed either British citizenship, an essential criterion of military service, or referred to themselves simply as "Canadian," although Canadian citizenship did not officially exist until 1947. Analyses by place of birth, parents' place of birth or citizenship, religion, and spoken languages combine to reveal some important differences among the nurses, but the overall lack of diversity exposes systemic biases against the enlistment of black, Asian, and First Nations women. In the United States, black nurses engaged in a protracted and highly politicized campaign to gain entry to the armed forces during the Second World War. Historian Darlene Clark Hine argues that the war was a "watershed" experience that ultimately led to the breaking of the colour bar in the United States.[108] In contrast, black Canadian women who wanted to become nurses had to train in the United States or elsewhere, and there was no parallel black nursing organization in Canada to mount a campaign for inclusion in military service.

Military recruitment policies among First Nations men reveal multiple forms of discrimination. For example, initial RCN recruitment policies required personnel to be of "pure European descent and of the White Race"; similarly, RCAF and army requirements stated that recruits were to be of "pure European descent with parents who were British subjects."[109] At the height of the conscription crisis in 1943, however, the Privy Council altered these requirements, permitting the recruitment of men of all racial origins.

Yet formidable barriers continued in the form of educational requirements and health standards that First Nations peoples still found difficult to meet. Given that, according to one study, 75 percent of First Nations children completed only one to three grades of formal schooling during the 1930s and few ever achieved junior matriculation (completion of Grade 12 in Ontario or Grade 11 in the rest of Canada),[110] the lack of educational opportunities would certainly have also prevented First Nations women from entering nurse-training programs.

According to the 1941 Canadian census, 72 percent of employed nurses were of British origin and 20.1 percent of French origin, with the remaining 7.9 percent from German, Italian, Jewish, Dutch, Polish, Russian, Scandinavian, or Ukrainian backgrounds. There were only seven "Indian" or First Nations nurses and thirty Asian nurses in the census, and no black nurses identified.[111] The military nursing profile was similar to the civilian profile. The vast majority of military nurses were born in Canada of either British or French backgrounds (92.6 percent) or born in Great Britain and immigrated as children to Canada (a further 4.7 percent). The remainder (2.7 percent) were born in continental Europe (Belgium, Denmark, Sweden, Italy, and Czechoslovakia), South America (Argentina and Peru), Asia (as missionaries' children in China), Russia, and South Africa.

But place of birth sometimes obscures a level of ethnicity that becomes more apparent when combined with analysis of parental birthplaces. Since one of the two variations for attestation forms did not request information on parents, 558 records (53 percent) did not provide it. Analysis of the remaining 494 records, which do include this information, indicates that only 60.7 percent of fathers and 63.8 percent of mothers were Canadian born, suggesting that approximately 40 percent of the nursing sisters were first-generation Canadians; 22.5 percent of fathers and 20.4 percent of mothers were born in Great Britain, indicating that the nursing sisters also had very strong British ties. Indeed Ethel Johns, editor for the *Canadian Nurse*, waxed eloquent on British professional and personal roots in 1940, ignoring the French-Canadian nursing heritage altogether and writing, "Although we Canadian nurses have distinct and vigorous characteristics of our own, our roots go deep into the rich soil of British tradition. The simplicity, the thoroughness, the devotion of the nurses in the Old Country are a continuing inspiration to us. This is the shining armour with which we may clothe ourselves in the day of battle."[112]

Although familial connections to Britain do not adequately explain such strong Anglo-bias within the nursing sisters population, they do partially explain differences in volunteer rates compared to French-Canadian and American nurses. Other factors, such as the dominant language used within medical units and questions of reciprocity (mutual recognition of nursing credentials between countries), also came into play. The Canadian armed forces medical units functioned predominantly in English after initial plans for francophone units did not materialize. As several nurses pointed out, francophone nurses were typically posted to Kingston for language training soon after their enlistment.[113] NS Gaëtane LaBonté was one French-Canadian nurse who claimed that she enlisted "quickly while my parents were away for the summer. When they came back, it was 'fait accompli.'" LaBonté and her francophone nurse colleagues were among those sent to Kingston, where, as she said, "It was very hard for us who spoke English in a limited way ... The nurses would give the lectures and they would stop. And then one of us would translate to make sure."[114] Her unit mobilized early and moved overseas quickly because the RCAMC wanted a French-speaking hospital unit ready to move to France when the opportunity arose. But France quickly fell to Germany, and LaBonté's unit spent the next two and a half years waiting in England, where "we thought the worst was over, as we had been transplanted very suddenly from our cosy French milieu to a completely different world in English ... I was soon called 'All Wet' because [the matron] would order me to sing that thing of a song that my generation never sang: *Allouette*."[115]

It is unclear whether Quebec-trained nurses initially had reciprocity to practise in England, as their provincial association had an associative relationship only with the CNA. But Frances Upton, president of the English professional nursing organization in Quebec, reported in 1942 that, "reciprocity has been established between our organization and the General Nursing Council for England and Wales, a fact we have hoped for many a long day."[116] Whether this delay actually deterred French-Canadian nurses from enlisting is unknown: opposition to conscription in French Canada during both wars may well account for at least some of the discrepancies in enlistment rates.[117] Demographic analysis does illustrate that the vast majority of military nurses who were born in Quebec, or enlisted there, trained at one of the two large English-speaking schools of nursing in Montreal: the Montreal General Hospital or the Royal Victoria Hospital.

Language may serve as another indicator of ethnicity, particularly the one that a respondent lists first when answering a question about what languages are spoken and read. Nurses' responses to the language question may have been contingent on what they believed to be at stake personally, and there was no formal assessment of language performance. Based on their self-reports, then, 85.5 percent were unilingual anglophones, 0.3 percent were unilingual francophone, and 10.3 percent were bilingual in French and English. At least 4.0 percent were multilingual, speaking languages in addition to English, French, or both: Danish, Dutch, Finnish, German, Icelandic, Italian, Norwegian, Polish, Russian, Slovak, Spanish, Swedish, Ukrainian, Arabic, Chinese, Flemish, and Czechoslovakian.

Religion is another variable loosely associated with race and ethnicity. The vast majority of military nurses reported themselves to be either Protestant (77.9 percent) or Roman Catholic (20.8 percent). In spite of discriminatory training-school admission practices, some Jewish women (0.4 percent) did acquire professional credentials and enlist in the armed forces as nursing sisters. NS Tritt applied at the Montreal General Hospital School of Nursing but found that it did not accept Jews, apparently because "they get married too soon." She reapplied successfully to the Reddy Memorial Hospital in Westmount, graduating in 1941. After working at the Jewish General Hospital to acquire the necessary two years' experience, Tritt joined the RCAMC.

Another notable aspect of homogeneity is the influence of class on the social construction of nursing. Although student nurses came from both working- and middle-class families, the nursing profession resembled other middle-class female professions regarding educational criteria for admission to training schools and the length of training programs.[118] Nurse leaders, in their push for recognition as a legitimate profession, had by the early 1940s raised the minimum educational criterion for admission to training schools to the junior matriculation level. At the same time, they achieved control over accreditation of schools of nursing, enabling them to regulate both the length and content of training programs. These two strategies effectively limited the profession to women who could afford both the time and expense of prolonged education, as they typically could not complete their training until they were twenty-three or twenty-four years of age.

Like race and ethnicity, class is a socially constructed and historically situated concept. It is one of several intersecting variables of difference and problematic as a category of analysis.[119] Although we lack clear criteria and means to determine class, it is generally understood as the "milieu within which one lives and from which one takes one's cues in almost all aspects of behaviour, but it is a milieu from which it is possible to escape and achieve some upward mobility."[120] Traditionally, sociologists have used indicators such as income, ownership of property, level of education, degree of occupational skill, and positions of responsibility or power to determine class. More subjective indicators include occupational ranking based on public opinion polls and ranking based on prestige in lieu of wealth or power. The most commonly used criteria, however, are: income, property ownership, education, and occupational status based on level of skill (professional, managerial, clerical, semi-skilled, unskilled, manual, or non-manual).[121]

Gender complicates class analysis, as women's experiences are not adequately reflected in the criteria traditionally used to determine class. The assumption that women "share" the family class position based on their father's occupation

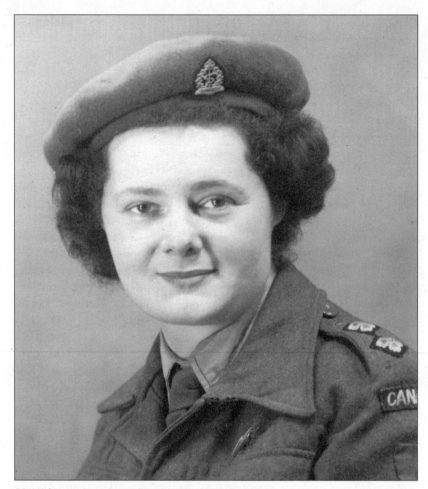

RCAMC Nursing Sister Estelle Tritt. *Courtesy Estelle Tritt Aspler*

has dominated past analyses of class.[122] But women's historians warn that, although this practice of shared class is sometimes useful, it is fundamentally imperfect since "the terms 'working class' and 'middle class' should be regarded as a guide to the status and power of women's families rather than as a reliable measure of women's ability to command resources or to share in full the values of male capitalist society."[123] The nursing profession tended to attract women with both the resources and family support necessary for an extended period of training: assets associated with middle-class families.[124] As McPherson contends, the gendered configuration of household resources was a more crucial determinant of class than the position of the male head of household, and she demonstrates that nurses came from a range of class backgrounds. Student nurses typically had a higher level of education prior to nurses' training compared to other working women, and yet working-class women were still well represented.[125]

Acknowledging the problems associated with the use of fathers' occupations as an indicator of class for women, I nonetheless adopted this approach to examine the class origins of military nurses. It is important to note, however, that these nurses were fully qualified professionals; the majority had at least two years of independent work experience prior to enlistment and at least 10.5 percent of them had either college or university education as well. Nurses were relatively privileged among working women, despite the Depression that left many of them barely able to live independently.

The Canadian census offers a comparison between the class positions of military nurses and the general population of the same period, in spite of the limitations with occupational census data in 1941.[126] The census categorized work into twelve main categories based on sectors of employment rather than social class indicators such as relationships to the means of production. For example, seven of the twelve categories included owners, managers, and labourers within the same categories of manufacturing, trade, construction, logging, mining and quarrying, personal service, and transportation and communication.

Personnel records asked if a soldier's father were living and, if so, what his occupation was. The formulation of this question resulted in a data gap if the father was dead, which was the case for 23.7 percent of the records. Deaths and files in which the occupation was not recorded constituted 43.2 percent of the records in this sample, while another 6.8 percent reported fathers only as retired, incapacitated, in the military, or unemployed, with no other indication of previous employment. Although the forms asked only if a soldier's mother were living, two nurses assertively added "housewife" as an occupation on the form. Data from the oral histories reveal that at least 34.8 percent of mothers had worked prior to marriage. Some also worked after marriage: one was a nurse, five were teachers, one was a grocery store clerk, and one was a factory supervisor.

Acknowledging these limitations, I adopted the 1941 census categories to examine the occupations of military nurses' fathers. In spite of socio-economic disruptions during the 1930s, the class backgrounds of nursing sisters remained remarkably stable, based on comparisons to both the Weir Report and McPherson's analysis of the civilian nursing workforce.[127] Among military nurses, 34.2 percent of fathers worked in farming, fishing, or ranching; 41.3 percent in professional, business, and clerical positions; and 23.8 percent in skilled, semi-skilled, and unskilled occupations; 0.7 percent were men of independent means. Thus, 23.8 percent of the nurses were from working-class families and 75.5 percent were from middle-class families.

The 1941 census considered nurses as professionals, categorizing them with architects, authors, clergymen and priests, dentists, civil engineers, judges and magistrates, lawyers, physicians and surgeons, professors, social workers, and teachers – regardless of fathers' occupational status. Class was, and still is, problematic in nursing because it intersects with gender, race, and ethnicity to privilege some nurses over others. "Nurse" was not a universal category but rather reflects a wide range of roles that nurses assumed: hospital bedside care, administration of hospitals and schools, independent practice in outposts, management of employee health programs in industries, private duty and public health, teaching in hospitals and universities. Although Second World War nursing sisters came from both working- and middle-class backgrounds, they often parlayed their education, expertise, and military officer status to reposition themselves on an individual basis during and after the war.

It is difficult to compare Canadian military nurses with other military nurses because very few studies have examined them demographically, except for aggregate data. Reading American, Australian, and British literature "against the grain," however, one gleans some comparative insights. Approximately 52,000 American nurses served with the United States Army Nurse Corps (USANC) during the Second World War, working in over 120 military hospitals and on more than 40 hospital ships.[128] Frequently described as "young in years, and in the service,"[129] American women recruited into the new USANC Cadet Nurse Corps program received an abbreviated training program wherein they could spend the last six months of their training in federal hospitals, thus helping to meet the quota for military nurses.[130] American nurses have been portrayed as younger than their Canadian counterparts and less experienced in terms of postgraduate courses and graduate nurse experience. Whereas Canadian nurses enlisted with extensive post-training courses in operating room techniques and years of nursing work experience, for example, the USANC did not offer formal operating room courses until 1944, and nurses became proficient primarily through "on-the-job" training.[131] And whereas Canadian military nurses were from a range of class backgrounds, American nurses who served on the South Pacific island of Bataan, for example, have been described predominantly as having "grown up on farms or in towns ... labored in the fields, made their own clothes, and read by lamplight, and they knew how to live lean, without amenities, and were accustomed to hard work. The Army had given them luxuries and a new life, and now it was time to pay the Army back."[132]

Like Canadian nursing sisters, all American military nurses were women. The service was also predominantly white, although black nurses lobbied for, and finally gained, admittance to the army during the conscription crisis when there were insufficient numbers of white volunteers.[133] Perceived as less-skilled workers and regarded by the American public as less desirable for the care of white soldiers, black military nurses reported that they were assigned to less pleasant cases such as prisoners of war. While Chinese-American, Puerto Rican, and Native American women were assigned to racially integrated units, Japanese-American and black nurses served in segregated units.[134]

Australian military nurses shared a strong demographic resemblance to Canadian nursing sisters.[135] Analysis of 3,477 Second World War Australian nursing sisters indicates that 92.6 percent were Australian-born and 83.6 percent claimed Protestant church associations. Approximately one-third of them were daughters of farmers, and at least 22 percent had working-class backgrounds. The average age was 28.5 years, with a range of 22 to 39, which was narrower than that of Canadian nurses. All were British subjects. Like Canadian nurses, they had to be unmarried on enlistment and resign on marriage, until policies changed during 1942. To date, there have been no other analyses of demographic variables, training, or experience for comparison.

Accounts of Second World War British nursing sisters, primarily the Queen Alexandra's Royal Army Nursing Corps, contribute valuably to knowledge of the larger international military nursing context. But lack of attention to demographic analyses limits our ability to generalize from these accounts, to make comparisons across national nursing services, or to synthesize from the experiences of thousands of rank-and-file nurses who made up the vast majority of military nursing services.[136]

The social, professional, technological, and military contexts of the 1930s positioned Canadian nurses as a readily available, feminine workforce who volunteered in overwhelming numbers for the armed forces. Nurses had a great need for work, and they were well-prepared with skills, education, and nursing experience, which they used to enhance their applications for military service. Reliance on the civilian profession to train nurses and provide them with credentials relieved the military of the burdensome tasks and costs associated with the enlistment of nurses only for the duration of the war.

With access to such a large pool of recruits, the two remaining issues for the Canadian forces were how to balance military needs with perceived civilian needs for nurses, and which nurses to select. Eligibility criteria set by the military established the basic parameters for who could become nursing sisters, although other factors helped shape the actual distribution of demographic characteristics within these parameters. Hospitals, along with the nursing profession, imposed additional official and unofficial restrictions on enlistment. But the nurses were also actively influencing their own appointments and resisting various barriers that threatened to prevent appointments. Enlistment, however, was only the beginning of military nursing service. The next challenge was how to transform civilian nurses into military nurses.

2

Incorporating Nurses into the Military

The military had little doubt regarding the value of nurses as professionals. Medical Officer T.S. Wilson objectified and quantified nursing sisters, writing in the *Journal of the Canadian Medical Services,* "Of especial importance in a surgical centre are the attached nursing sisters, whose services like that of a Thomas Splint in compound fractures of the femur, are often worth five to ten bottles of blood or plasma in the eventual outcome of a case."[1] Nursing sisters made a significant difference in the care of soldiers, while releasing non-commissioned men for combat duty. They enthusiastically filled every position in Canada and overseas, working in unconventional settings and taking on expanded roles "for the duration." But the military was highly ambivalent about admitting women to this masculine environment, especially to the active theatres of war. The postwar quotas of thirty army, thirty air force, and twenty navy nurses ensured their temporary status and restored military medical services as masculine terrain.

Nurses of both wars constituted an expandable and expendable feminine workforce. The Canadian Army Medical Corps (CAMC) had demobilized nursing sisters as soon as possible at the end of the First World War. When the Second World War began, the renamed Royal Canadian Army Medical Corps (RCAMC) once again had to transform civilian nurses into military nurses and incorporate them into the medical organization. While these nurses were well prepared as civilian professionals they were far less prepared as soldiers. Their nursing skills enabled them to take on new and expanded roles that emerged during the war, shaping decisions about where they could serve. They accepted dangers, risks, and military discipline as part of the adventure – as well as the price to pay for associated opportunities and benefits. It was gender, not nurses' abilities, that constrained their work – especially dominant discourses concerning women's roles and military women's safety.

Continuity and Change in Military Nursing
The second generation of Canadian military nurses built on the leadership,

tradition, and reputation of the first generation, who provided initial guidance at the beginning of the war in 1939. "Retired" nursing sisters began forming local units in Canada as early as 1920 and had established a national association of nursing sisters by 1932. The association was limited to nurses who had served overseas, however, and initially they met for mutual support (including social, health, and financial needs) and the promotion of military nursing.[2] The *Canadian Nurse* published some of the veteran nurses' brief personal accounts during the war and the interwar years, and at least two nursing sisters published memoirs prior to the Second World War.[3] Their personal stories and friendships continued to influence civilian nurses and student nurses during the 1930s, as well as new military nurses such as NS Jessie Morrison, who recalled, "We knew we had big shoes to fill."[4]

First World War nursing sisters provided leadership that bridged the two generations and ensured continuity of Canadian military nursing traditions. Both Matrons Emma Pense and Elizabeth Smellie had served during the First World War and with the interwar permanent nursing service. Smellie subsequently became the RCAMC matron-in-chief for Canada, while Pense served as the RCAMC matron-in-chief in England, although she was soon replaced by Agnes Neill.[5] In a Canadian Broadcasting Corporation radio interview announcing her appointment, "Miss Smellie," as she was always known, spoke of the special relationship between the two generations: "Now a word to the new nursing sisters – your predecessors offer you greetings and good wishes. I suppose you will have your own distinctions, as we did ... Don't be resentful if, as we veterans pass you by, we reveal extraordinary interest in your uniform and tell you we wish we were going again, because we do so, scarcely realizing how much water has run under the bridge since 1918."[6] At least five first-generation nursing sisters re-enlisted. They were between forty-one and fifty-four years old on re-enlistment, and served an additional four and a half to six and a half years each. Only one retired before the end of the war; the rest served at least a year beyond the 1945 Armistice.

But there were also differences between these generations of military nurses, based on changes in enlistment policies, military training courses, and new nursing service branches (changes based on technology and role differences are the subject of a later chapter). Initially, medical units organized, much as they had in 1914-18, as complete units mobilized from large hospitals associated with medical and nurse-training programs. But this policy became problematic during the Great War when civilian hospitals lost a large portion of their staff to the military, necessitating changes to the enlistment process. Winnipeg General Hospital staff mobilized first, as No. 5 Canadian General Hospital (CGH), with Toronto General Hospital staff forming No. 15 CGH. Ruth Littlejohn, a Winnipeg General nurse, had to "take over the teaching of classes for the student nurses on maternity" in 1939 when the army "stripped the hospital of nurses and physicians" and "there

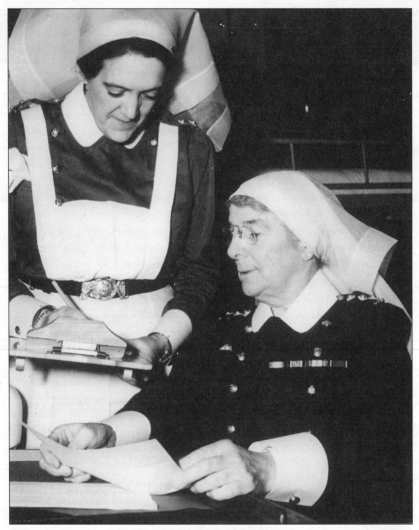

RCAMC Nursing Sister M.N. DeVere and Matron Charlotte Nixon, on No. 46 Canadian hospital ship, *Lady Nelson*, April 1943. A veteran military nurse of the First World War, Matron Nixon re-enlisted at the age of fifty-four to supervise Canada's first of two hospital ships during the Second World War. *College and Association of Registered Nurses of Alberta Museum and Archives, Mary Macleod Collection*

were no experienced nurses on the wards."[7] *Canadian Nurse* editor Ethel Johns wrote that hospitals were feeling the effects of the withdrawal of "key" nurses for military duty by early 1941. Elizabeth Smellie, who had also been a vice-president of CNA, reiterated the need for good relationships with the civilian profession and subsequently modified recruitment policies to integrate nurses from across Canada within the different medical units.[8]

Defence Scheme No. 3 (1938), the basis of Canadian war preparations, recommended proportional representation by population in attempts to deal with sociopolitical issues such as recently high levels of unemployment, national manpower requirements during "total war," and conscription. The unemployed demanded equal access to military jobs, but the distribution of labour within Canada had to be considered as well.[9] Proportional representation also influenced the mobilization of medical units. Nursing sisters of No. 10 CGH and No. 12 CGH were the first nurses recruited under a new policy made by Matron-in-Chief Smellie at the end of 1942 to replace the practice of mobilizing medical personnel as groups from civilian hospitals. Smellie reported to the matrons' conference at Ottawa that "from now on all units are representative of different sections of Canada, not of individual localities."[10] In another example, the *Lady Nelson*, Canada's first hospital ship, was staffed by twelve nursing sisters specifically selected in pairs to represent six regions across Canada. Once units had a full complement of nurses, additional nursing sisters enlisted as "reinforcements" to replace those who resigned or supplement staff during periods of heavy casualties, moving between units as needed.

The second area that changed was military training for nurses. Although nursing sisters received varying levels of training, programs gradually became more formal than the lectures one First World War nurse described as talks to "fill the sisters' time at sea."[11] Some army nurses reported having little orientation – and what little there was focused primarily on recognizing ranks, using titles, and understanding organizational structures within the military. Others received two weeks of classes and drills, a trip through an improvised gas chamber to test their use of the ubiquitous gas masks that they would have to carry throughout the war, and a period of work within a military hospital in Canada. This served as a probation before promotion to first-lieutenant and coveted overseas postings. These nurses wrote qualifying exams that included questions on the *King's Regulations and Orders for the Canadian Militia (KR)* as well as on nursing duties, such as, "What is your duty with regard to the admission of a patient to your ward, death of a patient, and patient's kit?" and "Discuss the responsibility of a matron in charge of a general hospital with regard to nursing sisters' quarters and domestic economy, confidential reports, nursing sisters on sick list, neglect of duty by N.C.O. in charge of ward."[12] Still other nurses underwent both oral and written examinations, as prescribed in *KR*, paragraph 787. NS Estelle Tritt explained that, at Kingston Military Hospital, "they handed us the 'King's Rules and Regulations' to study when we had time ... Then I had to write an exam with the *KR* camped right beside me. But I passed ... learned how to order meals in military hospitals ... account for all the cutlery. This is what we were taught – to account for all the cutlery, the dishes, this and that."[13]

Several nurses described additional field training, route marches, and field manoeuvres (or schemes) lasting up to ten days at a time. For one, NS Evelyn Pepper described her training as "Learning how to march, salute, read a map, pitch a tent, take it down, put it up again, live in it and like it, eat out of a billy-can, drive anything from a motorcycle to an ambulance, fire revolvers and 303's, practice Judo techniques on our fellow-officers, plus a general orientation to army terminology and procedure, bulged our training days and hardened our muscles." By 1943, the RCAMC had an official "Qualifying Course for the Nursing Service," described as a four-week course that was necessary for promotion.[14]

A few nursing sisters received no military training. NS Frances Oakes, for example, was one of the first nurses in the Royal Canadian Air Force (RCAF), in November 1940. She went overseas before the RCAF developed a three-week training program known as the "School of Aviation Medicine Course in Aviation Nursing" and presented at Havergal College, in Toronto. But most RCAF nurses who enlisted after December 1942 attended one of twelve such courses. NS Jean Wheeler, with the South African Military Nursing Service, explained that she did not have any "army training" because she was "just going to nurse after all." Betty Riddell served with the United States Army Nurse Corps, where she found the situation similar because "we knew how to nurse." She had no military training in preparation for her postings in the United States and Papua New Guinea.[15]

Royal Canadian Navy (RCN) NS Dorothy Surgenor blamed the tenuous position of navy nurses, who were considered "support" personnel, for her lack of training: "I didn't even have a basic training. I just went from nursing to nursing. And this stood up very sharply because one day, [six] of us were supposed ... to be a colour party for launching a corvette. And we didn't know anything about marching, much less saluting or anything else. So for two days, our patients instructed us on how to do this, because nobody really knew ... We weren't really part of the navy ... We were not given any pre-instructions. We had to learn from the patients because they *loved* teaching the nursing sisters ... We were in the navy but not part of it."[16] NS Kay Christie also felt nurses were not fully accepted members of the military. According to her, nursing sisters were typically added to the contingent of men rather than integrated within the contingent. She referred to herself and May Waters as the "plus two" component of the Hong Kong contingent: "We were always 'plus two.' You know, there were 96 men officers plus two [nursing officers]."[17]

Whereas all of the First World War nursing sisters had served with the army, Second World War nursing sisters served with all three branches of the Canadian armed forces, as well as in the South African nursing service. The RCAMC was the only nursing service at the beginning of the war. When the RCAF and RCN formed separate nursing services, Matron-in-Chief Smellie continued to provide initial leadership, facilitating continuity in policies, uniforms, pay, and benefits among the different service branches.

Matron-in-Chief Smellie epitomized both continuity and change through her leadership of the RCAMC nursing service and, indirectly, the other two military nursing services. She brought previous experience from the First World War, tempered by interwar roles with the Victorian Order of Nurses and the Canadian Nurses Association, to the diverse contexts of the Second World War. As matron-in-chief, she became the highest-ranking woman in the armed forces, the first woman to serve as a full colonel in any modern military. In addition to early leadership for RCAF and RCN nursing services, she super-vised the formation of the military Women's Division, the Canadian Women's Army Corps, in 1941.[18] She also reinforced an idealized image of military nurses while reassuring the public of nurses' femininity, in a 1940 nationwide radio broadcast: "A nursing sister, no matter where she is, still represents the spirit of nursing and Canadian womanhood. Beyond rules and regulations, there is an individual code to abide by on or off duty. One thing we know – the Canadian nurse will be well taken care of – the Army sees to that."[19]

Nursing Sisters as an Expandable Workforce

Changes in the technologies of destruction, transportation, and communication during the Second World War influenced the type of medical and nursing care required as well as who gave this care, and in what settings. Massive burns from tank and plane warfare (which had only been introduced by the end of the First World War), more extensive head, chest, and abdominal trauma (due to more destructive weaponry on both sides), and the ongoing dangers of extensive wound infection all led to highly invasive surgical interventions based on innovations since the first war. Important "firsts" included massive use of blood, blood products, and intravenous fluids as well as experimental reconstruction of body parts and the introduction of penicillin. The treatment of psychiatric and stress-induced syndromes was also significantly different from that of earlier wars. Each set of changes relied, to some extent, on the availability of nurses who could assume expanded roles. In addition, the nature of large-scale campaigns during the Second World War involved the rapid movement of troops over vast distances, requiring care to be given on or near the frontlines. Transfusions of blood and plasma given in the forward areas to treat shock, for example, made a significant difference in the survival of casualties, permitting their evacuation and subsequent care behind the lines. As the war progressed, military and medical policies moved nurses forward as part of small mobile field units that followed the troops closely, sometimes under enemy observation and within range of their weapons.

Location was one factor influencing the type and size of medical units, and therefore the characteristics of nurses' work. Military hospitals in Canada functioned primarily as sick bays, screening and immunization units, and trauma centres for casualties resulting from training accidents, particularly the Commonwealth Air Training Program, wherein young men learned to fly planes. Other sites included experimental stations for chemical and biological warfare, such as the station at Suffield, Alberta; hospital trains; prisoner of war and internment camps; and convalescent and rehabilitation hospitals.[20] Overseas, there were hospital ships transporting casualties between North America, England, and the Mediterranean in addition to stationary and mobile medical units in England, continental Europe, the Mediterranean, South Africa, and Hong Kong. Within each location, postings and nurses' work varied according to the particular service branch – army, air force, or navy.

The largest cohort was the RCAMC nursing service, with at least one hundred medical units in Canada, three military hospitals in Newfoundland (considered an overseas posting), and thirty-three medical units in England. In addition, RCAMC nursing sisters moved with their units to North Africa, Sicily, Italy, France, the Netherlands, Belgium, Germany, and Hong Kong. As the senior medical and nursing service, it was the army – and not navy nurses – who staffed the Canadian hospital ships (the *Lady Nelson* and *Letitia*) and sick-bay quarters of the *Queen Elizabeth* and *Queen Mary*, transporting soldiers, prisoners of war, and war brides, and thus exacerbating rivalries between the nursing services. Some RCAMC nurses also participated in patient evacuations from the continent to England after D-Day on Dakota and Sparrow airplanes. Others staffed military hospital trains within Canada. Attached to regular passenger trains, hospital trains had specially designed and furnished cars accommodating sixteen to twenty-eight bed patients in addition to "sitting" patients.[21]

Two RCAMC nursing sisters, May Waters and Kay Christie, went with the Canadian contingent to Hong Kong at the end of 1941 – although it was not what they had envisioned as military nursing when they enlisted. Christie, wanting to go overseas, had had Jamaica in mind when she volunteered for a semi-tropical posting. When offered a tropical posting and given only five minutes to deliberate her decision, she accepted a "secret" overseas posting to an unknown destination. Christie travelled alone to Vancouver by train with mounting trepidation, instructed not to talk to anyone en route: "My heart just dropped when they said Vancouver. I thought, you don't go to England (or Jamaica) by way of Vancouver. But I had said I would go and it was too late."[22] She and NS Waters, who boarded the same train at Winnipeg, discovered in the middle of the Pacific that they were headed to Hong Kong with the Canadian troops, posted to a British military hospital there. Exactly three weeks after the troops arrived, Japanese soldiers attacked Hong Kong as well as Pearl Harbor. On 26 December 1941, Waters and Christie became prisoners of war when Japanese troops took over the hospital, and they endured hardships and privations for the next twenty-one months.

A small number of RCAMC nursing sisters remustered with the establishment of the two new nursing services. Twelve of them joined the RCAF in November 1940. The director of Medical Services (Air) administered the

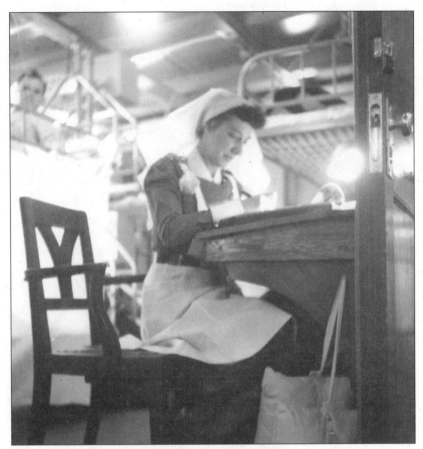

The RCAMC was responsible for the sea transport of soldiers from any of the Canadian armed forces branches. Thus RCAMC nurses, not RCN nurses, worked on the two Canadian hospital ships. At Naples on 29 January 1944, RCAMC NS M.B. Meisner was serving "at sea" on the *Lady Nelson*. LAC/Frederick G. Whitcombe/DND fonds/PA-163659

air force nursing service for more than two years, with consultation visits by Matron-in-Chief Smellie, until the RCAF appointed Jessie Porteous as matron in April 1943 and principal matron (RCAF) with the rank of squadron leader a year later. At the end of 1944, there were about a hundred RCAF air training stations with hospital facilities or infirmaries across Canada and Newfoundland, ranging in size from units with only a few beds to the 700-bed hospital at St. Thomas Technical Training School in Ontario. Nursing sisters staffed units of twenty-five or more beds and medical units of the Royal Air Force training schools operating under the British Commonwealth Air Training Program in Canada. Outside the Dominion of Canada, nursing sisters were stationed at RCAF hospitals in Gander, Newfoundland, and Goose Bay, Labrador, as well as in England at station infirmaries for No. 6

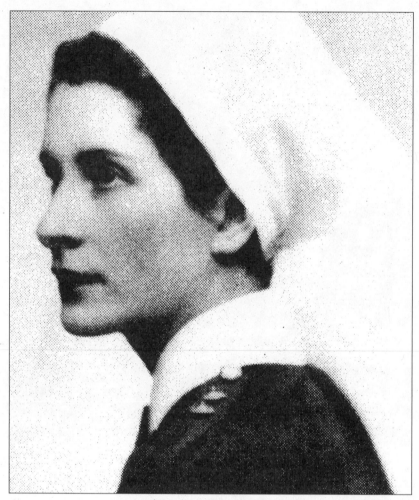

RCAMC NS Kay Christie was one of only two Canadian military nurses to serve as prisoners of war. *Royal Canadian Military Institute Museum*

Bomber Group (Northallerton), No. 3 RCAF Personnel Reception Centre (Bournemouth), RCAF Repatriation Depot (Warrington), and the specialized plastic surgery wing for Canadian burn patients at East Grinstead. Six nurses completed an air evacuation course at Bowman Field near Louisville, Kentucky, during 1943. They became part of RCAF No. 6 Casualty Air Evacuation Unit, flying casualties from the continent to base hospitals in England during August 1944 and evacuating civilian patients from Newfoundland and Labrador to larger medical facilities in emergencies. Four nurses, who joined No. 52 RCAF Mobile Field Hospital's advance party, were probably the first Allied women to land in Normandy after D-Day in June 1944.[23]

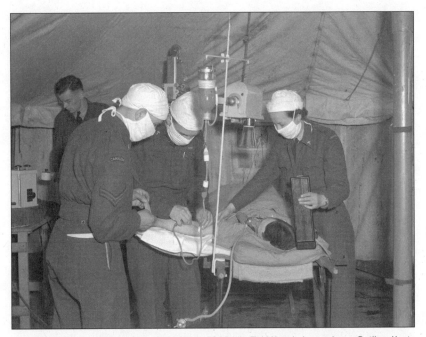

In preparation for the D-Day invasion, RCAF No. 52 Mobile Field Hospital moved near Detling, Kent, for increased experience in resuscitating and evacuating casualties. Unit members such as orderly Donald Bunce, MO G.R. Hall, and NS Wyn Pitkethly, shown here on 16 August 1943 in England, put this valued expertise into action later in Normandy, only thirteen days after D-Day. *Canadian Forces Joint Imagery Centre, PL-29967*

Three RCAMC nursing sisters remustered with the formation of the RCN nursing service in November 1941. As she had for the RCAF, Matron-in-Chief Smellie provided interim leadership for RCN nursing sisters, until the appointment of Matron Marjorie Russell almost two years later. RCN nurses served at nine land-based naval hospitals: the HMCS *Naden* at Esquimalt, British Columbia; the HMCS *Stadacona* and RCNH *Rockhead* at Halifax, Nova Scotia; the RCNH *Ste. Hyacinthe* at Ste. Hyacinthe, Quebec; the RCNH *Cornwallis, Protector,* and *Shelburne* in Nova Scotia; the RCNH *Avalon* at St. John's, Newfoundland; and the HMCS *Niobe* at Greenock, Scotland. They also served at several clinics and special units: the *Donnacona* at Montreal; a special treatment centre for tuberculosis at Ste. Agathe, Quebec; the *Tecumsah* at Calgary; and the HMCS *Conestoga* at Galt, Ontario, where they were responsible for training members of the Women's Division as medical assistants.[24]

Because the navy was a fighting force with no mobile hospital ships of its own, RCN nursing sisters did not serve at sea. As NS Surgenor explained, there were few survivors of naval battles, and sick-berth attendants could provide most of the first aid required at sea. Navy hospitals in Newfoundland

and Labrador were strategically located in relation to German submarine activity while also providing a much-needed resource for the local civilian population. The majority of patients were survivors from the Battle of the Atlantic and merchant seamen. The only nursing sister death from enemy action during the Second World War, among all three services, was that of a RCN nurse who drowned during a submarine attack on a civilian ferry, the *Caribou*, which was sunk in the Cabot Strait off Newfoundland.[25]

South Africa was another strategic location on the main evacuation routes between England and the Middle Eastern theatre (since the Mediterranean route was unsafe for transport and became a second battle zone), and between England and the Far Eastern theatre (China, Burma, and India). The South African government received special permission from the Canadian government in 1941 to recruit 300 Canadian nurses for its military hospitals to address a perceived shortage. NS Jean Wheeler believed that the shortage was partially related to policies prohibiting black nurses from caring for white patients and partially to the government's reluctance to divert white nurses from civilian to military hospitals.[26] Canadian nurses in the SAMNS enlisted through the RCAMC and wore the RCAMC uniform, but they served without commissions and with the South African military responsible for their transportation, pay, and postings. At least 301 Canadian nurses served in South Africa during the war. They left Canada in three main groups and several smaller sailings to complete the draft and supply replacements. Matron Gladys Sharpe was the liaison officer between the Canadian, British, and South African governments. SAMNS nurses signed one-year, renewable contracts to serve primarily in British military hospitals located in South Africa. The largest was a thousand-bed hospital at Baragwanath, near Johannesburg, where Canadian nursing sisters constituted most of the nursing staff. They were also posted to military hospitals at Durban, Pretoria, and Pietermaritzburg. At the end of their contracts, two-thirds of them signed on with the SAMNS "for the duration," with subsequent postings to Egypt, North Africa, and Italy.[27]

Not all the SAMNS nurses were happy with their conditions of service. When they learned that they had to pay for their own accommodations in South Africa and that the cost of living was higher than in Canada, some protested the discrepancy between their pay and that of the RCAMC nurses. When she discovered how little her monthly pay of £13 would cover, and that it was one-third the rate for RCAMC nurses, NS Marguerite McLimont wrote, "We shall have to cut our living to our pay."[28] Other SAMNS nurses could not manage with the lower rate. NS Angela La Croix returned to Canada in February 1943, for example, enlisting with the RCAMC a month later because she had financial responsibilities for her widowed mother.[29] After the war, the Canadian government passed an Order-in-Council to "top up" South African war service gratuities and extend equal veterans' benefits to these nursing sisters, in partial compensation for their lower rates of pay during the war.[30]

Diverse geographical settings required diverse organizational structures as the medical services adapted to the ever-changing needs and contexts of the war. Almost all nursing sisters, with the exception of 1.0 percent who served only with the SAMNS, began their work in district military hospitals and troop-training camps across Canada. While 25.1 percent of them remained in Canada for the duration of the war, others had postings abroad, often in multiple theatres. Thus, at least 68 percent served in England, 31.4 percent in continental Europe, 18.2 percent in the Mediterranean, 7 percent in the North Atlantic theatre, and 4.3 percent in South Africa, in addition to the two nurses at Hong Kong. They worked in a variety of settings, moving wherever their skills were needed.

The RCAMC organized units initially as "field ambulances," following the same "chain of evacuation" developed during the First World War. A field ambulance was actually a system for collecting and evacuating casualties to different levels of treatment based on the stability and treatment needs of the casualties. It evolved functionally, and, according to a 1941-42 reorganization plan, each ambulance was to be fully mobile and consist of one headquarters plus two stretcher bearer units without other attachments. Medical officers and stretcher bearers provided the first level of assistance at regimental aid posts located near battle sites. They managed basic first aid and treated minor illnesses, initiating evacuation to the next level as necessary and moving constantly with the battle. With no capacity to keep or treat casualties, they did not require nurses at this level.[31]

From regimental aid posts, casualties went to various field dressing stations, field surgical units, and casualty clearing stations. Dressing stations initiated a triage system of priority for care: rapid diagnosis, essential emergency treatments, sorting and labelling casualties in order of priority for further evacuation, and documentation of care given. They were sometimes differentiated as "main" and "advanced" dressing stations – the term "advanced" referring to their position relative to the frontline, not to any specialized level of treatment. Surgery and nursing care were initially unavailable until patients reached casualty clearing stations and stationary hospitals, but this changed during the war with the addition of small specialized units in forward areas.

Between the Dieppe raid in 1942 and the invasion of Sicily and Italy in 1943, the RCAMC participated in various training schemes in the United Kingdom, such as Exercise Spartan during the spring of 1943. Lessons learned during these schemes led to changes in the delivery of medical services. For example, instead of transporting casualties over long distances to surgical care safely behind the lines, as in the First World War, the emphasis shifted to taking surgical care forward to the casualties.[32] This required the addition of small specialty teams, more mobile than complete hospital units, who could work on or near the frontlines doing emergency surgeries, transfusions, and fluid resuscitation. The efficacy and efficiency of these units depended greatly on nursing sisters such as NS Patricia Moll, who was with No. 1 Field Dressing Station in Italy, which was set up two and a half miles behind the frontlines but ahead of Canadian artillery and in sight of German patrols.[33]

The two smallest specialty units were field surgical units and field transfusion units, which attached to various field dressing stations as needed, forming combined units known as advanced surgical centres. Once the centres ceased admitting casualties, the field surgical unit and the field transfusion unit moved off to another field dressing station, leaving regular personnel to recover and evacuate the casualties, who by that point were post-operative. Field surgical units were totally self-contained, with a generator, water tank, and sufficient linen, equipment, and personnel for thirty to forty operations as well as vehicles to transport the unit. Based on the British Army's experience in the Middle Eastern campaigns, and tested by Canadians in Sicily and Italy, field surgical units had two surgeons, two nurses, an anaesthetist, and two orderlies on staff.[34] Ten such units were in operation with Canadian troops in Italy and northwestern Europe. Although it remains unclear if nurses were posted to field transfusion units, they did work in the resuscitation wards of field surgical units, where transfusions were administered. NS Pepper and other nurses frequently described the tangle of infusion lines that resulted as intravenous fluids and blood products hung from ropes strung along the tops of tents, impeding movement within the hospital tent wards.[35] Within such newly formed and reorganized units, nursing sisters encountered a variety of new technologies and modified others. As NS Elsie Barr wrote, "much of our expertise (savoir faire) was acquired by encountering a problem and rising to the occasion."[36]

RCAMC physician W.R. Feasby assessed the effectiveness of nurses in these units, writing that "without the excellent post-operative care provided, the work of the surgeons would have been of little avail however far forward they might have been positioned."[37] One field surgical unit in Italy attributed to "better nursing" the decline in mortality rates from 15 and 16 percent to less than 10 percent.[38] At least one medical officer was sceptical about having nurses with field surgical units. He wrote to the *Journal of the Canadian Medical Services* that "in this particular set-up there have been 6 Nursing Sisters – four on the wards of the FDS [field dressing station], and one with each surgical team. It has been of value I think, but I can well visualize situations where it would be impossible to have the nurses with us, and for that reason have not departed very far from our previous routine. Certainly the nursing on the wards has been excellent, and having our own girls has, if nothing else, improved the morale of the patients – in fact we have been criticized for spoiling them!"[39] This medical officer refused to consider nurses as anything more than temporary assistance, to the point of denigrating their substantial contribution to patient outcomes as mere "morale building."

Because the presence of nurses in forward units was both new and contentious, nursing sisters had to negotiate their relationships with other members of the unit carefully. NS Helen Bright, at a field surgical unit in Belgium, wrote for example that, "During this slack time, we had the opportunity of becoming acquainted with the orderlies with whom we were to work and to feel our way into the unit which had never had nursing sisters before."[40] The war diary of No. 5 Casualty Clearing Station claims there were "early doubts about this innovation," referring to the introduction of nurses during February 1944, but then notes acceptance based on nurses' performances: "Most of the FDS commanders are a little leery about having nursing sisters around, believing that their personnel may resent their presence. In this case, however, the personnel of the FDS are very pleased to have them. Nursing orderlies have done considerable work and have considerable experience, but they have 1,000 questions to ask that only a nurse can answer. Realizing this, the nursing sisters have been putting on lectures and demonstrations for them."[41]

In an attempt to avoid placing nurses in forward areas, the RCAMC assigned nursing sisters to train "other ranks" – that is, non-commissioned men – as nursing orderlies, also known as medical orderlies, medical assistants, or ward orderlies. Training began with a class of 80 men at Camp Borden in October 1943. Such training lasted three months and qualified 489 orderlies over the first year. The "most promising" of these orderlies received an additional sixteen weeks of instruction in operating room technique and went to work at field surgical units and casualty clearing stations. Although orderlies certainly played important roles, both physicians and nurses were keenly aware that orderlies could not substitute for fully trained professional nurses in terms of patient outcomes.[42]

The majority of RCAMC nurses served overseas in large Canadian General Hospital (CGH) units, with a capacity for 600-1,200 patients each. Out of twenty-six RCAMC medical units all together, eleven remained in England for the duration of the war; the rest converted to field hospitals and moved to the Mediterranean in 1943-44 and northwestern Europe in 1944. When medical units moved to an active theatre of war, they often doubled in size to accommodate the number of casualties. Reinforcement medical officers and nursing sisters joined such units as required and as available, while regular personnel worked extended hours to complete surgeries and evacuate patients in preparation for the next round of admissions. To extend bed capacity, patients could be treated on stretchers, just inches off the ground. As NS Jean Dorgan wrote, "The fact that we had 200 beds meant nothing. When we ran out of beds we used stretchers."[43]

Nurses also served in smaller 200-600-bed Casualty Clearing Stations (CCS). Active during the Battle of Britain although the unit would not move to the continent until 1944, Matron Agnes MacLeod's CCS consisted of "an orderly room tent, an admission and discharge tent, a medical service

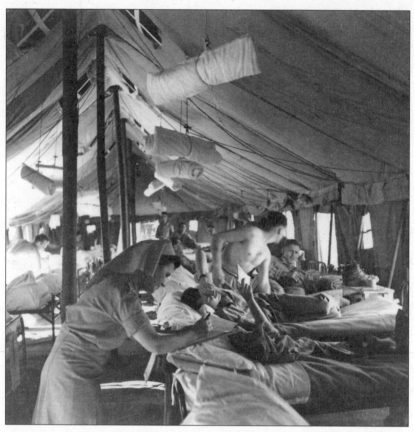

Tented hospital units, such as RCAMC No. 15 CGH at El Arrouch, Algeria, during August 1943, served as a major evacuation point for casualties from the Sicily and Italian campaigns. Located in northern Africa during this period, it could adapt for the increasing number of patients and provide more stable facilities for surgery and prolonged recovery periods than forward mobile units could do while in active theatres. There, NS D. Mick had plenty of experience dealing with sirocco winds, desert heat, and very limited water supplies in addition to caring for casualties. *LAC/Frederick G. Whitcombe/DND fonds/PA-141498*

tent, a surgical service tent, support services, and patient tents – in all well over fifty tents." She noted that patient turnover was rapid because they kept only short-term cases that would recover quickly and evacuated the rest.[44]

CCSs had evolved during the First World War in response to needs for increased mobility of medical and surgical care. But their size had become increasingly cumbersome as the Second World War progressed and theatres of war expanded over larger areas. Newer, specialized units could better fill mobility requirements, and CCSs therefore shifted their focus to the immediate post-operative care of patients and stabilizing casualties in preparation for evacuation. The RCAMC scaled CCSs down to essential components and

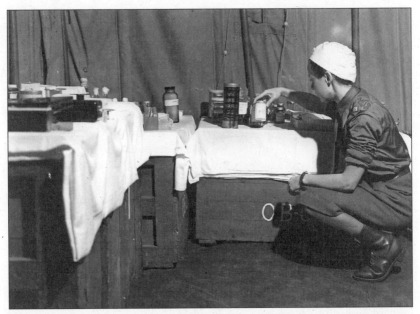

One of the challenges of mobile units such as RCAMC No. 6 CCS was the storage and rapid packing/unpacking of essential surgical supplies and instruments. While still in England during October 1943, this nursing sister used all available resources, including packing crates, to organize her supplies. *LAC/Lieutenant C.E. Nye/DND fonds/PA-213779*

reduced them in size to between 100 and 200 beds by 1943. They were then positioned in pairs in close proximity to the frontlines, where they admitted patients in an alternating system popularly known as "leap-frogging." One unit would fill to capacity at a time, allowing the other unit to stabilize and evacuate its patients, and then move ahead of the receiving unit and reverse roles. They were typically located approximately five miles behind the front, moving forward whenever the distance to the front approached fifteen miles. They were often situated near a small Canadian Stationary Hospital (CSH). Hospitals, not to be confused with CCSs, FDSs, FTUs and so forth, were designated as either Canadian General Hospitals or Canadian Stationary Hospitals, though both were in fact mobile. They managed lower-priority casualties and sick soldiers while also serving as a pool of nursing reinforcements for the more forward units. As mobile units, both CCSs and CSHs adapted to whatever existing facilities were available: schools, convents, barns, bombed-out factories, chateaux, or canvas tents. NS Pepper was one of eight nurses at No. 5 CCS, which leap-frogged with No. 4 CCS at least eighteen times in Italy. She and another nurse were left behind by their unit as it moved forward, to continue caring for soldiers until they could be evacuated. At one point, they were on their own for four to five days with only a driver, cook, and seventeen patients.[45]

Hospital ships, trains, and sometimes air ambulances were used to evacuate casualties who required more than two weeks' recovery time back to England. There, CGHs and other specialized medical units continued their treatment. Prior to the summer of 1943, the main admissions to CGHs were casualties from the Battle of Britain and the Dieppe raid, as well as training accidents in the United Kingdom, and personnel for minor surgeries or illness. Later, they received casualties evacuated from the Mediterranean and northwestern Europe who had on-going needs for surgery, convalescent care, and rehabilitation. Burn patients, for example, required months and sometimes years of reconstructive surgery performed as a series of meticulous, progressive steps to graft and rebuild eyelids, mouths, noses, ears, jaws, and other essential body parts.[46] Most of this was done overseas, partially to spare the families as well as the victims of some of the impact of their injuries and partially, to avoid media attention to the effects of war. Personnel with venereal diseases constituted another patient population that increased over the course of the war and required months of treatment in CGHs before penicillin became available in 1943.[47]

Not all patients were Canadian or Allied troop casualties however. Medical units also treated prisoners of war (POW), both in Canada and overseas, as well as some civilians. Nursing sisters cared for more than 150 children during the bombing of Coventry, and 69 children from Birmingham received treatment at No. 1 Canadian General Hospital in Marston Green during 1940.[48] NS Margaret Fletcher wrote home about two sisters, seven and eleven years old, treated at No. 2 Casualty Clearing Station in the Netherlands: "The little one had to have her arm off at the elbow, & the sister had two holes in her posterior chest, & a chest full of blood – more grenades. I had the job of making a pincushion out of the poor little souls, and couldn't speak a word to them. I never felt such a heel in my life."[49] NS Betty Nicolson described a local family in Sicily, who sought help from the only medical service available to them: "We had a peasant in the [operating room] once when I was on duty. And we heard a lot of moaning and groaning coming up towards the hospital. It was a group of Sicilians pulling a donkey, pulling a wagon. And obviously, a family all moaning and groaning. Their father had been out in the field tilling, and he had gone over a mine. And they were bringing him up to our hospital, of course. We knew though, when he came in, that there was nothing we could do for him. But we set up an intravenous anyway and just waited."[50] Similarly, in Newfoundland and isolated training camps across Canada, RCAF and RCN nursing sisters often served as health care resources for whole communities. Some of the first RCAF air evacuation flights involved nurses on "mercy flights" to take patients to larger medical centres, and RCN nurses even became involved with "well baby clinics" for civilians in their local settings.[51]

Initially, the military based their projected requirements for nurses on First

World War experiences with staffing. Military plans called for a medical service with bed capacity equal to 10 percent of the overall troop force. Medical units functioned with a relatively small nursing component in comparison to civilian hospitals of similar sizes, but decisions about teamwork and using both "other ranks" and recovering soldiers as nursing assistants made these patterns work.[52] For example, twenty-four-hour coverage for a static 600-bed hospital typically required eighteen medical officers, a principal matron and a matron, fifty nursing sisters, two physiotherapist aides, one dietician, and seventy nursing orderlies. A 1,200-bed hospital required a minimum of eighty, and more often 100 nursing sisters, although actual staffing varied according to the number of casualties and level of acuity.

Rather than being static organizational structures, medical units were fluid in size, staffing, and function; they were also contingent on needs and resources. In England, for example, small groups of nurses worked with specialty teams in units that grew into large specialized hospitals. Twenty nurses worked with Dr. Wilder Penfield, the well-known Montreal neurological surgeon, at the Hackwood House site of No. 1 Neurological Hospital, while five nurses worked with the Canadian plastic surgery team at Park Prewett. These two units merged as the Basingstoke Neurological and Plastic Surgery Hospital in 1943, which held 600 beds by 1944.[53] Field hospitals expanded with tents and low-lying stretchers. General hospitals sometimes operated as casualty clearing stations, and casualty clearing stations sometimes downsized to operate as advanced surgical centres or field dressing stations. NS Kellough described No. 5 CCS in the Netherlands, as generally having "about fifteen Nursing Sisters" but sometimes "up to twenty," some of whom they lent out as needed.[54]

Staffing requirements depended on the setting, number of casualties, intensity of war activity, and the prevalence of contagious diseases – as well as whose perspective was solicited. Military authorities claimed that nursing sisters enjoyed better working conditions than nurses in civilian hospitals, and some nursing sisters were inclined to agree. But they also described episodes involving long hours of continuous work, a large volume of admissions and evacuations, and frustration with assembly-line care.[55] NS Helen Mussallem judged military nursing to be much more fragmented than civilian nursing: "In the Army, it was just a question of, I don't like to use the word, but sort of patching them up and get them ready for more war, or patching them up and sending them back to Canada."[56] NS Frances Ferguson described coping with an influx of casualties at No. 6 CCS in France: "The highest number of nurses I think I remember in the CCS, was eight. We were supposed to be a 20-bed unit and we got patients in all during the day. We got some at night, too ... We had patients in the bed, under the bed, head-first if they had something wrong with their feet, and feet-first if there was something wrong with their head ... At one time we had about 56 patients in a 20-bed unit. So what do you do with them? They were all in need of a lot of help. So that means with eight nurses on, to cover for 24 hours, they've got to go pretty hard. So we went as long as we could walk and it was daylight. We were on the go."[57] NS Margaret Roe also recalled working hard: "I remember being so tired coming off night duty, you'd walk past the dining room going upstairs to your room … We'd just plod upstairs, and we were just so tired, we didn't want to eat. You felt nauseous."

As one strategy to cope with the workload, nurses taught medical orderlies and recovering patients to assist them and then supervised their work. In the army, they trained other ranks, and in the navy and air force, they trained Women's Division personnel as well. The training began informally, but as the number of soldiers increased, so did bed capacity and, therefore, the need for more assistants. Beyond the obviously modified level of training, there were other significant differences between medical assistants and nursing sisters. Like the physicians, nurses were civilians first and soldiers second, while the other ranks were soldiers first and medical assistants second.[58]

Medical orderlies (or assistants) extended the eyes, hands, and feet of the nursing sisters. As NS Pepper wrote, "Our 'boys' … had come from farms, businesses, shops, school rooms, construction work, and numerous other occupations far removed from the teachings and routine of a health institution … Most of the instruction was accomplished on the job." However, they were also "alert, watchful learners," many becoming "expert and highly reliable" as they dealt with "dust, heat, stench, and the scarcity of water."[59] NS Ferguson recalled that, "They weren't cooks or cleaning men or anything else. They were on duty with us, and they helped us watch the intravenous and anything else we needed done." But orderlies could also be problematic and sometimes less than enthusiastic about their assignments. NS Louise Jamieson had to have the ward sergeant enforce the work list on her ward; she also had to "watch the back rub bottles," containing alcohol, to prevent the orderlies from taking them. NS Tritt felt the assistants required careful supervision, given their limited training. As one example, she asked an orderly for some sterile supplies during a surgical procedure: "So he brought out this big pillowcase, and we said, 'What's that?' He said, 'Oh, I sterilized them and then I opened them, and put them in this pillowcase.'" He hadn't realized that he had recontaminated the sterilized equipment.

Patients were expected to work during their recovery period, and the medical services depended on this work to offset the quota of nurses and orderlies posted per unit. NS Littlejohn recalled posting patients to the ward "duty roster," while NS Bayly also explained that as soon as patients could move around, they were expected to make their own beds and help on the ward in general.[60] NS Margaret Mills labelled this work as doing "Joe Jobs," which included cleaning sinks, sweeping floors, and the like.[61] But dependence on patients' labour could work against the nurses. NS Joan

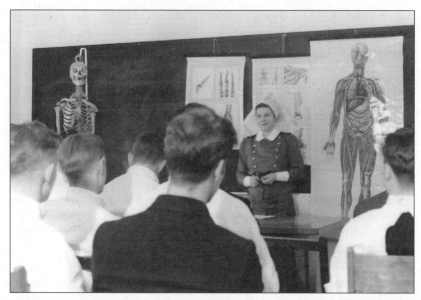

Military nurses were highly valued for their teaching expertise as well as their nursing skills. RCN NS Waterman, for example, gave lectures to medical assistants at the RCNH *Avalon* at St. John's, Newfoundland, 22 May 1942. These other ranks were important resources on the medical units, extending the number of casualties that could be handled. *LAC/DND fonds/PA-137822*

Doree claimed there were never enough nurses at Basingstoke Hospital: their quota was based on the expectation of assistance from "up-patients," but her unit didn't have many patients capable of providing assistance because of the number of serious burns cases treated there. As the war continued and Canada experienced military manpower shortages, Doree also noted that medical units lost personnel to combat duty: "We had fewer orderlies because they were taken away to carry a gun, they were so desperate for soldiers."[62] Despite these problems, medical orderlies and recovering patients did keep the number of military nurses relatively low, although the degree of success in substituting less well-prepared workers for fully trained nurses in the forward units was far more limited than in CGH units. Nursing sisters were able to parlay their higher level of technological skills and knowledge into new roles and responsibilities as an expandable workforce when serving closer to the frontlines, where fewer healthcare personnel were available.

By 1943, the military was grouping patients with special needs together with staff who had specialized skills into particular units such as such as No. 1 Neurological and Plastic Surgery, the RCAF Plastic Surgery Wing at East Grinstead, No. 15 Canadian General Hospital for VD patients, or No. 14 Canadian General Hospital for psychiatric patients. As practitioners in these units treated larger numbers of patients with, for example, head injuries, chest trauma, extensive burns, and more psychiatric problems than ordinarily encountered in civilian practice settings, they developed expertise in dealing with these problems. One such specialized group was the maxillo-facial surgical team, which dealt with injuries requiring reconstruction of the jaw and/or face. This team included a surgeon, a medical specialist, an anaesthetist, and several nurses trained in specific techniques associated with skin grafting and treating muscle contractures that occurred with scarred tissue. Other teams developed expertise in areas such as chest or head surgery.[63]

As the staff worked together within these small units, they came to know and value each other's roles and expertise. NS Hallie Sloan called it "a true apprecia-tion of each others' skills – that we knew what the surgeons and physicians did was absolutely vital. And what we did was absolutely vital in carrying out those orders. Because everybody wanted everybody to get better, or to at least be comfortable before they died." Personnel in such units developed standardized practices for efficient handling of large numbers of casualties that eliminated the need to wait for individual medical orders. NS Wannop never received the post-ing to Europe that she desired, because her expertise with burn patients kept her at Basingstoke. As she explained, "When a big push would come and patients would be brought in, you were pretty much on your own. But by this time, you pretty well knew what to do ... The doctors were so busy ... They used to come around once a day and check everything, and if there were any questions. And then you carried on, and if you were concerned about something, you know, you could always call them. But they gave you a lot of responsibility ... I was told that because it was such a unique hospital and the work was specialized – that you couldn't do it in the field. And that's why they kept us there, and flew the patients back to us."

Gender, Danger, and Public Perceptions

Military nursing was not without dangers, although both media of the time and historical accounts have represented nurses as working only in traditional roles and within safe settings, well-protected by the armed forces. The literature has perpetuated historical silences regarding military women in general and nurses in particular. As NS Mary Bray wrote about her submission to one anthology, for example, "We were asked to recall the fun times but indeed there were more sadness and horror of what the war was all about."[64] The military actively campaigned to prevent nurses, and indeed all troops, from speaking or writing about their experiences during the war, censoring the mail to prevent informa-tion leaks to the "enemy." From NS Pepper's perspective, "It was certainly a man's war. Many situations were quite unnatural for women. For example, obeying security rules when writing home was difficult: You mentioned only the mundane happenings, when you were just *dying* to tell your family all about the last combined operations field exercise of the whole Corps ... Imagine not being allowed to mention, either by name or unit, the boys from home whom

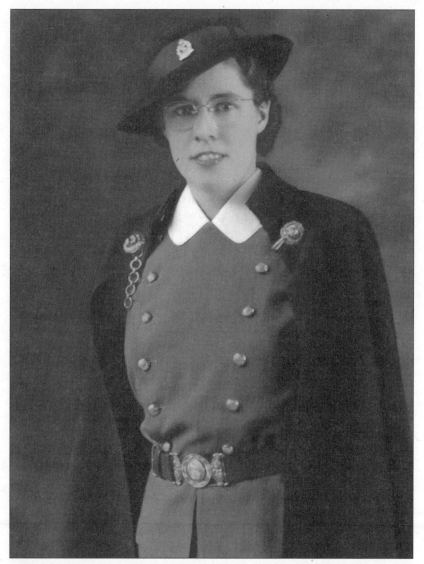

RCAMC NS Eva Wannop remained in England at the specialized burn unit located as part of No. 1 Neurological and Plastic Surgery Hospital at Basingstoke, in spite of her desire to join a unit going to the continent, because of her skills and knowledge in the care of burn patients. *Courtesy Eva Wannop*

you were caring for! Also, the fact that at sun-down every nursing sister in the Italian theatre of war had to don long trousers and cream herself with anti-malarial ointment rather than an exotic perfumed product would have made interesting reading in letters sent home. As a result of these security regulations, we padded our letters and made it all sound like real fun."[65]

Nurses' training, from their earliest student days, had already socialized nursing sisters to confidentiality regarding patients. Many of them internalized the additional constraints of military censorship, to the extent that they still hadn't talked about their experiences fifty or sixty years later. Some had personal reasons for silence or declaring topics off-limits, like NS Fletcher, who wrote to her brother, "Mind you – there will be lots that I won't talk about, because things that happen in Eng[land] & the continent just wouldn't be accepted in Victoria – just as the odd drink wouldn't be accepted by some of our relatives."[66] Other nursing sisters were clear in interviews that they would not discuss certain topics. Regarding personal relationships between physicians and nurses within medical units, for example, NS Van Scoyoc replied, "It went a little bit beyond family! We'll leave it there."[67] Several nurses were very uncomfortable with criticisms of the military or physicians; at least two requested to have statements they had made deleted from their accounts.

For the most part, nursing sisters were "excellent soldiers" in maintaining official silences during and after the war. Wartime journalist Lotta Dempsey called them "a silent service among women ... who tell nothing. That reticence has become a part of their work and their life in the Army."[68] It wasn't until 1999 that NS Carter wrote about several "near misses" she had during the bombings in England. Stationed with No. 1 CGH at Marston Green between Coventry and Birmingham, Carter "learned to control her fear" while bicycling to the hospital from her billet in the dark when summoned during night bombings. Recalling that one bomb fell close enough to throw her from the bike, she wrote, "I never told anybody at the hospital about it, as too much was happening."[69] In other cases, silence proved costly: NS Mussallem recalled one nurse who returned from Italy in a catatonic state with severe psychiatric problems.[70]

Public reticence to associate combat and risk with military nurses was partially related to maintaining public support of the war, but there was also deep denial on the part of society that nurses were an essential part of the military machine.[71] Nurses made the machine more efficient by returning men to combat, more acceptable by assuring the public that competent care was readily available for casualties, and more normal by showing that women could serve safely. Their silence and relative invisibility also meant that some nursing sisters never received needed counselling or support, either during or after the war. Some spoke about feeling restless, unsettled, and unable to make decisions following the war. Some struggled through years of unhappy relationships and/or dysfunctional family situations. Still others continue to cope with painful memories and losses. NS Ruth Littlejohn frequently referred to feeling "scattered," at a "crossroads," and at "loose ends," while NS Mary White described a deep unhappiness with the military both in general and in particular, for lack of counselling services during and after the war.[72]

A four-page *Canadian Nurse* article included photographs of RCAMC nurses serving in Sicily, repeatedly delivering the message that there was little distinction between military and civilian nursing – that nurses served in familiar, safe environments, and that the most advanced medical care was always available for Canadian troops.[73] One photograph shows a nurse relaxing in front of a tent while washing dries on the clothesline, much like a domestic scene or a camping holiday. Another shows a room filled with hospital beds neatly lined up, much as they would be in any civilian hospital of the period. A third photograph portrays a group of nurses sitting in front of a "beautiful piece of tapestry" with a tea service on the table in front of them. Each image reinforced messages of safety and normalcy in military nursing. A letter from Matron Edith Dick to the *Canadian Nurse* also assured her civilian colleagues that "we live surprisingly normal lives over here."[74]

These discourses, like Matron-in-Chief Smellie's earlier assertion that the army always protected its nurses, promised more than was realistically possible. Nursing sisters' accounts and records reveal more deaths, injuries, hardships, and exposure to danger than are generally acknowledged. The literature reports that only one nursing sister died as a result of "enemy action" during the Second World War. RCN NS Agnes Wilkie was returning from Sydney, Nova Scotia, to St. John's, Newfoundland, on the ferry SS *Caribou* when a German submarine torpedoed and sunk it. Wilkie and her companion NS/Dietician Margaret Brooke hung onto a capsized lifeboat for over two hours in the cold, rough waters of the North Atlantic. According to Brooke, "There was about a dozen of us. We clung to ropes. The waves kept washing us off, one by one, and eventually Agnes said she was getting cramped. She let go, but I managed to catch hold of her with one hand. I held to her as best I could until daybreak. Finally, a wave took her. When I called to her, she didn't answer. She must have been unconscious. The men left tried to reach her, but she floated away." Brooke was rescued, and Wilkie's body was recovered for burial with full naval honours.[75]

At least eleven other Canadian nurses died while on active duty in addition to NS Wilkie: four died in motor vehicle, bicycle, or airplane accidents; seven died from disease or infection (see Table 2.1).[76] The RCAMC statistical records reported the deaths of only army nursing sisters: they show the deaths of nine nurses and one occupational therapist who served as a nursing sister. But at least two RCAF nursing sisters died, one in a training accident and another from a medical disease. And although the "Books of Remembrance" held in the Memorial Chamber of the Peace Tower on Parliament Hill list seventeen names of nursing sisters who died "during or after" the war, one death resulted from disease two years after the war and the remaining names are not corroborated by other sources.[77]

Perhaps the most poignant death involved a nurse who developed septicemia from an infected thumb at No. 8 Canadian General Hospital. She received treatment with a sulfa drug and blood transfusions while unsuccessful attempts were made to secure doses of a new drug for her. Penicillin was still in early

Table 2.1

Canadian military nurses' deaths due to enemy action, accidents, and disease, 1939-45

	Service	Date	Age	Place	Cause
Marion Bell	RCAMC	26 Sept. 1940	29	England	Biking accident
Frances Spafford	RCAMC	8 Mar. 1941	28	England	Coma, unknown cause
Frances Polgreen	RCAMC	11 May 1943	32	England	Septicemia
Ruth Ashley	RCAMC	6 June 1943	28	England	Brain tumour
Nora Peters	RCAMC	12 Aug. 1944	34	Italy	Motor vehicle accident
Vera MacDonald	RCAMC	22 June 1945	26	England	Motor vehicle accident
Frances Cooper	RCAMC	26 Oct. 1945	35	Vancouver	Uremia
Gladys Fitzgerald	RCAMC	30 Dec. 1945	35	Ottawa	Bacterial myocarditis
Frances Gannon	RCAMC	15 Mar. 1946	43	Calgary	Cerebral haemorrhage, hypertension
Agnes Wilkie	RCN	11 Oct. 1942	–	Newfoundland	Drowning, result of enemy action
Jessie Margaret McLeod	RCAF	29 Apr. 1941	39	Dartmouth, NS	Cerebral meningitis
Marion M. Westgate	RCAF	27 Oct. 1943	26	Regina	Flying accident

Sources: Based on data extracted from Department of National Defence personnel files, archival documents, and medical journal publications.

stages of testing, with only very small amounts produced at the time she needed it. It would emerge from the war as a "miracle drug" but too late for this nurse.[78]

Wartime motor vehicle accidents were quite common, especially in England, where blackout conditions prevailed and many roads were heavily damaged from bombing. Motorcycles – referred to as "Hitler's secret weapon" against the Allied forces – were particularly notorious as a cause of injury and death among enlisted men.[79] Frequent "mess" parties, and the alcohol served at these events, compounded risky driving conditions. Bicycles were also a very popular form of transportation and recreation, given the extent of gasoline rationing, but they were also unfamiliar to the many nurses who described riding their first bicycles in England. Those who had ridden bicycles in Canada were unfamiliar with the hand brakes on British ones. There are numerous accounts of biking adventures and accidents. NS Helen Morton, for one, required head and facial stitches after her accident: "It was at night you know – I didn't have any lights and I shouldn't have been riding the bicycle at night. I ran into this thing [a truck]. A man drove us back to the hospital and then they sent an ambulance to get the bicycle."[80]

Other dangers were associated with travel to and from postings, on- and

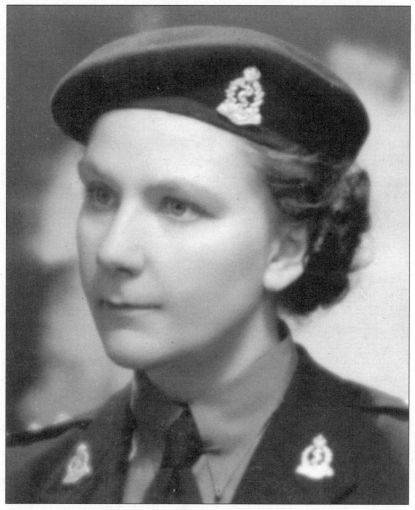

RCAMC NS Pauline Cox was one of the nurses on the *Santa Elena* when it was torpedoed in the Mediterranean Sea while en route to Sicily. *Courtesy Pauline Cox Walker*

off-duty activities, training demonstrations, and combat. Ninety Canadian nurses, plus five other nursing sisters and four Red Cross workers travelling with No. 14 CGH, required rescue when their ship, the *Santa Elena*, was torpedoed in the Mediterranean en route to Sicily in 1943. NS Pauline Cox was on the *Santa Elena* when, at the end of the evening meal, around 6:00 p.m., an aerial torpedo hit the stern of the ship:

> Right away the ship sank in the stern part. And went down quite a bit, but we were still alright. So then, they had us get to our [lifeboat] stations. We had

practised that before. We had a Philipino crew who ... had never even tried to use them. So they hadn't any idea how to get these boats out and how to do it. So it was quite a mess ... Finally mine landed on the water and we had to row over to the Monterey which stood by ... The rest of the convoy went and put up a smoke screen ... you had to bring the boat along side the ship, and as the waves took your boat toward the ship, one person would grab the net. They had a tremendous net on the whole length of the ship, and you had to climb it. And so, that was not easy. Anyway, we managed. All of us got out. There was just one of the girls who couldn't make it. So they sent down one of these, sort of like a sling, and were able to put her into that. And then they got her up. Anyway, we got up ... and some of the boys there would heave us over. And our faces were black. All you could see were black faces from the smoke screen. Nobody recognized anybody ... The girls picked up by the destroyer ... said they were grabbed out of the boat. They didn't touch the ground at all. They were passed from one soul to another, into the destroyer and down [deep into the ship].[81]

The Canadian destroyer SS *Monterey* picked up one group of nurses and delivered them to Naples while the rest went to Philippeville in North Africa courtesy of an Allied ship. They lost all their personal belongings as well as their hospital's equipment. Both NS Cox and NS Marjorie MacLean described the strafing during the attack. Cox said, "It was like July the 1st standing on that deck and watching all this stuff going up. That's what it reminded me of, fireworks, a tremendous amount of stuff went up." MacLean remembered that, "when you got out and away from the [ship], you could still hear some of the shooting going on. It was a beautiful night, warm and everything. I don't think it was more that a couple of hours before the other [ship] picked us up."[82] NS Nicolson was a reinforcement on her way to Sicily with No. 5 CGH in the same convoy. According to her, whenever aircraft attacked the convoy, the nurses were ordered below deck. She questioned the wisdom of this order: "I wondered if that was a good thing or not, in case we had been hit. I mean there were lots of us, but anyway, we were below."

When the nurses of No. 5 CGH landed four miles from the front on the ninth day of the invasion of Sicily, they surprised military leaders, who were not expecting the arrival of women during an assault. Their supply ship, carrying both medical supplies and personal belongings, was blown up as they were landing from a transport. NS Nicolson recalled that "they were horrified because there were nursing sisters there. And it was the first time ever in any British or Allied war that nursing sisters had been landed on an assault area. And he didn't know what to do with us! It was kind of exciting ... They got us into trucks and moved us a little farther up, to Syracuse. We went in at Augusta. So they got us away from that harbour where the other ships were coming in and landing ... They didn't know what to do with nursing sisters. We weren't supposed to be there at the beginning!"

Nurses experienced bombing, strafing, and accidents both on and off duty. NS Morton remembered the regularity of bombing at Bramshott, England: "That first September we were bombed several times every day. And we could set our clocks by the time the Germans would come over. We got so [familiar with the bombing missions, that] we could recognize their machines – the sound of their machines. And they'd come at exactly the same hour every night, to bomb London."[83] NS Sloan humorously recalled that night-time bombings in Europe forced hard decisions: "At night, the firing in our area was heavy, and although the tracers and flares were beautiful to behold, the rattle of shrapnel through the trees was frightening. Our Colonel issued hospital beds for all sisters, and instructions to hop under the bed with bedroll once the firing started. Since moles, field mice and lizards inhabited the area under the beds, we had to make a choice between the shrapnel and the livestock. Usually we ended up on the bed with tin hats covering our faces and enamel wash basins over our stomachs."[84]

At least fourteen RCAMC nurses were wounded in training accidents and by "friendly fire."[85] Three were injured during a grenade demonstration in England, two suffering phosphorus burns and one requiring plastic surgery to seventeen wounds on her body. Another nurse spent two months in the hospital with a fractured skull and shoulder sustained in a jeep accident that killed her companion.[86] NS Jean Scrimgeour was the only survivor among five pedestrians hit when a passing jeep ran over a land mine in Italy.[87] And although NS Sloan suffered a fractured spine in three places when she fell off a railway handcar in Canada, she was still able to serve in England and Europe after D-Day.[88] In Catania, Sicily, the nursing sisters of No. 5 CGH lived on the top floor of a sanatorium converted into temporary military hospital facilities. The building was located just below Allied batteries, with the nurses' mess on the balcony of the top floor. During an air raid on 2 September 1943, "friendly fire" fell on the balcony during dinner – injuring twelve nurses and three orderlies with shrapnel. Two nurses required evacuation to North Africa and one to England.[89] NS Kellough was at No. 5 Casualty Clearing Station near Nijmegan, the Netherlands, where the nurses billeted in local homes. On one occasion, her commanding officer collected all the nurses in the middle of the night, gathering them safely at the hospital just as German troops entered the town.[90]

My research revealed many more non-fatal injuries: fractured arms, legs, spines, and skulls along with wounds requiring surgery, stitches, hospitalization, and rehabilitation. These casualties never made it onto official wounded lists, although nurses often spent days or sometimes months in recovery. Discourses concerning women, safety, and male protectiveness contributed to making such injuries invisible. Women were supposed to be protected, far from frontlines. Invisibility was also consistent with the image of nurses as sacrificing mothers or angels who selflessly cared for patients with infectious diseases such as tuberculosis, diphtheria, or influenza, willingly exposing themselves to risk.

Still other dangers lay in store. Rough seas and submarine threats required strong stomachs and considerable courage among those serving on hospital ships. Even when in port, the ships could still come under threat. The hospital ship the *Lady Nelson*, for example, made several trips to the Mediterranean during 1943, retrieving patients from Sicily, the Italian mainland, and North Africa and delivering them to England and Canada. During one trip, while nursing sisters were ashore at Philippeville, planes bombed the harbour, sinking a British ship and killing 400 people while damaging the nearby *Lady Nelson* as well.[91] NS Littlejohn and her group felt compelled to return to the ship for immediate duty. Finding that the *Lady Nelson* had moved out into the harbour for increased safety, they argued with security personnel and finally persuaded an American captain to take them out to the ship. There, they climbed up a rope ladder in skirts and gloves while carrying purses, demonstrating that nurses could blend "feminine" and "masculine" behaviour as necessary. Littlejohn said, "When we walked into what had been the dining room, I wish you could have seen the look of astonishment on the doctor's face. 'What are you doing here? How did you ever get here?' I replied, 'We haven't climbed up ladders on the farms for nothing. We've been up lots of ladders before.'"[92]

Adverse weather presented a different set of challenges: a North African sirocco blew down hospital tents and dispersed patient documents across the desert, and extremes of heat and cold made caring for patients in tents and makeshift buildings with missing windows or doors miserable, dirty work. Heavy rains called for rubber boots in place of nursing shoes. NS Eleanor MacGregor described the North African heat as so intense that nurses slept under wet towels to cool down; later in the season, NS Pauline Cox recalled the cold conditions in Italy: "We got so cold. Ethel and I went on night duty when the first unit opened up with 140 patients. It was so cold, that's when I put a hot water bottle on one side and put a string onto a hot water bottle [for my] back in order to keep warm. We were freezing to death! It was awful. We worked all night with hot water bottles hanging around [our necks]. We were not very handsome, I tell you!"

Other occupational hazards included malaria, tuberculosis, infected wounds, lice, fleas, scorpions, electrical equipment, occasional belligerent patients and POWs, exposure to toxic substances, and more. At least one nursing sister required hospitalization after receiving a severe electrical shock from a gauze cutter in an operating room.[93] Malaria was endemic to the Mediterranean region, and all personnel were supposed to take preventative measures including anti-malarial drugs. According to NS Cox, "We were on Mepacrine from the time we hit Italy till we left. And we were all as yellow as ducks' feet ... Everybody was supposed to be on it, but of course, the boys up the line never bothered to take it half the time. They would come down with [malaria]." NS Kellough remembered a sign on the mess table reading, "Have you had your mefloquine today?" NS Morton reports having to swallow daily doses of the drug in front of her commanding officer. As NS MacGregor explained, if personnel came down with malaria, "It was considered a self-inflicted wound." NS Carter claimed mepacrine made her hair lose its curl and fall out.[94] Other nurses also recalled that their teeth turned black in this theatre of war, an effect they attributed to using heavily chlorinated water to make tea; NS Kellough confessed that new staff thought the nurses strange looking with yellow skin and black teeth. To control lice and fleas as well as the diseases they carried, soldiers' clothing was impregnated with DDT (dichloro-diphenyl-trichloroethane). DDT powder was also issued for personal and patient use.[95] NS Cox recalled using DDT liberally: "I remember always shaking some in to my bedroll. We had these little bedrolls – that was our bedding in Italy. And we used to open the thing up and shake this stuff in. I mean, when you think of the amount of DDT that went in to those bedrolls! We must have been completely saturated in the stuff! Anything was better that those fleas that you'd get!"

The most difficult conditions facing nursing sisters were probably experienced by NS Kay Christie and May Waters, who were prisoners of war. They were the only two Canadian military nurses working with British nursing sisters of the Queen Alexandra's Imperial Military Nursing Service (QAIMNS) and voluntary aid detachments (VADs) at the Bowen Road British military hospital in Hong Kong when Japanese forces attacked the hospital on 8 December 1941. The hospital itself was under attack for eighteen days, taking 111 direct hits that damaged two of the three floors. Nursing staff from Bowen Road also served at small auxiliary hospitals on the island. At one such hospital, St. Stephen's Boys School, horrendous atrocities were committed against patients and personnel. There, medical officers and patients were shot and bayoneted, QAIMNS NS Molly Gordon and six VADs were raped, three of the VADs were subsequently beheaded. Christie recalled Molly Gordon's account to her:

I will never, never forget the look in her eyes! ... Molly wasn't young, she must have been in her late 40's, just a little woman ... The Japs took a lot of the men's bodies, the ones they had killed, and dragged them across the corridor and into a small room, and put the bodies in there. Then they dragged mattresses in and put them on top of the bodies. And then they went at the nurses ... They took [their Red Cross arm bands] off and wiped their faces with them, and then they stripped them and they went after the nurses. And Molly said it wasn't just one Jap per person, she said it was just a series of Japs on you. And what they were really afraid of, was that these women would be infected, [with] something like venereal disease ... Eventually, in a day or so, they got them [the women and bodies] back.[96]

Christie and Waters knew about these atrocities and wondered what would happen to them. They were on duty Christmas night, when "each time footsteps approached the darkened ward, we'd wonder 'Is this it?'"[97] The Japanese arrived on Boxing Day, ordered the hospital to surrender, put up barbed wire, and declared it "Prisoner of War Camp A." Japanese soldiers maintained constant surveillance in the wards and dormitories, day and night, carrying guns with bayonets while running their fingers up and down the blade. Christie recalled unnerving experiences of being watched during patient procedures, waking up at night with a guard standing in the doorway, and observing "every method of torture" used as punishment.

According to the Geneva Convention, nurses were not supposed to be taken as POWs, but Japan did not sign or recognize the agreement. For the first eight months after capture by the Japanese, Christie and Waters remained at Bowen Road, caring for casualties as well as they could with dwindling supplies. In August 1942, all female nursing personnel were loaded onto trucks and taken to a civilian internment camp, Stanley Camp, on the other side of the island, where the Canadians lived behind barbed wire with 2,400 other women. At the camp, NS Christie and Waters were confined to a nine-by-twelve-foot room with a third, civilian nurse for another fourteen months.[98] They eventually acquired the barest of furnishings, sharing one enamel basin for washing purposes and scrounging an assortment of parts to create a makeshift "hot plate" to prepare their meagre rations. The Japanese refused to recognize women as officers or grant them the few officer rights that would have provided minimal pay to use on the black market to supplement their daily rations of 8 ounces of cooked rice, 3 ounces of flour, ¾ ounce of "flesh" (meat or fish), and some indigestible "greens."

In March 1942, the Japanese announced their intention to pay "the two nurses that had the two stars on their shoulders" an officer's allowance corresponding to that of Japanese officers. The two stars indicated a lieutenant's rank in the RCAMC (hence officer status), and while the two Canadian nursing sisters carried that rank, British nursing sisters did not and were not included in the offer. According to Christie,

> [The QAIMNS] Matron got mad and said that if they wouldn't pay her Sisters, well they weren't going to pay us either, which was very foolish because we could have bought some things we could have shared. But, no, she wasn't going to have anyone paid if her Sisters weren't paid – they finally slapped her face, she'd argued with them too much ... Our Canadian officers [the men] established a fund and they gave the three Padres, and May and myself, 25 military yen a month [from their pay]. A military yen has no real value but we used to be able to get a bit of stuff with it. That's why May and I had money ... and that's the only way we managed, because it would have just been dreadful.[99]

Over the years following the war, Christie wrote and spoke further of their physical hardships – poor diet, weight loss, vitamin deficiencies, visual deterioration, lack of clothing, difficulties associated with personal hygiene – as well as the psychological hardships related to lack of privacy, many restrictions, and daily uncertainty. She and Waters received only one Red Cross food parcel, and Christie received only three letters (delivered a year after they were written) during the entire experience. Her family remained misinformed of her situation; the official report was "missing, presumed dead," and an escaped prisoner reported that she had indeed been killed. But she described enforced idleness and hunger as the most difficult aspects of this period. A group of local civilian nurses from Hong Kong were responsible for operating a small hospital for those interned at Stanley Camp, but the local nurses did not want military nurses working with them. After eight months, however, they acquiesced because they needed night-duty relief. During the fall of 1943, the Canadian government was finally successful in arranging for the repatriation of Christie and Waters as part of an American-Japanese prisoner exchange. The Japanese did not release the British nursing sisters or VADs for two more years. According to Christie, "We were told that the Japanese were out to humiliate the British, and they did." She clearly differentiated, however, between Japanese soldiers and Japanese civilians, making it clear that the latter were not involved in these activities.[100]

The suddenness and violence of the Hong Kong defeat reinforced the dangers of posting women to active theatres, and increased anxieties regarding nurses' safety in the military. At the same time, articles and letters published in newspapers downplayed the risks. The armed forces implemented policies that were ostensibly for women's protection: restricting their off-duty activities; setting up barriers in and around the postings in the form of fences, mandatory escorts, and guards; and issuing frequent "confined to barracks orders." NS Jean MacBain called fencing "the greatest drawback for all of us ... We (nursing sisters) were not allowed out unless accompanied by an armed escort. 'Don't fence me in' was our theme song." NS Rendall recalled an incident while in North Africa involving theft more than physical danger: "One night when we were all sleeping the Arabs came into our compound. And some of our girls had their clothes hanging out on the line (they'd washed them). The Arabs came and just took everything. They even went through a couple of the tents and grabbed the things off the poles where the girls had their clothes. They took a shirt; maybe another one got a skirt. So our outfits were kind of incomplete for a little while ... [After that incident,] our compound had the barbed wire around and we had the guards all the time."[101]

Nursing sisters were valuable resources, and, as was the case with other scarce medical equipment, precautions were taken to preserve them. The military divided them up for transport, for example, so that at least some might survive in case of an attack during travel. NS Van Scoyoc, with No. 6 CCS, recalled how "we were set up so that when we moved, there was one nurse in each truck. In case we would be shelled, we wouldn't lose all our supplies or all our staff."[102] Near Caen, France, according to NS Rita Murphy, nurses were ordered to sleep in "slit trenches" dug about twenty inches into the ground, as a precautionary measure against anti-personnel bombs "so we would be available in case of disaster."[103]

While military nurses characteristically displayed a healthy sense of adventure and a good measure of humour as well as determination to outlast the war, some of them developed physical responses to sustained danger and the conditions in which they worked. NS Sloan, for example, developed a nervous tic related to psychological stress resulting from the intense bombing she experienced while serving in Belgium:

> It was a horrible time. I developed a tic – it was very embarrassing. It happened so often. My arm shot out: jerk, jerk, jerk. That was in Antwerp where the Germans were trying to get the harbour, the use of the harbour, because it was the best harbour on that North coast ... Although they said that these things [the V-2 bombs] crashed in Antwerp every 20 minutes, they never did hit the port facilities. They were difficult to control, their projectory [sic], I guess you call it. But they were frightening because they were devastating. They made no noise and made these terrible, terrible concussions ... In the last hours in Antwerp, they hit a theatre and we got 1200 casualties from the theatre – civilians. And it was very bad. But that's where I got the tic.

Medical units frequently set up in vacated facilities, and nurses had the job of preparing space for patient care – another potentially dangerous, as well as distasteful, job. In Rome, for example, they found toilets "filled to the brim," plumbing and electricity destroyed, live grenades in drawers, as well as "an arm under a mattress and a leg up on a shelf."[104] NS Elizabeth Burnham described the stress within her unit: "We were put up in one large ward, fifty-five of us, the beds having just been vacated by the Germans ... Heavy shelling kept on all night which didn't make us feel very relaxed ... I think we were a bit overwhelmed by the constant shelling." She added, "Alone on the roof on night duty with many shell-shocked and mental patients, I often wondered about our safety in this wartime nursing."[105]

During the invasion of Hong Kong, NS Christie struggled between her own fears and the requirement to obey orders to lie under the patients' beds during bombing attacks in order to be available for the most helpless patients who could not be moved to safety:

> The nursing sisters had orders, from the DMO [district medical officer] that we

must – each must get under the bed of the sickest patients … to look after them. We were to look after the patients but, you know, I couldn't see much sense in that because we all might get a couple of floors of the hospital come down on top of you. But then to get a big iron bed, and a patient and a double mattress come down on you! … I had been lying in the space between two [beds]. I could look after two patients and not get the whole thing down on top of me. But somebody must have told, and so next day there was a notice posted: ALL NURSING SISTERS, and ALL was underlined about ten times, WILL GET UNDER THE BEDS OF THE SERIOUSLY ILL OR DAMAGED PATIENTS.[106]

As nurses were increasingly integrated into the military, their position as non-combatants became less clear, and medical units became strategic components of battle plans. Prior to one major offensive at Cassino, Italy, in November 1943, the medical units concentrated under camouflage instead of prominently displaying the Geneva Red Cross symbol. The nurses became suspicious that this was not really a "rest period," when, according to NS Pepper, they watched and listened to battle plan discussions as the "traffic" increased daily. Likewise, when in March 1945 No. 3 CGH, No. 1 CGH, and No. 4 CCS moved from Italy to join the European invasion, they moved first to Marseilles and from there to the Netherlands in secret, stripped of all identifying insignia. This was particularly problematic for nurses, who had to be kept out of sight and confined to barracks to avoid disclosure in Marseilles as a large group of women, moving together, and in uniform.[107]

In addition to physical and psychological dangers, nurses often experienced personal and professional dissonances. They spoke ambivalently about sending patients back to combat units and seeing the same soldier readmitted two or three times. At a casualty clearing station near Nijmegan, where NS Bayly worked, "There were quite a few Scottish regiments around us that had casualties and they started a cemetery beside the hospital. There were perhaps two or three there, when we came. And then, the whole area was filled. And they'd play the bagpipes and the 'Last Post.' Well, it went just right through you, you know. You listened to it. So after the war, I burst into tears if I heard it for quite a while. That was one thing I couldn't stand for a long time … We had a chap attached to us from the Graves Commission, for a short time. And the poor fellow, I never knew his name. We called him 'Graves' all the time."

NS Betty Herringer explained that "You expected, but hoped against hope, you would not find your friends among the badly wounded and severe casualties."[108] Yet, when a nursing sister was killed in a jeep accident in Italy, her friends "had to dress her in her uniform, fix her hair, get a casket and arrange for burial," in addition to forming the Honour Guard.[109] NS Lettie Turner felt most unprepared for the civilian suffering and starvation and for nursing prisoners of war who carried photographs of their families

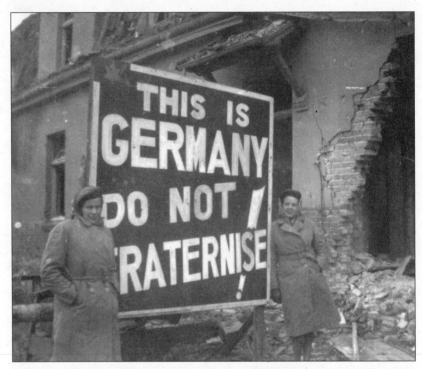

As medical units followed the rapid movement of troops across northern Europe after D-Day, personnel participated in events such as the liberation of Holland and Belgium. Nursing sisters such as RCAMC NS Pauline Lamont and NS Muriel Hillman also moved into Germany as part of the Army of Occupation. There they encountered reminders such as this one near Groningen during the fall of 1945, that they were in enemy territory and were not supposed to fraternize with local people. *Courtesy Pauline Lamont Flynn*

and children – putting, as she said, "a different face on war."[110] For NS Van Scoyoc, the most haunting memories were associated with a casualty clearing station posting after VE-Day, when her unit received patients from a nearby concentration camp: "A lot of the time, we had to give them morphine. Because they were so ill-nourished, it was so painful for them. And a lot of them never made it back to their country. It was very sad ... When I was in Holland, I remember that at night we would often hear screaming. And we thought it was a psychiatric hospital, a Dutch psychiatric hospital. That it was the patients that were screaming. But afterwards, we realized we were quite near Belsen [a German concentration camp], and it was probably the people from Belsen we were hearing. But we didn't know it. We didn't know it until we got home, really."

Treatment of POWs presented its own challenges for nursing sisters. Penicillin was a scarce resource, usually held in reserve for the very worst cases and for allied soldiers. When a surgeon ordered NS Fletcher to give penicillin to a POW, "I just looked at him; we had had hate drilled into us for so long – that anything German was evil. I said, 'Do you mean to say you're going to take that penicillin away from our boys who need it and give it to that man?' He looked at me and said, 'Sister, you damn well do what you are told and don't try to play God.'"[111] Some nurses described Germans who refused care, spat in their faces, or unnerved them with looks of hatred during treatments.[112] NS Bray, at No. 3 CCS when the unit took over a German casualty clearing station in France, admitted that professional bonds did not necessarily transcend national boundaries as when the "German nurses glared at us and we glared back."[113]

It was relatively rare for nurses to speak about fear, stress, revulsion, grief, pain, and horror. In most accounts, including my interviews, nursing sisters preferred to tell or write anecdotes about off-duty social activities and novel living conditions, or memories of soldiers' bravery in facing wounds and death. To some extent, such reticence reflected their training as nurses, which stressed discretion and self-sacrifice. Added to this was the common harshness of military life and the expectations associated with their status as military nurses. As journalist Lotta Dempsey wrote of the Canadian nursing sisters, "Trained not only in hospital routine, first aid and care of the sick but also in discipline and service, they take to the rigors and strict routine of military life without qualms."[114]

Nursing Sisters as an Expendable Workforce

Like their forerunners of the First World War, second-generation nursing sisters constituted an expandable workforce during the war and an expendable one at the end of the war. Almost everyone expected them to return to civilian life, understood primarily as assuming roles in hospitals, private duty nursing, or at the "hearth."[115] Department of Veterans Affairs counsellors perceived demobilizing military nurses either as women destined primarily for matrimony or as well-qualified professionals who would need no assistance to find employment, especially during the nursing shortage that had emerged and increased since 1943. As one counsellor wrote on a nursing sister's file, "Eventually marriage must be given a place in this winsome lady's figuring."[116] Overall, nursing sisters were eligible for more and better veterans' benefits than their predecessors had been – although their options were usually limited to stereotypical women's roles recommended by the counsellors at discharge interviews.

The Second World War lasted longer for many nursing sisters than for the regular troops, as they continued to care for recovering casualties and ill personnel as well as refugees and civilians released from concentration camps through most of 1946. Nurses continued as members of the active service and then as part of the army of occupation while medical units gradually downsized and closed throughout Great Britain and continental Europe. The last overseas medical unit closed on 15 May 1946 – six years and nine months after the declaration of war. Military hospitals across Canada also closed as the care of soldiers with long-term medical needs transferred to Department of Veterans Affairs (DVA) hospitals, where several hundred nurses, including at least 12 percent of the sample in this study, were hired as civilian civil servants. From 1946 to 1947, seventy-nine nursing sisters served with the Canadian Army Active Force (Interim) while the military considered the size and structure of a permanent postwar nursing establishment.[117]

The postwar quota of thirty RCAMC, thirty RCAF, and twenty RCN nursing sisters resulted in permanent positions for only 2 percent of the Second World War Canadian military nurses, although, according to their discharge interviews, many more expressed a desire to remain in the military. Mirroring the recruitment of nurses during the war, attempts were made to maintain regional representation in the postwar nursing service. Fewer nursing sisters had enlisted from the western provinces, a fact that helped Saskatchewan native NS Sloan succeed in her application for a postwar RCAMC position. She spent the rest of her nursing career in the military, retiring as matron-in-chief of the combined Canadian Forces Medical Service in 1968. Other nurses had a less positive experience. When NS Margery MacLean returned from overseas, her superior told her, "The war is over. You will leave the service." She refused to accept dismissal, however, recalling, "We were about twenty-five of us, sitting there. And I said, 'I'm waiting for my boyfriend. I'm going to work!' And he said, 'All right, you can go up to the Military Hospital.' There were ten of us went up to the military hospital. The rest of them quit."[118]

The war had offered nurses a reprieve from the difficult working conditions of the 1930s, as well as opportunities to further themselves professionally and socially. When it ended, they were eligible for veterans' benefits, which many described as "opening new possibilities" for them.[119] The Post-Discharge Re-establishment Order, PC 7633, provided financial support for veterans who "were unemployed, pursuing vocational training or higher education, temporarily incapacitated, or awaiting returns from farming or other private enterprise."[120] The complex benefits program, know as the Veterans Charter, was explained in a brochure entitled *Back to Civil Life*. Although the program ostensibly treated men and women equally, allowing all veterans to make choices and participate in its administration, in reality women were disadvantaged by a program designed primarily around men's needs.[121] Few women qualified for the Veterans' Land Act, women's benefits were modified according to marital status, and DVA counsellors reinforced gendered occupational choices through their powers to recommend or deny benefits to individuals. Wounded veterans were eligible for further compensation with medical care, living allowance supplements, and long-term disability pensions.

Nurses usually qualified for three components of the package: a war service gratuity, re-establishment credits, and education allowances. Length of service, rank, and postings determined the amount of one's gratuity, with extra allowances granted for overseas postings. The basic rate was $7.50 per thirty-day period of service in Canada and $15.00 per thirty-day period of service overseas, and a supplement for each six-month block spent overseas. Gratuities for military nurses serving four or more years, with overseas postings, could constitute a substantial amount in the postwar period. NS Doris Carter, for example, received a gratuity of $2,052.50 for 57.5 months – almost five years – of service.[122]

The re-establishment credit, which was equal in amount to the basic gratuity, was considered an alternative to training or land-settlement grants. It could be used for housing, furnishings, tools, establishing a business, or purchasing insurance or a government annuity.[123] Education allowances were in the form of stipends for tuition and monthly living expenses for the duration of courses, but veterans had to meet the established admission requirements of the desired program. This often put educational programs beyond the reach of many of the Depression generation, who had left school without their Grade 12 matriculation, which was a requirement for university courses.[124] Thus nurses frequently chose certificate courses in nursing specialties offered by universities rather than university degree programs. Almost one-third of the nursing sisters had enlisted during the final year and a half of the war and therefore qualified only for small gratuities and pro-rated benefits. They were also among the last to be discharged, based on a "first in, first out" principle. When they were discharged, many found classes filled to overflowing at universities offering nursing certificates and degree courses.[125]

Nursing sisters found a variety of ways to shape their compensation benefits. NS Pauline Lamont and her veteran husband combined their disability, re-establishment, and education allowances, each making gendered choices. She received a small disability pension of $40 per month for her "war wound" – acquired when she had to "hit the ditch" when a convoy of military trucks forced her off the road while she was biking at night – until the army finally paid her pension out with $98 in 1950. She used her re-establishment credits to purchase a bedroom suite while her husband used education benefits to go to university.[126] NS MacLean bought a washing machine and furniture with her credits, in anticipation of her upcoming marriage.

The war service gratuity and education benefits were the two most significant programs for nurses, but access to them was conditional on the circumstances of discharge and the DVA counsellor's recommendation. The official discharge order carried great import, as its language worked to control soldiers' eligibility for benefits, medals and awards, gratuities, and re-establishment benefits. It could also affect their self-esteem and social standing.[127] I found no "dishonourable discharges" among my sample of nurses, but there were cases where nurses were "asked to resign," citing reasons such as "psychoneurosis" or "unsuitability for the military." As was discussed previously, nurses who married prior to 1943 had to resign their commissions and thereby forfeited all rights to benefits. Official records stated reasons for discharge in a variety of ways that were often ambiguous, such as permitted to retire, permitted to retire on compassionate grounds, permitted to marry, resigned, or, simply, demobilized. It was very important to qualify marriage with the phrase "with permission," in order to retain benefits. Pregnancy was another situation in which language could reveal or obscure a situation that would result in loss of benefits. Terms such as "physiological tumour," "absence of menses," or simply "unable to meet medical requirements" appear in records. Those in power made decisions about the contents of these personnel records that had potential consequences for a lifetime.

DVA counsellors also shaped nurses' options and choices. While many nurses were satisfied with the discharge process, others felt they did not receive adequate support or advice. NS MacGregor was not impressed: "I went for a physical examination and a lot of interviews. The officers doing the discharge procedure seemed much more interested in the amount of benefits I would receive than in what I would do with the rest of my life after over five years in the Army. I was given a pin to wear to show I was a veteran, and a ribbon to show that I had served overseas, defending the Empire."[128] NS Wheeler claimed that poor counselling forced her to live on her savings while studying at the University of British Columbia and waiting for veterans' credits to begin.[129]

A civilian nursing shortage began to emerge during the war, and by the end, there were many more vacant positions than nurses wanting to fill them. DVA counsellors and nursing leaders perceived returning military nurses to be a "solution" to the civilian shortage, and tended to assume they could or would want to return to civilian nursing rather than discussing their broader employment or education options. Almost all of the discharge summaries contained comments that nurse veterans would have no problem finding employment. With few exceptions, there was little or no support for nurses who requested career change. Even when nurses indicated they were not seeking employment, either because they had married or intended to marry after discharge, counsellors noted on their records that they could always "fall back on nursing if need arises in the future." Married nurses were encouraged to use their re-establishment credits for furniture or appliances rather than education. As one record put it, the nurse should "use her benefits to improve her home conditions."

Nursing was clearly perceived as the ideal feminine profession for the postwar world. According to the *Canadian Nurse*, "When we survey, specifically, the position of women in this postwar world, we recognize again that you are in a fortunate field – free from male competition. You contemplate a world in which no man wishes your job or thinks that your earnings cut him off from legitimate employment."[130] Society urged other women to relinquish paid work to returning male veterans and resume traditional feminine roles as wives and mothers. But nurses were needed at civilian bedsides, and the military released them as an expendable workforce, without concern for their futures.

Nursing sisters enlisted in great numbers, knowing well that they had "big shoes to fill." They experienced both continuity and change as the Canadian military medical units expanded across three service branches, seven theatres of war, a variety of practice settings, and new expanded roles. They moved forward to the frontlines willingly, as it became clear that professional nursing made a difference in outcomes of medical and surgical care. Dominant gendered discourses assured military nurses that they would "always be well taken care of" and serve in safety. Although nurses' experiences did not always correspond to these discourses, nursing sisters accepted a variety of dangers and risks as the price to be paid for their enhanced status, benefits, and work opportunities. They already knew "how to nurse" when they enlisted, although they had much to learn about adapting to the wartime conditions under which they would serve. But they knew almost nothing about being a soldier or the class-, race-, and gender-specific set of expectations that would shape them into both officers and ladies within the military.

Shaping Nursing Sisters
as "Officers" and "Ladies"

When Nursing Sister (NS) Kathleen Rowntree arrived in England with No. 23 Canadian General Hospital (CGH), she drilled and went for route marches, played softball, and spent the evenings in a "neat little pub" where there was a dance hall. "One morning I got called into the matron's office and told that 'jitterbugging' was not becoming to an officer. That was the first of a few trips to the matron's office, but I survived." Matron Gladys Sharpe warned NS Jean Wheeler and her group of South African Military Nursing Service (SAMNS) nurses that one port or one sherry was the limit, as they were "not to disgrace themselves" in their use of alcohol. And as NS Margaret Van Scoyoc, with No. 12 CGH in England, put it, "We certainly didn't want to be sent home! Conduct was a very important factor. Maybe we were too conscientious!"[1]

Hospital training schools had screened and socialized student nurses, with particular emphasis on discipline, obedience, hard work, and endurance in addition to emphases on femininity and nursing skills – training that resembled military routines and deference for authority in many aspects. The Canadian armed forces then recruited graduates of these programs for the nursing services, offering them working conditions far superior to civilian working conditions. Military nurses enjoyed full-time employment, food and housing, medical and dental care, a pay rate triple the average nurse's salary (and equal to military men of the same rank), and proximity to the military men serving overseas in addition to opportunities for adventure, travel, and meaningful acts of patriotism. It was not difficult, therefore, to recruit nurses for the military, but the presence of women in the ranks did raise anxiety levels for both the armed forces and the general public.

As historian Leisa Meyer points out, mobilizing women for the war effort without disrupting contemporary definitions of masculinity and femininity was a constant concern for civilian and military authorities alike. Her study of the American Women's Army Corps (WACs) during the Second World War suggests that the women of this service performed only those jobs associated with traditionally feminine roles and thereby relieved men for jobs associated with traditionally masculine roles – thus preserving social expectations on one hand while generating considerable anxieties over sexuality on the other hand.[2] Canadian nursing sisters also served in a highly feminine role as nurses and, as such, conformed to certain social expectations. But unlike the WACs, they were not constrained to the "usual" enactment of these roles associated with traditional practice settings. Indeed practice settings, particularly overseas and in active theatres away from conventional family and social constraints, required particular attention to the regulation of relationships between military men and women.

Some anxiety stemmed from the logistical issues associated with men and women living and working together in close proximity twenty-four hours a day. These issues included shared spaces and privileges in the officers' mess, separate ablutions facilities, and appropriate sexualities. Other anxieties arose from questions about how to supervise women within this male domain and how to avoid controversies that might threaten nurses' femininity or public support for the war. The military addressed these anxieties by ensuring that nursing sisters comported themselves as "officers" and as "ladies" according to gender-, race-, and class-based discourses that reinforced respectability while maintaining male military privilege.

Most nurses had already experienced a militaristic style of training as students. While not particularly eager to return to regimentation compounded by subordination as women in the military, they knew there were plenty of replacements for nursing sisters who either could not, or would not, fit into military life. At the same time, they found that the armed forces "turned a blind eye" whenever and wherever nursing skills were needed – permitting a degree of resistance to military authority.[3]

Nursing sisters, already well-prepared professionally, had to learn how to soldier and what was expected of them as military officers. During her orientation at Camp Borden, for example, NS Kathleen Dickey learned "that it was our responsibility to quickly learn, take this training seriously and not spoil the show for the sake of the men ... At this point most of us realized we were marching to war and often wondered just what part a nursing sister did play in the Army. As for nursing, we were learning nothing."[4] Historian Kathryn McPherson has analyzed nursing as "performance" and "nurse" as a learned role. Her analysis can be extended to military nursing, which was more than the adaptation of nursing skills to wartime contexts. It included the performance of specific behaviours and attitudes, with sanctions to enforce conformity.[5] Performance of their role required nursing sisters to juggle multiple intersecting identities. They had to challenge prevailing social expectations regarding masculinity and femininity, prove their hardiness as "one of the boys," demonstrate their worthiness as "officers," and ensure their respectability as "ladies."

Military rank and military uniforms were highly visible signifiers of the interplay between gender, race, and class in the shaping of women's roles. Military rank carried embedded expectations of nurses as officers, along with equality of pay and benefits. As relative rank, however, it was a gendered second-class rank lacking the power of command. When nursing sisters did receive the power of command and commissions in 1942, it was still restricted to authority over women and patients on medical wards.[6] In a similar manner, nursing sister uniforms carried embedded expectations of nurses as ladies, reinforcing prevailing social constructions of femininity. Journalist Lotta Dempsey linked the uniform to their work, role, and position within the British Empire: "The uniform they wear, designed for the job they do, is like the role they play. It is the King's Uniform."[7]

Reconstituting Masculinity and Femininity

Canadian nurses had enlisted as an integral part of the militia with relative rank since 1904, making them the first women military officers. British nursing sisters did not receive temporary "emergency" commissions until 1941 or become officers until 1942, and Australian military nurses received rank in 1943 but were not integrated into the military until 1951.[8] Yet, the Canadian military was careful to structure nurses' rank in ways that limited women's authority over men, marginalized them to the lowest officer levels with little opportunity for advancement, and created a second-class officer status through the use of alternate titles such as nursing sisters and matrons. RCAMC nurses typically enlisted as second lieutenants and moved through the ranks to first lieutenant, captain, major, and lieutenant colonel. RCN nurses followed a similar, but flatter, promotion system, with titles of acting sub-lieutenants and sub-lieutenants. RCAF nurses enlisted as pilot officers, advancing to flying officer, flight lieutenant, squadron leader, and wing commander.[9] But gender intersected with rank, shaping advancement differently for men and women. For example, while one medical officer at No. 1 Neurological Hospital advanced through the ranks from lieutenant to lieutenant colonel in only nineteen days, NS Hallie Sloan described her progress this way: "I went overseas as a Lieutenant Nursing Sister and came home as a Lieutenant Nursing Sister, and it took twelve years to get my Captain's rank."[10]

Nurses understood the importance of rank as well as the various ways in which it influenced their relationships with patients. As NS Margery MacLean said, "Your patients were more conscious of the fact that you were a lieutenant instead of a private ... They can't talk back to an officer."[11] NS Margaret Fletcher arrested a soldier for drunkenness on her ward.[12] NS Helen Mussallem wanted to avoid arresting a corporal, explaining, "If you were in charge as I was, and the 'boys' were misbehaving, the sergeant major would say, 'Corporal Mackintosh did this, this, and this and I want him put under arrest.' You'd have to go with your clips on your shoulder and say, 'Corporal Mackintosh, you have done so and so, you are now under open arrest (or closed arrest)' ... I didn't like that part of it ... But you had to do it that way. You were on duty and that was one of your roles ... I remember saying to the Sergeant, 'Try and talk him out of it.' He would answer, 'Sister, we've got to get on with this.'"[13] On at least one occasion, a soldier lost seven days' pay for leaving a ward without the permission of the nursing sister and then lying about it.[14] Sometimes nurses used discretion to bend the rules, as NS Eva Wannop did in England: "If a chap came in a little later than usual, we didn't report him. Because what difference did it make? He didn't do it on purpose. If he was a little late getting in, he'd just get undressed and go to bed, and didn't say anything. Because otherwise you know, the army was so rigid that they'd have him up on the carpet. Unless he did something wrong, and I don't think it was wrong to be a little late."[15]

Nurses of all three services were accountable to the director of Medical Services through a parallel administration system of matrons, principal matrons, and matrons-in-chief. The RCAMC had two matrons-in-chief due to the size of the nursing service – one in Canada and one overseas. Both the air force and the navy delayed the appointments of matrons-in-chief as interesting debates eventually developed regarding who would control nursing sisters and military nursing within these two branches. Matron-in-Chief Smellie quickly recognized the need for separate matrons for each service, as the size of each service increased and as the units expanded geographically. She requested the appointments, but Surgeon Commodore Archie A. McCallum, RCN medical director general, delayed Matron-in-Chief Russell's appointment almost two years, until September 1943, and Air Commodore R.W. Ryan, DMS for the RCAF, delayed the appointment of Matron Jessie E. Porteous almost two and a half years, until April 1943.[16]

Rank was extremely contentious for RCAF nurses. After the formation of a Women's Division with alternative rank structures, there were concerted efforts from within the RCAF administration to move nursing sisters into the Women's Division. The nurses fought the move with arguments that it reduced their wages to only two-thirds of equivalent male officers' pay and positioned them outside the medical services administratively. In rebuttal, one male officer complained that, "If full membership was granted to Nursing Sisters, they would be eligible to act on the Mess committee and vote on all matters raised at Mess meetings ... and that would not be desirable."[17] A brigadier and the Canadian Nurses Association became involved in the bitter fight until finally, Minister of Defence (Air) C.G. Power confirmed RCAF officers' rank and power of command within hospitals and medical settings for nursing sisters. Non-nursing medical personnel, such as dieticians and physiotherapists, however, were Women's Division personnel.[18]

The appointment of a matron, the head administrative position within the

RCAF nursing service at that time, was equally contentious, according to an exchange of memos and letters that reveal long-standing power struggles between nurses and RCAF hierarchy, in particular the Director of Medical Services (Air), R.W. Ryan. With the decision to form a separate nursing service during the fall of 1940, Major A.D. Kelly at No. 1 RCAF Training Centre (St. Thomas, Ontario) recommended the appointment of NS Ada Squires as matron to Ryan. Squires was "known to be competent, a good organizer, and a disciplinarian," but she declined the position because of family obligations. Kelly next recommended NS Frances Oakes, in November 1940, as equally competent but Ryan took no action – possibly because Oakes went overseas around that time, or possibly because she became involved in the resistance to moving nurses into the Women's Division. Ryan preferred to administer the nursing service himself with only occasional consultation by RCAMC Matron-in-Chief Smellie. But by May 1942 Smellie, stretched in her own responsibilities, officially asked for the appointment of an RCAF matron. In July, she recommended five RCAMC nurses for consideration but Ryan rejected all of them, stating he didn't want "to go to other services" and preferred his own nurses. Some reasons given for the rejection of candidates allude to discord among nurses and reveal gendered stereotypes. One nurse, for example, was considered strict but "only on matters of no importance ... She leads to discontent among nursing staff and some nursing sisters prefer to stay in their bedrooms rather than face dinner knowing what was coming to them." Another candidate was forty-nine and "has passed that very difficult and uncertain period of a woman's physiological life [read as menopause], and therefore, has settled down to a matronly routine." Air Commodore E.E. Middleton, in a memo to Ryan, declared he even preferred a civilian matron to a non-RCAF nurse.[19] As a result, Matron Porteous was not appointed until April 1943, after a change in command, when Air Commodore J.W. Tice became the director of Medical Services.

Apparently, underlying tensions in the RCAF ran deeper than rank, divisions, and the appointment of a matron. They included issues regarding saluting and drilling by nurses that were not resolved until 1944, and then only after the president of the Canadian Nurses Association became involved. Apparently RCAF nurses opposed the military practices of "paying compliments" by saluting and participation in drills and parades – arguing that the nature of their work kept them constantly on call to attend the sick. The air force and the nurses compromised in March 1944: nursing sisters would use an alternate form of paying compliments by "turning the head and eyes and bowing the head in the direction indicated."[20]

Saluting by nurses was contentious in the other nursing services, too. The salute was associated with masculinity, privilege, respect, and rank. As civilian nurses, nursing sisters had "paid compliments" in a hospital version of saluting – by rising when a physician or senior nursing staff entered the ward or room.[21] But they were far less comfortable receiving compliments or enacting authority associated with rank. For RCAMC NS Pepper, saluting was masculine behaviour that threatened nurses' femininity: "Saluting is very unfeminine. Saluting-on-the-march is even worse. When orders came that all nursing sisters were to salute their senior officers and return the salute of junior ranks, we were all upset. So much so that when three of the sisters saw a brigadier approaching, they exchanged a few heated words about who was to give the salute. Finally, the sister on the outside agreed to perform the honors. She did. Up came her arm. Off flew her hat. The brigadier retrieved it from Piccadilly Circus."[22] NS Frances Ferguson said, "I don't think we ever thought about rank. Except that we had to salute other officers. We learned to salute in a hurry. But it felt rather strange to have people saluting – going down the street."[23] RCN NS Marjorie Cowan wrote, "When we first became nursing sisters, we (at that time) did not return a salute; we were told to acknowledge a salute with 'a smile or a nod, but never a wink.' In due course, we had a class to teach us the correct naval salute."[24] Some nurses simply avoided encounters that might require a salute, like NS Betty Young and her friend, who decided to change directions and go down a side lane instead. As she recalled, "You'd get used to it. But the first time, it really bothered me."[25]

For the most part, nurses learned to drill and parade like other soldiers had to do. RCAF nursing sisters may have escaped these exercises, but RCAMC nurses did not. They could be both the pride and the despair of drill sergeants during these "toughening up" exercises, sometimes making the sergeants, whom they outranked, nervous. NS Margaret Mills recalled that "one sergeant used to take us out on route marches which was pretty strenuous for us and the sergeant was very nervous because we were all commissioned officers ... Little did he know we were more scared of him (I think) than he was of us."[26] NS Eleanor MacGregor drilled at the University of Toronto armouries with First World War veteran Sergeant Major Ed Miller, writing that "he was a very kind and patient man. He despaired of us. When a soldier stands at attention, there is no day light showing between his arms and his body. There was no way we could accomplish this, so he finally [acknowledged] 'Dames are built differently.'"[27]

In civilian settings, nurses were independent and relatively autonomous in private duty work, although they still acknowledged intrinsic lines of authority within physician and hospital hierarchies. Given their years of experience prior to enlistment, most nursing sisters found that the return to discipline and constant surveillance as military women was not an easy transition. At the beginning of the war, the armed forces appointed nursing sisters who had served during the First World War and older nurses with considerable experience in the administration and supervision of civilian hospitals, to be the matrons of newly mobilizing units. And when Canada received its own hospital ship in 1943, there were no nursing sisters with previous experience on hospital ships. So First World War veteran Charlotte Nixon came out of retirement at the age of fifty-four to serve as the matron of the *Lady Nelson*. NS Ruth Littlejohn worked on the *Lady Nelson* with "Ma Nixon," whom she described as "a bit out of touch" but well respected and fun loving, producing laughter when she appeared on deck during an air raid with a tin helmet on top of her veil.[28] When the big "pushes" of 1943 and 1944 began, new units formed and existing units enlarged, requiring the promotion of younger nursing sisters through the ranks to head up these additional units.

Not all matron-nursing sister relationships were as congenial as those on the *Lady Nelson*. NS Florence Jamieson served first in Canada, under Matron Gladys Sharpe, who had been director at the Toronto Western Hospital School of Nursing before the war. Jamieson gave examples of some of the tensions between nurses in her unit and Matron Sharpe: "She was measuring the length of our skirts and all that sort of business and probably expecting nursing sisters to conduct themselves in the same way that you were expected as a student and that created some problems ... It was brought to the attention of Miss Sharpe by a Western graduate who was older. I thought she deserved a great deal of respect for being able to talk to the group and realize that she was not performing the way they thought she should ... She gained a lot of respect for doing just that ... Well you see that didn't bother me because I was such a recent graduate. But for some of the nursing sisters who had been out earning a living ... it was very irritating to them."[29] Jamieson later volunteered for the South African contingent with Sharpe as the SAMNS matron and liaison officer between the British and South African authorities. Jamieson was put in charge of one group of nurses for the trip out of England, and found that she, too, had difficulty exerting her proper authority over peers. Attributing the problem to class differences among nurses, she found a way to leave the troublemakers behind on arrival in South Africa. As Jamieson described the situation, "Of the thirty-one, I found out that there were about five of them that were sneaking out at night, and going down and sleeping with whomever in the male category ... From the background that I was from, I just couldn't understand how anybody in a Canadian uniform on a British ship during wartime could do that. My education was being enlarged ... I tried different things and then I realized I was being very unrealistic ... I just gave up, because I thought it was like Miss Sharpe ... I was to proceed to Baragwanath Military Hospital in the state of Transvaal. So I had to choose twenty people from the thirty to go with me. So I left behind the five that were a problem."

NS Margaret Kellough served with No. 15 CGH until her promotion as assistant matron of that unit, and later as matron of No. 5 CCS. These promotions placed her in an uncomfortable position of authority over peers, and as she acknowledged, "You knew their best and not their best, and their work, and everything else. You had to be very impartial and I often knew what the girls were doing ... I often knew where they were going but I didn't say anything to anybody." When asked about specific disciplinary problems, Kellough admitted there were some but declined to talk about them. On one occasion, she lost an argument regarding marching orders for nurses in an Easter Parade at Oss, Holland. She had to rally the nurses to conformity, explaining: "I argued and argued with him because we were on duty and Number 4 CCS was at rest. Their Colonel hadn't asked them to march. I said to the Colonel, 'Well, there will only be a few of us, because the girls that are on duty can't go and the girls that are on night duty are sleeping.' So actually there were only nine of us and myself that could go in this march. And we had taken some marching drill and stuff, but we weren't that proficient at it ... So our girls were practically ready to revolt and I said, 'Look I've done as much as I can with the Colonel, we've got to do it, let's do it to the best of our ability.'"[30]

Gender, class, and rank intersected in the military to shape nurses' public behaviours, social activities, and personal appearance. While rank segregated nurses socially from the non-commissioned officers or enlisted men, it also reserved and enhanced their social status with all male officers – since military women were scarce resources. Paradoxically, rank positioned them in closer social contact to physicians than was typical in their respective civilian settings. As NS Van Scoyoc explained, "We were a minority and these were our first experiences of relationships with friends who were engineers, signals ... people outside the medical profession ... It did change our ideas of our relationships with doctors, in that we had always looked up to them as 'gods,' but they didn't spoil us ... These other people did – the officers from other units really spoiled us ... [The doctors] were left without female company ... We benefited by having other male officers around, and the doctors were sort of left out socially."[31]

NS Margaret Allemang found that military rank relaxed some of the traditional barriers between medicine and nursing: "In some ways, the Air Force was a more relaxed situation for me. And more informal, with much more socializing with the medical people. We'd always have coffee together in the morning."[32] Nurses with less professional and military experience tended to maintain more traditional lines of deference towards the medical officers. As NS Bea Cole said, "I think regarding the more experienced nurses, that there was a good comradeship between them and the medical officers. I wasn't exactly like a probie, but I ... must have been probably ten years younger than any of the medical officers."[33]

The responsibilities and privileges of rank permeated all spheres of activity: the hospital, the military unit, and civilian settings. NS Betty Nicolson put it this way: "When you are in the Army, and especially overseas, you were in the Army *all* the time."[34] NS Doris Carter learned "there were 'no mistakes' as such made in the Army" when she tried to explain that her posting was incorrect. She also learned, when reprimanded for having liquor in her personal possession, that "all my thinking would be done for me."[35] When NS Kitty Murphy's picture and reactions to a posting for Newfoundland appeared in a local newspaper, her commanding officer immediately issued a statement that "no authority was given to this Nursing Sister to state her views to the Press."[36]

Some nurses accepted the inevitability of military decisions affecting their personal and service lives, while others resisted policies and protocols. NS Evelyn Pepper didn't want to leave her CCS unit in Italy, writing, "I was sad to leave but quietly moved on. One always did as one was told. Unless you were of senior rank ... you were never a participant in the decision-making."[37] NS Mary Bower struggled with authority throughout her army career, as she explained: "There was the military protocol, you know ... I didn't really fit into that ever, I think, which was probably a problem to everybody." At one point, Bower's matron paraded her for "inciting the soldiers to riot." Bower spoke of her earlier upbringing and her association with labour and socialist movements in western Canada, which she felt raised suspicions about her activities in protests over soldiers' living conditions while serving with the RCAMC. Involvement with such working-class movements was inconsistent with officer rank and professional status. As Bower explained, "I think they would have loved to cut my pips off. And I walked into this ... The sergeant major came for me and he paraded me down to this room. I had no idea that I was going to be chastised or anything else. And I went in this room, and the matron was there, and my equals were sitting around in a circle. And the [commanding officer] of the hospital was sitting behind a desk. And the guy marches me up and salutes, you know, and stands there. 'Prisoner at the bar.' Me! And it was so stupid. He said I was ... inciting the soldiers to riot."[38]

Masculinity, as symbolized by military rank, remained a complex and contested aspect of the military nursing experience. As the first women in the armed forces, it was not always clear to nurses, or their male superiors, just how gender intersected with rank in the performance of military roles and responsibilities.

Remaining Feminine

Although rank might contain negotiable aspects, femininity did not. NS Mills referred to "being female" as nurses' chief contribution to the war effort.[39] They were expected to be the epitome of femininity as companions, dance partners, morale-boosters, and reminders of home and family – but always within the limits of respectability. NS Pauline Lamont described one display of nurses' femininity onboard a ship to England: "One day we heard the intercom saying, 'All Nursing Sisters report immediately to the port deck.' And so we thought, 'Oh boy, this is it. You know, we're needed.' And tore up and got on the deck. And the Captain was there smiling. And what happened

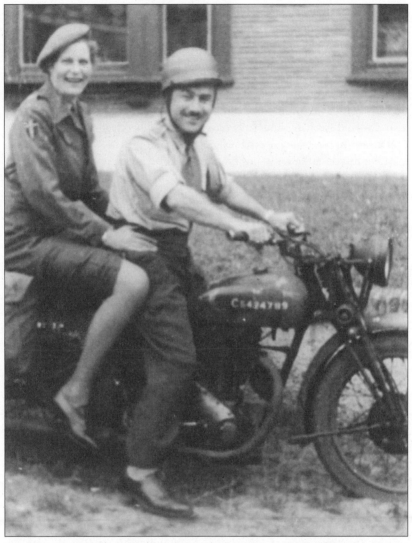

Lady-like deportment was essential for nursing sisters, reinforcing respectability as women within the military system and their status as officers. RCAMC Major/Principal Matron Edna E. Rossiter was certainly aware of these expectations when she and Major Pierce, both at No. 12 CGH near Bruge, Belgium, during April 1945, returned to the unit by motorcycle. She wrote on the back of this photograph, "The dignified Matron and Major Pierce (E.N.T.) coming home from the Officers Mess at Knocke. (We didn't start till it got dark for obvious reasons.)" *Hamilton Military Museum, 1998.006.002*

was, a Canadian frigate was right – very near us, and they had heard that there were Canadian girls on board. And they just wanted to have a look at us. So we all waved and yelled."[40]

Class-based femininity included, among other things, lady-like deportment at all times and in all areas of military nurses' service. As McPherson points out, "restraint" was the key element of ladylike behaviour, and much of student nurses' training during this period involved the inculcation of restraint into their practice and their lives.[41] The military provided plenty of opportunity to practise restraint. Along with "getting used to four-letter words, men, and Army life," according to NS Jamieson, learning to be a military nurse also involved knowing how to behave off-duty where there were abundant opportunities for drinking and engaging in sexual activities.[42]

Male officers frequently hosted parties and dances, inviting the nursing sisters, who then reciprocated with parties of their own. NS Estelle Tritt recalled how her matron used to post notices that read, "There will be a dance at headquarters. 'X' Nursing Sisters required," and expect the right number of nurses to sign up. If they didn't, she assigned them to attend as part of their duties. On social occasions like these, nurses could be chosen like chocolates from a box, as in NS Mary Bray's example, where "one day one of the officers came in to our Major and said, 'I would like to have six of your assortment!'"[43] NS Kellough referred to these social occasions as "emotional times," however, as nurses tried to fulfill dual roles as both nurses and companions to men, especially during brief lulls in the frontline action. She described the physical and mental stress of staying up most, or all of the night, and then going on duty with minimal or no sleep: "They would want parties and we felt that we were obligated to go to the parties because they would soon be going back into the line again ... We had to be up and at it in the morning ... They knew and we knew that some of them would come back as patients; some of them wouldn't come back. So it was an emotional time, but they had to talk to somebody."[44]

Orientation lectures reminded nursing sisters that, although they already knew how to relate to physicians and patients, they now represented the military twenty-four hours a day in both military and civilian settings. The officers' mess was a bastion of male privilege where the scrutiny of appropriate feminine behaviours was most evident. It was the main place for officers to relax and socialize away from enlisted personnel, and where they typically spent off-duty time. Nursing sisters, as officers, had access to this privileged area but were admonished to conduct themselves as ladies there. As NS Doris Taylor recalled, "You had to follow the rules or you weren't going to be there." The mess was "primarily men's domain," and nurses were not to wear out their welcome by "aimless sitting around ... drinking and chatting."[45]

Besides observing proper behaviour in the mess, nursing sisters were to avoid fraternizing with the "other ranks," criticizing the armed forces, or complaining in public places, and were to remember that "no lady ever drinks too much." Alcoholic beverages were readily available at dances and parties, but drinking to excess had its pitfalls. NS Van Scoyoc recalled an incident at

Petawawa, Ontario, when a colleague transgressed the boundaries of military hierarchy with negative consequences for her career: "One of the girls got drinking too much. It was a brigadier, and of course, they are very rank conscious, particularly in Canada. And she was talking about all his stars on his shoulder. And they said she had too much to drink. So she didn't get overseas." Sometimes the abuse of alcohol could be sufficiently problematic to warrant measures at the unit level. NS Amy White wrote home from HMCS *Niobe*, for example, that "we have had the bar removed from our ward room by mutual consent and serve coffee instead, every night at ten. The liquor was becoming too much of a problem."[46] Additional regulations covered carrying parcels and purses, smoking, make-up, nail polish, jewellery, gum chewing, hair style, loud talking, cleanliness, travel, uniforms, and shoes – but overall, as nurses were admonished, "our actions should be dictated by the laws governing the conduct of a lady."[47]

Advertisements in the *Canadian Nurse* reinforced the femininity of military nurses as well, portraying them as busy and hard working but always "fresh" and "achieving victory over odours" through the use of advertised products such as deodorants, tampons, and foot powder. One ad portrays a young nurse in battledress and tin helmet, caring for a bandaged but smiling young man in a bed, with a jungle scene framed in the window and a caption that reads, "Army nurses certainly have plenty to do these days, and still they must keep well groomed. That means attention to underarm freshness. MUM, the snow-white vanishing cream brings quick deodorizing victory over stale perspiration odor wherever it may arise."[48] Another ad portrays navy nurses with this message: "'Full speed ahead' is the order of the day for Navy nurses and there's precious little time for personal fastidiousness ... [MUM] goes into action quickly and stays on duty for long hours ... Signal for MUM during sanitary napkin time. And try it for refreshing hot, tired feet, too."[49] Tampax advertised its product under the heading, "Unprecedented times? Unprecedented problems" in reference to women's wartime work: "Working steadily with men in near proximity – often wearing close-fitting slacks or coveralls – with less opportunity for private retirement than in more leisurely or more domestic times – it is little wonder that so many have found in Tampax the ideal means for improving their hygienic habits, as an aid to uninterrupted activity."[50] Military nurses' feet sold foot powder in an ad portraying columns of nurses on parade, under the heading, "War Effort Speeded by New Success over Athlete's Foot" with a lead-in sentence that read: "Every nurse must keep her feet in most perfect condition to keep working and marching to victory."[51]

The most visible symbol of gendered rank and femininity in the armed forces was the nursing sisters' uniforms. The RCAMC uniform, patterned after the cherished First World War uniform, also served as the model for the RCN and RCAF uniforms, making it possible for military nurses from any of the three services to be readily recognized as Canadian nursing sisters.[52] NS Carter described the RCAMC uniform in a manner that emphasized its femininity: "There were three types [versions] of uniforms, each with an Alice-blue two-piece suit with two rows of small brass Medical Corps buttons down the jacket, a peplum, white stiff collar and cuffs, a leather two-inch belt with a lion's head brass buckle ... and a slim, slightly flaired [sic] skirt. One uniform was wool for winter dress affairs, one was silk for such events in summer, and one was cotton for work. Over the cotton uniform we wore a white cotton apron with a bib and straps, and the belt over the apron ... A white veil was worn with all these uniforms. A navy blue suit for 'walking out' was worn with a light blue shirt from Morgan's Boys' Department ... with navy blue tie, either wool or silk. We wore very smart navy blue brimmed felt hats by Stetson, with a ribbon band and the Medical Corps badge up front." Brown leather gloves, white scarf, brown "sensible" walking shoes or black "pumps" for social affairs, navy blue raincoats or greatcoats, a purse, a lace handkerchief for the jacket pocket, rank designations, and the Canada badge completed this outfit.[53] RCN nurses' uniforms were a darker "navy blue" with a maroon distinction cloth in the gold braiding and RCN insignia. RCAF nurses began their first year without military uniforms, except for a veil with the RCAF wings embroidered on the back, which they wore with basic white civilian uniforms. They continued to wear white uniforms for work but adopted an air force blue dress uniform based on the RCAMC model for dress occasions.[54]

Wearing these distinctive uniforms properly was a matter of pride and discipline and, for many nurses, they were more luxurious than the clothes they had been able to afford during the Depression. NS/Dietician Elizabeth Dean, for example, told how much she loved wearing them "because I'd grown up in Depression years and now I had all these uniforms."[55] They wore the dress uniform for all public functions, from the parade ground to weddings and dances, unlike some American nurses who seem to have travelled with evening gowns in tow.[56] NS Lamont associated self-respect, self-worth, and dignity with the nursing sister uniform: "I think we suddenly felt that we were valued, that we were respected. We were known by our uniform. We felt good in our uniform. People knew who we were by our uniform."

There were plenty of occasions to exhibit proper heterosexual ladylike behaviours, especially in England, when royalty and dignitaries visited medical units or hosted various teas, receptions, and cultural events where nurses represented the Canadian forces. NS Dorothy Surgenor recalled how RCN nurses had active social lives and were expected to be present whenever battleships came into port, whereupon they were "treated like queens" at the captain's table – almost the only occasion when the navy permitted women onboard ships. "You were somebody special ... You also dressed accordingly. I mean your uniforms had to be right, too. I mean you had an image to keep up."[57]

Admonished not to "disgrace" the uniform, and regulated to wear it on- and off-duty, nurses of all three branches had a constant reminder of the expected behaviours of a nursing sister. At HMCS *Stadacona* in Halifax, a policy that allowed the wearing of "civvies" on Sunday quickly changed when civilian feminine clothing proved too provocative. As NS Surgenor recalled, "In those days, you wore a white blouse usually, and a sweater. And it was fairly tight-fitting. I think we had about a month-and-a-half of Sunday dinners at the Admiralty house, when we got a message that we were not to wear civvies anymore on Sundays. The sweaters were too tight! We had to wear our uniforms."

As part of their cotton duty uniforms, nursing sisters wore bibbed aprons as well as veils. Beyond any utilitarian function, aprons were reminiscent of student training days and nurses' subservient, domestic roots. The gauze veils were reminiscent of the profession's association with religious sisterhoods and the charitable care of strangers performed by middle-class ladies. One songwriter portrayed Canadian nursing sisters in song as "Fairy Queens" who "waft care away in the battle clearing station" and "flit along the tent."[58] These symbols and metaphors were important tools that distinguished "respectable" military nurses from disrespectable "camp followers," women of sometimes questionable character who had followed armies during earlier wars, eking out a living as laundresses, cooks, maids, untrained nurses, or prostitutes.

Uniforms and veils were also visual reminders for nurses, patients, male officers, and the public alike. One officer, who was escorting nurses at night under London blackout conditions, allegedly remarked, "You know I'm not protecting you, you're protecting me [from prostitutes]."[59] The veil was a particularly evocative symbol. Nurses took great care to starch, iron, and wear it properly. NS Van Scoyoc described how "the officers liked to play a trick, to try to take our veils off. We were not properly dressed if the veil was pulled off or askew. It was considered a great misdemeanor." The veil remained a powerful symbol of nurses' association with the military: their rank and privileges, patriotism, and shared experiences in aspects of war that had been forbidden to other women. NS Lamont explained that after the war, veteran nurses who worked in DVA hospitals wore civilian uniforms but continued to wear the nursing sister veil. In her words, "We were so proud to have been in [the war]."

When posted to the active theatres, however, nurses stored the "Blues" and adopted British-issued khaki battledress. As NS Hallie Sloan wrote, "We packed our blue uniforms and white veils, donned khaki uniforms, berets, and high leather boots, and headed for Yorkshire for a toughening up period prior to D-Day." When tougher conditions prevailed, "[and] when the rains came ... everyone worked in gas capes, tin hats and gumboots, completely shattering the illusion of 'ministering angels.'"[60] The transition from Blues to khaki signified a transformation into "one of the boys," although there were

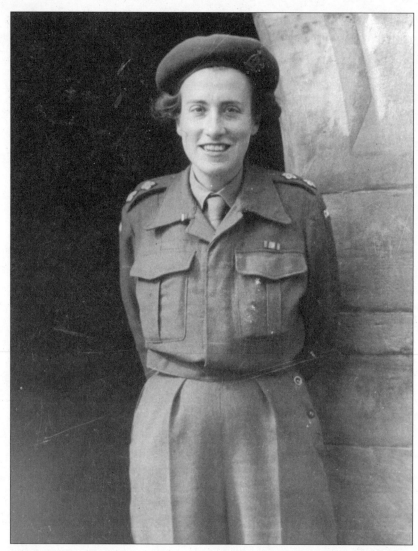

RCAMC NS Hallie Sloan, like other nursing sisters in active theatres, wore khaki battledress, which included both skirts and trousers for women. *Courtesy Harriet Sloan*

still feminine concessions such as khaki skirts during the day, while khaki bandanas and berets replaced the veil. Long pants were necessary protection against malaria-carrying mosquitoes after sundown, although nurses were not very pleased when required to wear them for dances. NS Nicolson called dancing in pants and heavy boots a liability.

NS Kellough, illustrating sexual fluidity and gender-bending behaviours during wartime, gave this example of dilemmas that arose: "We had to wear

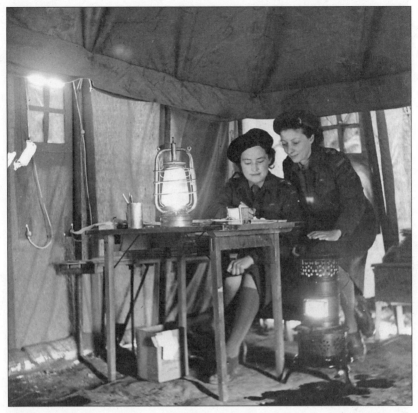

RCAMC NS Eloise MacDiarmid and NS Frances Caddy wore the battle dress skirt option while on night duty at No. 1 CGH at Andria, Italy, during February 1944. *LAC/Lieutenant Dwight E. Dolan/DND/PA-213775*

slacks on account of it being malarious [sic], and danced in our heavy boots. We said we looked very alluring with our mosquito cream on our face ... At the American hospital near us, their Colonel allowed them to wear skirts and we weren't. So one of my beaux or escorts, whatever you like to call him, he said 'If you wear those darn pants, I'm wearing a kilt.' I said, 'O.K., take out an American girl – she can wear a skirt' ... There were situations that you had to accept because the Orders came from the Colonel."

In other situations, the authorities questioned the wearing of khaki uniforms and trousers by women, especially when the nurses were travelling in public, where they represented Canadian womanhood. The wearing of trousers, along with other masculine styles of clothing, generated anxieties regarding masculinity and femininity, as well as anxieties regarding heterosexuality and homosexuality – particularly in light of the perception of "cross-dressing" as a manifestation of the "mannish woman," a euphemism for lesbian.[61] NS Tritt,

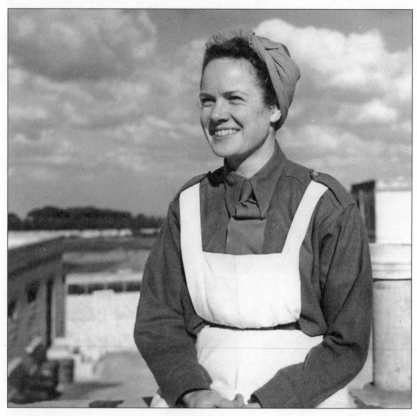

Like other RCAMC nursing sisters in active theatres where water was scarce, NS Elaine Wright discarded the white uniform veils for battledress khaki bandanas at No. 1 CGH in Andria, Italy, during February 1944, finding it made life easier under the conditions there. *LAC/DND fonds/ PA-213776*

nonetheless, felt that one matron was particularly "out of touch" with both nurses' realities and changes on the Canadian home front as well. When she was posted to No. 8 CGH in England,

> Matron MacDonald told us to travel in our battledress – which was the only thing, if you were travelling in an ambulance or in trucks usually. So away we went, to stop over in Brussels overnight at headquarters. And Matron Shaffner was quite shocked to see us in battledress. "How can you come in battledress to Brussels – a city? You wouldn't see women wearing slacks in Toronto or Montreal!" When I got off the train at Bonaventure Station [in Montreal after the war], there was my mother and my three sisters ... My three sisters were in slacks. So I felt like writing, "Dear Matron Shaffner, people are wearing slacks."

Battledress was also very practical for the living and working conditions. Water was severely rationed in some settings, such as Italy, and cleanliness became a challenge. Some nurses reported taking only sponge baths for four months or more, with the water serving double duty for laundry afterwards. NS Jean MacBain was especially glad for khaki, writing, "Khaki turbans kept our hair well hidden. Our shirts were also khaki so that solved our dirty shirt problem, it was such a neutral colour. We had only three shirts and not enough water to wash them so we rotated daily, hung them up to air and sprinkled them with Chanel No. 5. We had more of that than water."[62]

Nurses from the torpedoed *Santa Elena,* as well as nurses whose supply ship sank in Augusta harbour at Sicily, were extremely grateful for men's khaki clothing when all their possessions were lost at sea. There were limited amounts of small sizes, however, and the proportions were definitely masculine rather than feminine. Moreover, there was no women's underwear. NS MacLean requested her brother, stationed in England, to send an assortment of bras because there were none to be had in the army's stores. NS Pauline Cox grieved because she had big feet and her "nice new shoes" went down with the ship, but she managed to scrounge new ones from an American supplies dump. And only one woman had abandoned the *Santa Elena* with a tube of lipstick in her pocket, the only surviving make-up among the group.[63]

Unlike most of the units that had adopted khaki battledress, nurses of No. 5 CGH arrived at Augusta harbour on the island of Sicily, dressed as ladies instead of "one of the boys." According to NS Nicholson,

> We got into the harbour and got down off the ship. Down the ladders into the landing craft with our [vomit] bags, in case we were sick. And our helmet, and our knapsack, and all the rest of it – with our silk stockings still on, and our suits, and our fedora hats ... Skirts, of course! ... We were lucky nobody fell in ... We lost our supply ship. We didn't know at the time, but our supply ship went down with that bombardment. We lost all our equipment and our tropical gear that we were to wear. We were still dressed up as if we were going out for a nice walk in the country or whatever.

In unexpected ways, the nursing sisters' uniform helped Kay Christie and May Waters survive as Japanese prisoners of war. They were able to cut up their uniforms to make shorts, and their aprons to make "sun tops" as their clothing wore out during the twenty-one months of internment. Christie described using flooring to make slab shoe soles that she tied to her feet with strips of the blue uniform, like clogs. And when they were repatriated as part of an American prisoner exchange with Japan, she reported that, on the exchange ship, "the Canadians were so raggedy that we were called down first to the store. Everyone else could have either a dress or a skirt and sweater but because we were so poor, we could have more."[64]

As the uniform shaped soldiers, so did the uniform shape military nurses. Nurses were practically indistinguishable from fighting forces when in battledress.[65] This was sobering to those who realized how closely the medical services identified as soldiers. NS Irene Stephenson wrote about her experience after landing on the famous Mulberry harbour at Arromanches, France, after D-Day. The nurses came ashore in landing craft and then, she wrote, "It was into the trucks and across the dusty roads to Bayeux. I felt like I was about to save the world until we passed a group in a field and an elderly woman pointed to her bandaged knee and shook her fist at us. I guess she connected us to her injury somehow, and dressed in khaki battledress and steel helmets we all looked like soldiers anyway."[66]

Historian Mary Sarnecky attributes the low morale and disciplinary problems within the U.S. Army Nurse Corps partially to the lack of appropriate military nursing uniforms. Describing various versions of the uniforms as "sometimes confusing," often impractical, and "vested with much confusion, pain, energy, and emotion," she suggests that "morale frequently plummeted as a result of dowdy, baggy, or uncomfortable uniforms."[67] For most of the Canadian nursing sisters, in contrast, military uniforms were a source of pride, symbol of national identity, and visual representations of their status as officers and ladies.

Experiencing the Contradictions

There were at least three career-limiting life events that affected military women differently than military men: aging, marriage, and pregnancy. At the beginning of the war, the armed forces selected older, highly experienced nurses, who had additional expertise in administration, supervision, or teaching. As the "Report of the Committee on Nursing and Nurse Education in Canadian Hospitals" reminded civilian hospitals in 1941, "It must be borne in mind that there is a definite need for mature, self-disciplined women, experienced in leadership, to represent Canadian nurses overseas. Even in the so-called rank and file, military nurses are called upon to undertake supervisory duties and often under extraordinary conditions."[68] The armed forces clearly preferred to limit the number of nurses during this early phase. They filled nursing positions slowly and used nursing sisters to train medical assistants – putting their abilities in administration, supervision, and teaching to good use.

But the armed forces preferred these older, experienced nurses for another purpose, too – as "safe" women who could be entrusted with the control and supervision of younger, less-experienced nurses, both professionally and socially, as the number of younger nurses increased. The combined effect of training and postgraduate experience positioned nurses as older sisters or mothers in relation to the average soldier, whom they almost always referred to as "our boys."[69] These age differences partially desexualized the physical

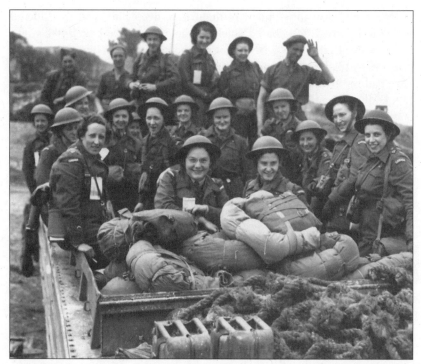

RCAMC nursing sisters of No. 10 CGH did indeed look like other soldiers during their landing on Arromanches beach, France, 23 June 1944. *LAC/Harold G. Aikman/DND fonds/PA-108172*

care of relatively healthy, young male bodies. One nurse recalled that, "the boys were proud of their Sisters – almost as if we were their own sisters."[70] Another nurse wrote, "Most nursing sisters had experienced young casualties of all nationalities, crying for 'Mum.' She was always there to talk, give him a smile, a pat on the shoulder or squeeze his hand."[71]

This preference also meant that military nurses were an aging population as the war continued over six years while the workforce remained remarkably stable. One-quarter of the nursing sisters served between four and six years, and almost one-half served between three and six years. Many nursing sisters were entering their mid-thirties and forties towards the end of the war. By 1943, there were sufficient numbers of nurses with enough military experience that the armed forces modified the age restrictions to include younger nurses with far less experience as the Allies prepared for large-scale campaigns in Italy and northwestern Europe.

Age restructuring had implications for nursing sisters with long service. At the end of 1944, the RCAMC recalled to England all the nursing sisters in Italy who were over forty years old. Meanwhile, the RCAF recalled back to Canada their nurses who were over forty. Known internally as "WOOFs" or "women of over forty," many of them were deeply angry at their forced withdrawal, which was based solely on age and not on their skills and performance in the field.[72] NS Dorothy Macham wrote in her diary, "I can't give any particulars but I think I am returning to England shortly. I guess I have had my 'fightin'. I will be sorry to go but I really think I am beginning to take these moves with a little less concern."[73] But another nurse was so angry that she resigned, stating as her rationale her unhappiness in "having been returned to Canada as over age for overseas duty."[74] It was also difficult for the younger nurses who arrived as replacements, as NS Bray wrote: "I'd missed out on all the pre-training and felt so sick at heart because I knew I was replacing an old stalwart type. And I felt really lost."[75] Sometimes the recall was disguised as a promotion, to a higher level of responsibility but at a unit in England or Canada. At other times, it was framed in terms of a need for military experience in the rehabilitation hospitals back in Canada. As NS Tritt explained, "We ... saw my old [obstetrical] supervisor, Arnodt, who was being sent home. And she heard that one of the other supervisors from Reddy [Reddy Memorial Hospital at Montreal] had just come over. And she was yelling, 'If McCaffrey is under 39 then I'm sweet 16,' because they were sending the older girls home at 39. One reason was, when the fellows came back from overseas and landed in Canadian hospitals with younger nurses, they weren't paying any attention to them, [saying,] 'After all, you haven't had our experience.' And so the older girls came back."

The RCAMC initiated another plan in November 1944, to return nursing sisters to Canada based on the date of their enlistment, compounding nurses' anger and accelerating the withdrawal of older nurses from the active theatres. NS Pepper wrote, "It seemed odd that it should happen at the height of what we now felt was our final campaign."[76] NS Constance Bond called the "first over" rule particularly disappointing because the new nurses "had taken our place where we should have been," just as the war was winding down.[77] When NS Dorothy Potts spent V-E Day alone after being recalled to Canada, she lamented, "I would have been there with them."[78]

The recall of long-term nurses and WOOFs disrupted well-established work teams in the field, removing the most experienced nurses, ostensibly because the military thought younger women were needed closer to the front. And as numerous statements from nursing sisters attested, it also prevented long-serving nurses from gaining closure so near to the end of the war. It is unclear why the military suddenly implemented these policies. The abundance of civilian nurses on enlistment waiting lists, as well as the large number of nursing sisters requesting overseas postings, made it possible to exchange older nurses for younger but still experienced ones. But there is no evidence that older nurses were less capable or less willing to serve on the frontlines. Yet the military had determined that their age was a liability, instead of an asset signifying nursing expertise.

Marriage was another liability for women in the military. Although marriage policies of the armed forces were consistent with the prevailing social expectations for middle- and upper-class women to resign from paid work when they married, the increasing need for experienced nurses and their resistance to these policies made obligatory resignation unenforceable. NS Eleanor Jones, for example, married secretly in March 1942. When her husband died in a training accident seven months later, she was charged with "Conduct Unbecoming to an Officer" and "Conduct Prejudicial to Good Discipline," and paraded before a brigadier, who gave her an official reprimand for marrying without permission. A subsequent series of interviews with her adjutant "always left me in tears." Although the policy changed in 1943, the reprimand was still on her file at discharge years later.[79] As the number of resignations related to marriage increased, a policy change permitted married nurses to remain in the service. This change allowed the armed forces to retain military nursing expertise, just in time for the campaigns in Italy and northwestern Europe. Marriage was still a career-limiting move, however, because married nurses could not serve in an active theatre: they had to remain in England when their units left for the Mediterranean, and those who married after leaving England had to return there.[80] These regulations were consistent with prevailing discourses regarding the need to offer even more protection and safer environments for married women, ostensibly related to their potential for child bearing but ignoring that unmarried women could become pregnant as well. They also relieved public anxieties and ensured continued support for keeping married women in the military.

Pregnancy was a third liability facing nursing sisters. It differed from the other two in that it terminated, not just limited, a military career. Whether married or unmarried, women bore the primary consequences of pregnancy. Yet the proximity of so few women to so many men made a certain degree of sexual activity, and the consequent threat of pregnancy, inevitable. NS Patterson described the military situation as "a female paradise" where "there were all kinds of men. And even the most unattractive person was really 'rushed.'" NS Anne Farries referred to the military as "an abnormal way of life": "You were over there mixing with married men and single men, and all of them were lonely, but the married men were perhaps the loneliest of all. There were a lot of affairs going on. If nurses got pregnant, they were sent home."[81] Some personnel relied on the anti-malarial drug mepacrine (also known as atabrine) as a means to prevent pregnancy. The drug was mistakenly reputed to cause sterility in men, and as NS Irene Henderson noted, it "proved not to be a birth control pill either, to the surprise of many!"[82]

My sources indicate that at least 6.5 percent of Canadian military nurses were pregnant on discharge, and pregnancy was the chief reason for all nurse medical repatriations, as was the case for female military personnel in general.[83] Unmarried pregnant nurses were not uncommon, and undoubtedly some marriages resulted subsequent to pregnancy. But pregnancy rates definitely increased after the policy change permitting married nurses to retain commissions. They increased again in the months after V-E Day as the war wound down, and women had less reason to avoid pregnancy in order to remain overseas. Nurses returned to Canada, designated officially as "walking wounded," having a "physiological tumour," or just plain "pregnant." NS Mary Nelson's physiological tumour was born on Armistice Day.[84]

Pregnancy became sufficiently problematic during the war, however, that the army decided to test women prior to overseas embarkation. NS Jean Ciceri recalled that, "One morning, throughout the two huts, you could see long lines of specimen bottles. A few nurses didn't get to go overseas."[85] Meanwhile, according to a 1944 memo from the London County Council Public Health Department to the RCAMC regarding Friedman (pregnancy) tests, since "rabbits are scarse [sic] and expensive," the army was "to avoid excessive numbers of tests."[86] One nurse managed to conceal her pregnancy for eight months until it was no longer feasible to return to Canada prior to giving birth. A civilian physician delivered the baby, who was then placed for adoption, and the nurse was discharged as "not well adapted to military service."[87]

For the most part, nursing sisters were required to restrain if not conquer their sexuality. Nurses were encouraged to develop a desexualized subjectivity during their training years, whereby they learned through complex and often contradictory processes how to care for the bodies of strangers (and men in particular) within the bounds of respectability.[88] But a military need for nurses to serve in dual heterosexual roles, as nurses and as women, added another level of complexity to nurses' sexuality. The guiding principle of "the conduct of a lady" applied to appropriate sexual relationships, enforced by "boarding out" (discharge) and loss of benefits as consequences for misconduct.

Data from this study contain veiled references and noticeable silences related to sexuality and pregnancy. The majority of nursing sisters described extensive and active social lives as well as the great disproportion in numbers of men and women, easy availability of male escorts, and camaraderie with medical officers. Most nurses either denied or avoided discussions about unwanted sexual behaviour and/or same-sex relationships. As NS Sloan explained, for example, "I've had the medical officers put their arm around my shoulder and talk to me about a patient or something. Or you're sitting at the little six-foot folding table in the so-called office and the guy comes around and sits on the bench beside you, and puts his arm around you, and talks to you about a patient or something. Well, if that's harassment, we had that. And they'd come by and give you a pat on the bum and say, 'Come on, let's go.' Or give you a slap on the back and say, 'That's a good job.'"[89] But NS Fletcher occasionally expressed annoyance with British officers in her letters home. As she wrote after one dance, "These damned Englishmen have only two ideas in their heads, & the first one is to get tight, & let the second one follow. I left the party in disgust at 11 P.M., & know of three other girls who simply walked off & left their partners. I know that our lads aren't angels, & we wouldn't ask them to be, but at least they have a little finesse about the whole thing."[90]

Many nurses spoke and wrote about the large number of weddings towards the end of the war, as well as their own marriages to men they had often known for a very brief time. NS MacGregor's second military marriage occurred within a month of being introduced to the man. NS Bower was in several relationships in which she almost married men she had known for a very short time, including the man that she did finally marry. She described experiencing many difficulties with military discipline and lifestyle, her general unhappiness overseas, incidents of sexual harassment, and a need for counselling that might have prevented her disastrous decision to marry.[91] Yet other relationships, formed just as quickly, lasted for long lifetimes.

Nursing sisters occasionally referred to friends, lovers, and husbands whom they had lost during the war. But they seldom spoke outright of sexuality, or how war and the military may have constrained or facilitated relationships. Those who did speak or write confirmed the blurring of social conventions related to sex, married officers, sexual "teasing," harassment, abortion, venereal disease, and same-sex relations. For example, NS MacGregor described a nurse named Dorothy, who just "radiated sex" and "would stand at the foot of the bed while Purdy [another NS] was trying to take out stitches from an appendectomy, and do a lot of very seductive wiggling. The patient reacted the way any healthy young man would react, and be terribly embarrassed while Purdy (muttering unkind things about Dorothy) tried to finish the job."[92] NS Carter related an incident at No. 1 CGH, where the matron and a number of nurses petitioned for the removal of a colonel who "made passes" at them. Carter also claimed to have known lesbian nurses in units where she worked.

But class, in the form of their status as officers, intersected with gender, constructing nursing sisters as sexually unavailable to the enlisted men. NS Fletcher described one such experience in a letter to her family. During a quiet night shift, she dressed in an "evening dress" for the benefit of the duty sergeant, explaining the scenario this way: "[The sergeant] was rather homesick & longing for a feminine female instead of one with a Sam Brown belt & a couple of pips – so he asked me if I would please get dressed up in it & just show him what a Canadian girl looked like in a Canadian evening dress. By that time it was 3:30 A.M. & nobody [was] very sick, so I sent him into the kitchen, & climbed into the whole thing, shoes & all. His only remark was, 'This is the first time that I have ever wished I was an Officer.'"[93]

Numerous accounts reflected on nurses' difficult position as single women living and working closely with married men, who were the majority of military medical officers. The war lasted for six years, and many of these women had enlisted during their prime marriageable years. Some felt too old to marry once the war ended, or left relations with married men behind them on return to civilian lives. Others lost significant relationships through death during the war and were unable to acknowledge or grieve their losses for a variety of reasons. Matron Macham explained that, in the case of her male friends, "When they returned home, most of them returned home to wives and families where they had been from (whom they'd been away from), in some cases quite a number of years, and so you lost those friendships."[94] NS Margaret Fletcher decided that she was too old to marry, adding, "I shall miss all my Army friends very much, & no doubt be most awfully lonely when they all go back to their wives. But it has been fun borrowing them from time to time. We have had a lot of fun & no one has been burned."[95]

The military nurse role was not always easy to perform. Nursing sisters had to simultaneously prove themselves to be as tough and hardy as the boys, as responsible and authoritarian as the officers, and as feminine and sociable as civilian "girls." But above all, they had to perform the role of respectable ladies. Rank and uniforms symbolized these expectations in a highly visible manner, constantly reminding nurses how to behave. The military learned over time to deal with the logistics of having nursing sisters in the ranks, turning the occasional blind eye to indiscretions and lapses in discipline. For their part, nurses accepted the gender- and class-based constraints of military life as the price to pay for the opportunities, income, status, and visibility they gained during the war.

The armed forces accepted nurses primarily because medical technology legitimated their presence in this military-medical-technological system. Their daily work consisted of salvaging men as key human resources to achieve military objectives, rehabilitating them for civilian life if salvage was impossible, or providing as much comfort as possible to them as they died. Despite their nursing experience, they had never encountered such massive numbers of traumatic casualties, such extensive wounds and burns, or the rapid pace of triage and evacuation that would come to characterize military nursing work during the Second World War.

Legitimating Military Nursing Work

To date, most accounts of nursing sisters have been inadequate and even contradictory. Most Canadian military histories depict Second World War nursing sisters primarily as "morale builders," and contemporary media accounts played down military nurses' work by portraying them largely as tea drinkers, shoppers, tourists, and brides.[1] Military medical accounts, although paying scant attention to nursing sisters overall, have attributed a reduction in morbidity and mortality rates to the availability of more nurses and better frontline nursing care during the war.[2] This chapter examines the received knowledge from the perspective of nursing sisters, for whom war was legitimate nursing work.

As the Canadian armed forces divisions became more actively involved in the war after June 1943, there was a correspondingly larger number of Canadian casualties. The respective medical branches made changes in the delivery of medical and nursing services in response to the volume of casualties and the types of care required by soldiers. They reorganized the number and size of hospital units, increased the mobility of specialized units while locating them closer to the frontlines, and experimented with the nature of the work as well as who could perform it.

Nurses were situated in a medical "no man's land" where tactical planning for military campaigns included the advanced positioning, staffing and equipping of medical units, where treatment decisions became military strategies, and where the "top secret" classification of medical developments gave allied forces advantages over their enemies. Medical and nursing services, through such close association with military objectives, took on a stronger national identity and less of a neutral position – threatening their claims to non-combatant status. Many nursing sisters referred to their participation in the war in terms of patriotism, with pride and acceptance of the militarization of care as both productive and normal. But there were, and still are, nursing sisters who questioned their participation in this process.

Nursing sisters enjoyed an elite professional status among nurses during the war, based partially on their closeness to the frontlines of combat and the frontiers of medical technology. As NS Margaret Allemang said, "If you'd been to the front, you were special."[3] They capitalized on opportunities to build further technological expertise and to become essential to the military-medical-technological system, but, as we will see, the postwar civilian profession was either unable or unwilling to accommodate this newly acquired expertise. For the most part, nursing sisters welcomed expanded roles and responsibilities as a way to legitimate their presence in the military, although it is unclear if these opportunities actually let nurses "out of the cage" of gendered civilian nursing practice, or merely "moved the cage," replicating civilian dynamics among the same physicians and nurses who had staffed civilian hospitals and then enlisted with the military medical services.[4]

Nevertheless, opportunities for expanded roles were contingent on geographical setting, the availability of medical officers and medical orderlies, and the social construction of new medical technologies as either women's or men's work. There was more flexibility and autonomy closer to the frontlines (and further from civilian practice in Canada), where patient acuity was higher, where there was less competition from other skilled personnel, and where risk taking was more accepted. Frontline nurses reshaped medical technologies as shared practices by integrating nursing perspectives into the use of these technologies, and when there were no technological solutions they relied on their own expertise to care for soldiers. When their skills and expertise were no longer required by the military, a small number of nursing sisters returned to civilian practice but the vast majority did not. Nonetheless, they influenced the workforce by their absence, as hospitals and healthcare agencies had to seek alternative ways to meet increased demand for nurses during a period of nursing shortages.

As a military-medical-technological system, the medical services were similar to other large technological systems with multiple actors and diverse interests at stake. It included a wide array of individuals, organizations, political entities, universities and research laboratories, regulating policies, and regulatory bodies, as well as industries that stretched across the Allied countries.[5] Donald Avery comes close to calling military medicine a military-medical-industrial complex in his analysis of Canadian science during the Second World War, but he stops short of using this term, acknowledging that medical science constitutes a gap within his research.[6] The lines distinguishing civilian and military applications of technology are neither clear nor absolute.[7] Decisions regarding medical research, the use of medical technologies, and the delivery of medical care during the Second World War were contingent on complex negotiations among various actors, within unequal power relationships and large societal systems.

Medical research and technology were important adjuncts to the concept of "total war" – the mobilization of all aspects of civilian society towards the international war effort – assuring the public that soldiers had access to the latest and best in medical therapeutics as well as expert medical personnel. In actor network terminology, nursing sisters were "enrolled" by the armed forces as an essential part of medical care for soldiers, and as agents of the state to "win the war." They, in turn, "enrolled" the military and the state to achieve their own objectives as nurses and women. The Canadian nursing profession participated both directly and indirectly in the war. The Canadian Nurses Association (CNA), for example, played a significant role from the very beginning through the publication of *Canadian Nurse* articles in support of the war, calls for civilian nurses to stretch both human and non-human resources during the war, investments of CNA funds in war bonds, and "a gift to the Government of Canada" in the form of funding to equip three mobile field surgical units (consisting of operating tables, instruments, and sterilizers).[8] In addition, nursing sisters mobilized their professional skills for the war effort, allowing the use of increased medical technology ever closer to the frontlines and legitimating their presence within the male military domain of war.

Nursing in the Context of Medical Technology

Two major debates dominate the literature on the social history of technology. One frames technology as an impetus for either stability or change, while the other frames technology as either a liberating or oppressing force. Historians of technology, medicine, and nursing have typically framed the Second World War as a "watershed" or critical period of medical-technological innovation, followed by a proliferation of medical technology linked to increased postwar prosperity, hospital insurance plans, rapid expansion in the number and size of hospitals, and rapid population growth after the war.[9] Military medical histories have, for the most part, followed this lead, focusing on specific artifacts or innovations associated with the Second World War such as penicillin, sulphonamides, anti-malarial drugs, and sodium pentothal; saline, glucose, blood and plasma infusions; gas gangrene and typhoid inoculations; splints, surgical techniques, and plaster of Paris casts; triage and the chain of evacuation, to name but some.[10] Few accounts have considered these technologies from the perspectives of social history or history of technology.[11] We know little about the transfer of medical technology to nurses during this period, how technologies may have shaped their roles and responsibilities, how nurses negotiated changes to their work, or what differences these changes made to soldiers or the military overall.

Nurses engaged with medical technology in historically specific ways. Prior to the 1880s, for example, medical and nursing technologies consisted primarily of domestic artifacts, botanical remedies, and treatments commonly available and familiar to lay people and professionals alike.[12] With the rise of Western medical science between the 1880s and the Second World War, nurses sought professional status based on claims as a scientific discipline with a specialized body of knowledge that differentiated trained nurses from untrained caregivers. Leaders in the nursing field emphasized the scientific principles of antisepsis and asepsis in relation to sterile procedures, surgical techniques, and patient-care environments. They taught scientific skills of precise measurement, such as taking temperatures, measuring fluid intake and output, and calculating medication doses. And they began to systematize nursing procedures under the rubric of scientific management.[13] Nursing sisters parlayed these scientific skills and knowledge into coveted work as military nurses.

Thus nursing sisters were already familiar with a good deal of medical technology. As students and then as graduate nurses, they had used a variety of implements, mastered hundreds of procedures, and adapted patients' environments for the prevention of illness and the pursuit of healing or of a peaceful death.[14] Graduate nurses such as NS Edna Rossiter, for example, had "poured" or "delivered" chloroform by mask for obstetrical deliveries at the Royal Jubilee Hospital in Victoria in the 1930s – all the while hoping the physician might arrive in time for the birth. She described her use of various types of plasters, stupes, fever sponges, as well as the application of heat, cold, and chemicals – work made "much more physically strenuous without antibiotics."[15]

The Canadian Hospital Council became concerned about increasing technology in hospitals during the 1930s, passing a resolution to delegate certain roles to specially trained graduate nurses based on "the shortage of interns and the increased use in modern medicine of various clinical procedures."[16] In response, the CNA decided to survey clinical procedures that nurses were already performing in 130 hospitals across Canada, publishing the results along with the questionnaire and descriptive data in 1941 as the "Report of the Committee on Nursing and Nurse Education in Canadian Hospitals." It provides a good snapshot of the state of Canadian civilian nursing technological skills at the beginning of the war. The survey asked hospitals to indicate which of ten listed procedures nurses were doing at their hospital, what level of qualification nurses required to perform the skill, and how nursing personnel coped with any additional workload. The report presented the data according to hospital size and whether or not the hospital had interns available. Findings indicated that most general duty nurses did not typically perform the ten technological skills included in this survey, and student nurses never carried out these procedures. Hospitals that did delegate such responsibilities to graduate nurses usually required them to acquire extra training beyond their basic programs. And the decision to delegate was contingent mostly on a perceived intern shortage or no intern program. According to the report, larger hospitals did not typically assign these duties to nurses, medium-sized hospitals relied increasingly on nurses with special preparation, and the smallest hospitals (those without interns) were grateful for any available graduate nurse who would agree to perform them.

When the Canadian Hospital Council and CNA met jointly to consider the survey results, nursing leaders protested the shifting of these new responsibilities to nurses without increased staffing. In addition to perceiving these extra responsibilities as a workload issue, they argued that these procedures and technological skills were medical acts and as such they were beyond nurses' scope of practice, raising concerns over legal accountability and hospitals' liability. The CNA stopped short of refusing the delegation of such technological procedures to nurses and instead restricted delegation to nurses who were "carefully selected and trained," and to hospitals without adequate intern service – which was 90 percent of those surveyed.[17] Although the Canadian Hospital Council and CNA eventually reached agreement, the Canadian Medical Association subsequently refused to endorse the recommendation. And since hospital administrative boards were dominated by physicians, hospital policies governing nursing practice were slow to change.

Many contemporary sources claimed that the Second World War imposed an unacceptable burden of medical technology on civilian nurses and hospitals; however, as the CNA survey shows, delegation was already a contested issue before the war. The war did shape where, when, and how medical technologies were introduced in support of military objectives, but it did not instigate radical changes from earlier nursing practice. Most of the surveyed technologies became part of standard military nursing practice during the war: blood pressures; intravenous infusions, including blood and blood products; intramuscular injections; taking blood samples; changing ordinary (as well as not-so-ordinary) dressings; serving as first surgical assists; and more.[18] Nursing sisters used these opportunities to develop further skills and expertise while becoming essential to the military medical system.

One aspect of my demographic analysis of the 1,052 military nurses in this study included their training and education prior to enlistment. They graduated from 183 different hospital training schools and four baccalaureate nursing programs (for a total of 187 schools), with the largest number of nurses from the Montreal General Hospital (6 percent), the Toronto General Hospital (5.5 percent), and the Royal Victoria Hospital at Montreal (5.1 percent). Five hospitals graduated 1.9 to 3.4 percent of the nurses each, while the remainder (70.4 percent) graduated from 179 hospitals, of which twelve were hospital training schools in the United States and one in England. Clearly, no single hospital supplied any large proportion of military nurses. Neither did nurses come primarily from large teaching hospitals. Indeed, at least 69 hospitals had only one nursing sister representing their training program. Nursing sisters represented a broad cross-section of Canadian nurse training programs, and it is reasonable to assume that their procedural skills were similar to those surveyed by CNA at the end of the 1930s.

Becoming Essential to the System

Military nursing during the initial stages of the war closely resembled civilian nursing practice except for the preponderance of young male healthy patients. Like their civilian counterparts, nursing sisters prepared patients and equipment for procedures, assisted physicians and surgeons during procedures, and cleaned up after procedures.[19] They assisted with large-scale immunization projects, sick room (or infirmary) services in response to a high incidence of communicable diseases such as mumps and diphtheria, and the pre-operative/post-operative care of patients undergoing remedial surgeries like the repair of hernias or dental extractions. These activities maximized the number of available volunteer soldiers and delayed or minimized the need for conscription. The nursing sisters gradually moved overseas to England, where they waited for assignment to field units in active theatres of war. There were relatively few changes to practice during this phase: traditional roles and relationships shifted from civilian to military settings without substantial changes.

Circumstances of war brought graduates from a large number of Canadian nursing schools together in units of mixed personnel, breaking down traditional rivalries between schools and facilitating identity as a national nursing service. Several large urban training programs, and their graduates, claimed superiority of training over other schools. Graduates of these schools dominated recruitment during the first year, much as they had during the First World War. But Fanny Munroe admonished readers of the *Canadian Nurse,* "It must be recognized that there is no one best way of doing things; that no one hospital is better than all others; that no one school is superior; that no city or province can claim superiority over another. Thinking nationally and not locally will bring a willingness to admit that new ways can be good."[20]

NS Pauline Cox was posted to one of the first integrated units to go overseas. According to her, nurses used the trip to England to get to know one another professionally as well as socially. NS Joan Doree and Ruth Littlejohn served on the *Lady Nelson* as part of a unit selected purposefully to represent as many provinces as possible. They were selected in pairs with preference given to "self-reliant, good nurses ... [who had] a good friend to go along because of the close quarters" onboard ship.[21] Littlejohn recalled that the first voyage was a training run where they had to rethink all of the procedures, adapting not only to one another but also to the conditions onboard a ship – minimal space and equipment, perpetual and unpredictable movement, and swinging berths, and so on. Blended units provided nurses with opportunities to share procedures, techniques, and knowledge from their diverse training backgrounds. They frequently recalled learning from one another, especially from Saskatchewan nurses, who were known as "Depression-trained" and famously innovative. Younger and more novice than most in her unit, NS Harriett Sloan said, "I was a reinforcement. That unit had been in England

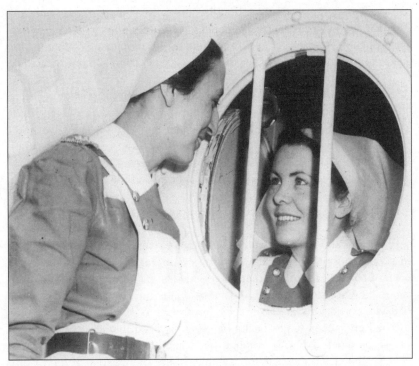

RCAMC NS Elizabeth Bateman and NS Yolanda Carr were two of the nurses selected to serve aboard the *Lady Nelson* hospital ship, where relationships between personnel had to endure the strains of living in such close quarters. *College and Association of Registered Nurses of Alberta Museum and Archives, Mary Macleod Collection*

a long time where they had lots of time to look after accidents and things – experience I hadn't had. But they were wonderful teachers. I thought I knew everything about nursing when I finished [school] and I found these ladies from Saskatchewan, who had worked for 'peanuts' and maybe board and room, could they nurse! I learned more from those nurses than I ever learned, I think."[22]

In addition to forming mixed units, the RCAMC implemented a policy of nurse exchanges in 1943, partially in response to nurses' requests for postings to active theatres and partially to ensure a more experienced workforce as younger nurses enlisted in preparation for major offensive campaigns. NS Elizabeth Pense alluded to the dual purposes of these exchanges, saying, "We were moved around for experience ... for the experience you could bring in, and the experience you could take out."[23] The policy had less positive results when personnel exchanges disrupted cohesive teams, however. For example, NS Margaret Fletcher complained in a letter home that the army had "gone nuts" because recent exchanges reduced the overall level of competency within her unit.[24]

Most nurses reported an unusual level of mutual support and teamwork compared to previous civilian experiences. With time and experience, a critical mass of competent and confident military nurses developed, facilitating the delegation of medical technologies to them. NS Pauline Lamont remarked:

> We suddenly became self-confident. We knew that people relied on us, trusted us, and that brings out the best in everybody. We also weren't too afraid to try new methods and new techniques, and we had to improvise a lot. And we weren't … supervised so minutely as civilian nursing … I hadn't seen any of [these wounds] before: shrapnel, abdominal wounds, terrible tank burns, amputations. You know, chest, all kinds of injuries … I did dressings and things I had never seen before … We were given trust. We were given responsibility. And we knew we could do it. And when we came back, we knew we had done it.[25]

Physicians and surgeons were accustomed to working with student nurses in civilian hospitals, where there was a constant flow of novice learners giving bedside care. They therefore gained a greater appreciation within the military medical units as to what graduate nurses knew and did at the bedside, particularly at the smaller forward units and on specialty teams focused on specific types of injuries such as head injuries, chest injuries, burns, or shock. NS Eva Wannop noticed a big difference at the plastic surgery unit at Basingstoke, for example, where she was one of four or five nurses working closely with a physician, anaesthetist, and a dentist. She felt that she was given more responsibility and autonomy:

> I do know that there was a lot that you catered to the doctor in civilian life but there was none of that there … They used to come around once a day and check everything, and if there were any questions or that. And then you carried on. And if you were concerned about something, you knew you could always call them but they gave you a lot of responsibility … You see we were such a small unit that Colonel Gordon used to, once a week you know, we would gather together and have talks … He was very helpful – but we were such a small unit.[26]

United by a common goal to "win the war," military medical units challenged traditional divisions of labour found in civilian practice. Nursing sisters frequently referred to the camaraderie and trust experienced among the staff. Small units in forward areas located near or in battle zones afforded many opportunities to teach and delegate new skills while developing associated knowledge for monitoring and providing supportive care in relation to the skills. Meanwhile, mass casualties provided a large volume of patients in need of similar procedures, allowing learners to consolidate newly acquired skills. NS Nicolson reflected on the acquisition of new skills:

When we were in the Army, you really ... had to think right on the spot [how] to do things. And you certainly did do things that you ... just never did in training, or in the hospital situation ... And you never hesitated. You just did [them]. You improvised lots of times ... Something had to be done so you did it, in other words. Regardless. And even if you weren't just sure, you did it anyway, to the best of your ability ... There were so many other people relying on you too, you know. So military nurses were a little different I think.[27]

But expanded roles and responsibilities were contingent on geography. When nursing sisters from forward units returned to England or Canada, for example, previous constraints were reimposed. NS Lois Bayly proceeded to carry out medical orders as she was accustomed to doing in her casualty clearing station (CCS) in Europe, saying "I just did it automatically because I had been [used to] doing it ... starting the intravenous and the Wangensteen."[28] She was warned that, while in England, it would be necessary to wait for a physician to do these procedures.

Younger nurses, enlisting near the end of the war, perceived fewer differences between civilian and military nursing practice. There were several reasons for this. They were seldom posted overseas or to frontline units because senior nurses had priority for these postings. When novice nurses did arrive overseas, matrons placed them at larger base hospitals and in more central ward areas where experienced military nurses could support and supervise them. These nurses were also less likely to experience collegiality or camaraderie with medical officers as older nursing sisters had. There was a significant age gap between the reinforcements and the original nurses, who had been older on enlistment and had already served four to six years.[29] Age and experience differentiated the two cohorts socially and professionally.

In addition, younger nursing sisters perceived less change between civilian and military nursing practice because training schools had already begun to modify curricula based on wartime experiences.[30] Nursing programs took advantage of federal funding to develop courses such as "Developments in the Field of Medicine, Given Emphasis in War Time" and "Some Aspects of Nursing Care in War Time," offered at the School of Nursing of the University of Toronto in 1943 and 1944 respectively.[31] Nursing textbooks reflected revised content related to war and changing medical technologies. For example, the J.B. Lippincott Company described their books as having "many new and important wartime additions," including material on sulpha drugs, poison gases, shock, and immunization, while the Macmillan Company of Canada promoted revised nursing textbooks as relevant to "wartime and post-war time needs."[32]

In addition to geographical setting, the gendered nature of work influenced who did what in the medical services. Work was typically perceived as women's work once it became standardized and simple enough, when it required meticulous attention to detail or fine hand work, or when it required a large labour force. The military medical services added yet another contingency to decisions about nurses' work – the availability of medical officers and orderlies. Nurses could replace physicians in many roles whenever these medical officers were needed in surgery or at regimental aid posts, or when the medical technologies became labour intensive and/or inconvenient to perform. Nurses could also replace orderlies when the latter were reclassified for combat duty. NS Lily Clegg served with No. 2 CCS, where, as she said, "During a big battle the nurses just went from one patient to another ... We finally had to give blood transfusions because we didn't see the surgeons at that point so we had to learn right then and there to put up and handle and change our own intravenous."[33] NS Constance Bond described how nurses learned from each other as necessary:

> When the doctors were really busy in France, we had to start intravenouses, but we hadn't had that training. But two of the nurses had been in England for a year before ... and they were taught there because the British nurses could start intravenouses and so they taught us ... Because when the doctors were in the operating room all the time, you just had to start them [IVs]. And often it would be plasma. I don't know that we ever gave blood. I think that was done in the operating room. It would be started [there] anyway.[34]

In gender-bending role reversals, military nurses shifted some of their more traditional domestic roles to the medical orderlies/assistants while retaining key technological roles as nurses' work. Orderlies did a "remarkably efficient" job under the guidance of nursing sisters, relieving them of many routine tasks such as bathing, feeding, and transporting patients so that the nurses could focus on medications, dressings, skilled assessments, and "morale." But orderlies could not replace nurses, as personal anecdotes and mortality statistics soon showed.[35]

Blood transfusions and the administration of penicillin provide two good examples in which socially constructed roles were transferred from physicians to military nurses, legitimating the nurses' work on and near the frontlines and making them essential to the larger technological system in the process. Both technologies are widely acclaimed for reducing mortality rates and salvaging soldiers for further action on the frontlines. Both involved elaborate technological systems that required international collaboration, huge scientific and monetary investments, and social acceptance as essential components of the war effort.[36] Initially, physicians administered and monitored both technological procedures. They experimented with the rate and volume of blood products as well as the formulation, route of administration, and dose of penicillin – along with potential application in various medical conditions. Once scientists and physicians standardized most aspects of the technologies, the military needed a reliable workforce to capitalize on potential benefits from the technologies. A comparison of transfusion and penicillin illustrates similarities and differences regarding military nursing practice changes.

Allied forces used a very limited amount of whole blood experimentally during the First World War, transfusing it by syringe directly from a donor to a recipient. Transfusion science and the use of blood in the treatment of shock evolved during the interwar period, although coagulation issues and blood compatibility constrained its use in civilian settings. During the Spanish Civil War (1936-39), Norman Bethune demonstrated that whole blood could be collected, stored, and transported for later use.[37] Then, during the early 1940s, Dr. Charles Best and the Connaught Laboratories of the University of Toronto in a collaboration between the National Research Council and the Canadian Red Cross, conducted extensive research on the production of dried plasma from whole blood, enabling its transport overseas, where the Allied forces began to use it in massive quantities. Dried plasma could be reconstituted and given without prior typing or matching, simplifying administration and reducing compatibility risks.[38]

With the rise in casualties and reorganization of the medical services (1942-43), surgical care and transfusion moved forward from CCSs to the frontlines in an attempt to reduce death rates resulting from shock and infection. The military used medical orderlies, trained to assume nursing roles on these forward surgical teams, until it became clear that nurses made a significant contribution that lesser-trained personnel could not equal. Field transfusion units operated as small mobile teams attached temporarily to regimental aid posts, advanced surgical centres, field dressing stations, or CCSs as needed. Specially designed metal containers that carried the plasma and all essential equipment for its administration resolved many of the technical difficulties. As NS Sloan pointed out, nurses considered this self-contained unit as much a miracle as the transfusion itself because they didn't have to clean it: "There was a whole service devoted to blood transfusion and they brought all the 'giving' equipment (and the [plasma]). And we just had to hang it up and give it. What was wonderful – we didn't even have to clean any of it afterwards (the tubing or anything). We just threw it back in the packing cases that the new blood came in. It was marvellous." The development of this special container reduced the procedure to a relatively simple task of inserting a needle into a vein, making it easy to administer transfusions even at regimental aid posts.[39]

Surgical centres and CCSs soon added whole "resuscitation wards" to their units, typically a room or tented space located next to operating rooms, X-ray machines, and laboratory and dispensary areas. NS Teresa Woolsey described her resuscitation ward as a small area "drip[ping] with bottles and tubes" and equipped with whole blood, plasma, oxygen, Wangensteen drainage, suction machines, and minor surgical trays.[40] According to NS Helen

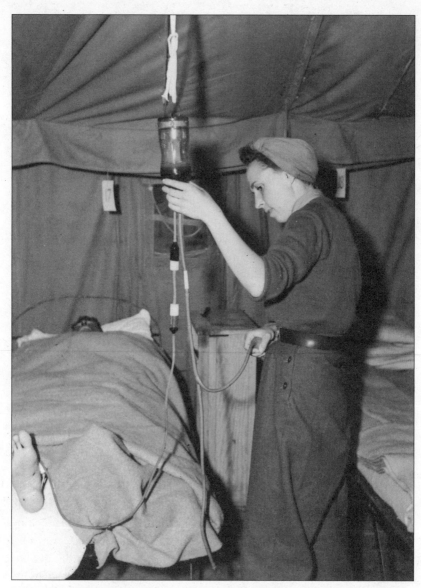

RCAMC NS B. Rankin administered blood transfusions to many wounded soldiers, such as this one at Montreuil, France, on 10 September 1944. Like other resuscitation units, she hung the bottle of blood on a rope from the top of the tent. *LAC/Lieutenant Frank L. Dubervill/DND fonds/PA-128234*

Bright, "the first and foremost thought and duty was to keep all tubes and bottles working."[41] As the use of blood and plasma increased during the war, resuscitation wards reached capacity sizes, and transfusions became routine nursing procedures, no longer limited to specialized nurses or areas of care.

One medical report noted that all patients requiring abdominal surgeries or amputations or who had compound fractures of the femur (thigh) got routine transfusions preoperatively – such cases typically represented about 80 percent of patients treated by the forward units. Each case received an average of five or six bottles (550 cc per bottle).[42] NS Fletcher, writing home from No. 6 CGH in September 1944, described her work as "just keeping an eye" on transfusions:

> It is most interesting here at this field hospital. We get cases straight from the advanced dressing stations. The bad ones only are kept here, and the rest sent on to a Base Hospital like 16. They all come to my recussitation [sic] ward from Admitting – & from there they clear through our O.R. or a Field Surgical unit that is attached to us … At the moment we are using good Eng. blood on our friends the enemy – but they are just as sick as our boys, & pretty glad to get taken care of. One is due for surgery P.D.Q. & I'm just keeping an eye on his transfusion while I write.

A month later, at No. 2 CCS, Fletcher was getting the "boys" ready for surgery during a particularly busy period and wrote: "Well, resuss started to boom & little Margie was on the run. They all get Penicillin, anti gas, anti Tetanus & transfusion routinely."[43]

At times, nurses embodied the technology, becoming a physical part of it. NS Frances Ferguson described the use of rubber bulbs as hand pumps to infuse blood at a rapid rate, and nurses as blood donors:

> We also gave intravenouses and blood transfusions … It was almost a case of pumping it in sometimes … with a bulb. This just made it go a little faster but there we were, using blood and trying to discover if we were over transfusing … You know, it had to be ordered properly. But it was a matter of saving a life. And we did it in a hurry, too. But I don't think I ever remember us having any bad reactions. Maybe we were fortunate … Anybody who knew they were 'universal' [blood type], was vulnerable [as a donor]. I was universal but I never gave blood. I wanted to, I had offered to, but I never did … But we all knew our blood type anyway, so I don't think they took time to cross match. As long as you were universal, you felt fairly safe giving it.[44]

The value of whole blood transfusions in the treatment of shock from blood loss was well known, but during the Second World War, plasma gained recognition for its osmotic properties and ability to reverse shock in burn patients as well.[45] NS Wannop worked extensively with burn patients for almost five years during the war. She recalled treating them with plasma and intravenous fluids, doing their blood work, monitoring the results, and charting fluid balances as nurses moved beyond tasks such as inserting needles into veins and infusing blood products, to building assessment and monitoring skills, interpreting changes in patients' conditions, and making decisions regarding their care. According to her, "That was one of the first things after we treated them for shock, we'd do the blood work ... Then we'd go from there. And the doctors were so busy that they would, you know, leave it to us when to start the Penicillin ... and oh, we'd take cultures when they'd first come in, just to see, you know, what the organisms were. And then, when they'd get them ready for operations, they'd leave it to us to tell them when they were ready for the operation."

Penicillin, like transfusion, emerged from the war as another life-saving miracle but one portrayed as a "weapon of war" used to "kill" wound infections as well as a military "top secret" that gave Allied advantage by reducing deaths from infections and salvaging manpower for combat.[46] Penicillin was not available before the war, and it required considerable research before Allied military medical units conducted clinical trials with it during the invasion of Sicily (October 1943). However, nurses did have experience with sulphonamides: another promising group of drugs that included prontosil, neoprontosil, and sulfanilamide, in use since the mid-1930s to treat infections.[47] Medical knowledge remained limited regarding the therapeutic ranges of these drugs, and they were known to have substantial toxic side effects that required careful techniques and monitoring such as those NS Wannop illustrated through her description of putting powdered sulfanilamide directly onto burns:

> You see, everything was new and experimental, and we didn't know what the saturation dose was for the sulfanilamide, so we would have to watch very closely ... You dusted [the wound] with the sulfanilamide and then you would put what they called a "tulle gras" on. Tulle gras was vaseline on a little net gauze. And we'd put [a gauze soaked with saline] on top ... And you'd change the saline gauze, not the tulle gras, but you changed the saline solutions. I think it was twice a day anyway ... practically all their body ... The orderlies didn't [do dressings]. They would help in the bath but not for the dressings. We did the dressings.

The sulphonamides – along with salvarsan for treating syphilis and atebrin for preventing malaria – represented a conceptual shift in thinking about "chemotherapy" (in this case, referring to the use of pharmaco-therapeutics in infections) that ultimately led to the new penicillin family of drugs.[48]

The story of penicillin is fascinating and multi-faceted. Governments, universities, and commercial interests collaborated in an intensive effort to produce sufficient quantities of the drug, waiving patent rights until the end of the war. The military had top priority for access to the drug, with civilians next and prisoners of war last. It has been referred to as "a technical triumph wherein scientists were heroes, doctors were holy men, and the 'man' who controlled its distribution was a god."[49] From Alexander Fleming's discovery in 1929 to Howard Florey's demonstration of its use in 1935 and large-scale clinical trials in 1943, penicillin was carefully guarded and controlled. Not until March 1945 were there sufficient quantities for both Canadian military and civilian needs. Germany attempted to develop the drug with little success during 1942-43 while Japan initiated a research program based on translated medical publications in February 1944, followed by limited production at the beginning of 1945.[50]

Penicillin produced dramatic effects. After NS Fletcher attended lectures on penicillin given by Professor Florey himself in London, England, she wrote, "We had never heard of penicillin ... We had our lecture and he showed us pictures; we simply could not imagine that he was telling us the truth. He showed us pictures of what they had been doing in the Mediterranean and it was absolutely astounding. So time and a half went by and we were allocated a little bit of penicillin for our worst cases."[51]

Military rates of wound infections and venereal diseases (VD) accelerated the development of penicillin – based on the likelihood of rapid recovery in these two patient populations and the significance of that recovery for the war effort. The first recorded use of penicillin by an RCAMC unit in a forward area was on 11 January 1944 at No. 2 Field Surgical Unit in Italy, where its use was initially restricted to cases of gas gangrene. VD was responsible for great numbers of medical admissions, and it required extensive treatment over a three- to four-week period, resulting in the loss of valuable human resources during this time. Left untreated, syphilis had devastating long-term results for military pension funds, as well as for society. During the Liri Valley campaign in Italy in June 1944, the shortage of troops due to a high incidence of VD was so severe that it justified the expense of penicillin because of their return to active duty within a matter of days. Thus, VD patients were quickly given priority for the drug. One army sapper (engineer) recalled the amazement of his unit when a member returned to duty after only three days of VD treatment with penicillin instead of spending the usual month in hospital.[52]

Penicillin was clearly experimental regarding the dose, form of administration, and indications for use. Physicians injected it directly into wounds, chest cavities, joints, veins, and muscles; they "dusted" it directly into wounds with a device called an insufflator; they experimented with giving it orally and rectally.[53] NS Helen Mussallem, an operating room supervisor in England, described physicians and nurses as learning about penicillin together, admitting:

> We didn't know enough about it and when we injected it into the men, they used to say, "Oh, please, I'd rather do without it." So we had this one badly wounded leg and we scrubbed it so well – the debridement [removal of infected, damaged tissues] was fairly successful. So we just poured the penicillin into it ... It was supposed to be injected but it was very painful. Those brave young

men could hardly take it. And I am not sure whether it was, I guess it was, good penicillin then or not. You see, we never knew. That was the trouble with that situation – you never knew what happened [afterwards] ... As I say, we misused it by pouring it into wounds. And I don't know whether that was good or not. We thought it was a good idea ... We didn't know a lot about penicillin then. It wasn't the same quality of course, as later. Impure penicillin.[54] .

During its early use, penicillin commanded particular attention and care. A special Canadian Penicillin Team introduced the drug to medical units in Italy, and a fact sheet about the drug included this caveat: "If penicillin should fall into your hands and you do not know how to use it do not 'play about with it.' It is extremely difficult to produce and supplies are inadequate."[55] Because the drug was perceived as scarce and valuable, some medical units decided not to give it to prisoners of war, but some nurses described giving it anyway – surreptitiously.[56] Some units even considered various ways to recover unused penicillin excreted through the urine, according to NS Tritt: "When it was first brought in, it was used very sparingly because there wasn't enough to go around ... We had to save the patient's urine because there was some thought of reclaiming the penicillin."

Once clinical trials established standard formulations, dosages, and intramuscular injection as the most effective method of administering penicillin, the drug had to be given every three hours, day and night, to maintain a therapeutic blood level. That's when penicillin became nurses' responsibility: "Regulations demanded it must be given by a qualified surgeon by injection and every three hours, day and night. It proved a major task ... as the surgeons just would not respond to calls after they were asleep and who could blame them!"[57] The medical units employed various strategies to deal with the increased workload resulting from these injections. Matron Evelyn Pepper, for example, added extra nurses to her CCS staff in Italy because of the workload. So that doses weren't missed during evacuations, yellow tags tied to the outside of soldiers' uniforms identified those who needed injections en route.[58] As NS Lamont said,

I just remember being aware that this was some miracle drug. We made it up in our own pharmacy. It was sort of grey colour ... And then quite often, we'd take a 10cc syringe because [time] was tight when you have 20 beds on each side, all wounded ... So you'd just go down the row. They all knew what was coming ... I think most of the patients, 90 percent all got penicillin. But on the other hand, I don't think everybody would have it because it wasn't that plentiful yet ... When the convoys came in, each man had on his tag, a description of his wound, if he had been given morphine, etc., if he had had penicillin ... I remember that we had to keep track of the penicillin (as much as we did morphine, practically) because it was so precious.

Nurses assigned to give penicillin for an entire shift earned titles like "Penicillin Queen" or "Penicillin Mary" from patients, who sometimes wrote poems about them. These nurses frequently described using one large syringe (10 or 20 cc size) to give 1-2 cc doses to multiple patients – with or without changing needles, based on a perception that penicillin was "self-sterilizing." Those who changed needles found it challenging to resterilize needles between patients when equipment and time was limited and water for sterilization was often scarce. Nurses barely completed one round of injections before it was time to begin the next round. Orderlies assisted by sterilizing needles and waking the men prior to the injection so they would not "come up fighting" from a deep sleep. Thus, military nurses became very knowledgeable about the administration of penicillin and, as NS Margaret Kellough reported, sometimes taught civilian physicians after the war.[59]

Blood transfusion and penicillin became part of nursing practice based on frequency of use and the need for a skilled labour force with a constant presence at the bedside. Military nurses enabled the use of these technologies, extending them to the frontlines and demonstrating their ability to expand practice roles. But the transfer of such skills to nurses also required a social reconstruction of this work as appropriate for women to perform.

Technology as "Dirty Work" and "Women's Work"

The sociological term "women's work" refers to work associated with the body, manual dexterity, repetition, and a need for meticulous attention to detail. In their research, Jocalyn Lawler and Margarete Sandelowski extend the concepts of women's work and body work to traditional hospital divisions of labour, referring to work performed *on* patients' bodies and *with* nurses' bodies as the primary tools. The term has links to "dirty work," or work that may be "designated dirty" due to inconvenience, relative invisibility (and therefore low status), or unsatisfying characteristics as repetitive, exhausting, routinized, stressful, or physically dirty. Most often these terms carry derogatory connotations, problematizing nurses' work by its association with physical care of the human body.[60]

From these perspectives, military nursing constituted body work and dirty work, based on the centrality of soldiers' bodies and physical care. Nursing sisters cared for mangled and burnt bodies with multiple wounds, missing limbs and other body parts, and exposed lungs and intestines; faces without features or lower jaws; whole wards of colostomy patients; and much more. In addition to such trauma, these bodies were just as likely to be filthy and lousy. Conditions were only slightly better farther back from the line, where patients arrived with foul-smelling casts and wounds filled with maggots after ten to thirty days of the Trueta method, which intentionally left wounds enclosed, without exposure for cleaning over extended periods. It is difficult to imagine work more stressful than forty-eight to seventy-two hours on duty in wards or operating theatres during a major battle, or working under enemy fire. It is hard to imagine work more repetitive or routinized than the assembly-line care necessary to admit and evacuate 1,200 casualties, all within twenty-four hours.[61] Although the interviewed nursing sisters agreed regarding the awfulness of war-torn bodies and wastage of youth, they clearly had different perspectives from sociologists about body or dirty work. They never described their work in derogatory or demeaning terms; they were doing what they had enlisted to do, and working where they wanted to be working. Two examples of such tedious, repetitive work included caring for malaria patients and dressing various types of wounds.

Malaria was a major cause of morbidity in the Mediterranean theatre in spite protective clothing, mosquito repellents and nets, and liberal use of DDT and prophylactic drugs such as mepacrine. In Sicily during the month of August 1943, for example, there were 1,184 actual or suspected cases. Diagnostic laboratories were unable to keep up with demands for diagnosis, calling it "an epidemic of serious proportions."[62] Diagnosis through microscopic examination of patients' blood was critical for treatment decisions, as not all fevers were caused by malaria, not all mosquitoes carried the particular causative agent, and not all forms of malaria were treated in the same manner. NS Doris Carter describes nurses' diagnostic and treatment roles in her memoir. She points out the importance of accurate diagnosis for both the immediate treatment with medication and the long-term implications to soldiers:

> We did blood smears to find the special microparasite that causes the disease, which is left in the body from bites by the anopheles mosquito ... A drop of blood was taken from a patient's finger, put between glass slides, and placed under a microscope. This was done when the patient's temperature was high – 103 degrees or more – and during a chill caused by the activity of the parasite. We had to be accurate with the tests; if the diagnosis was positive, the patient was put on medication specific for malaria. Besides, such a diagnosis could also affect the patient's future medial coverage and pension, when he returned to Canada.[63]

When interviewed, Carter described the process as labour intensive and unpredictable work that also required nurses to make decisions regarding the test and the outcomes: "We'd have one microscope, and we'd have about four little glass slides, and we were always taking a little drop of blood ... Then when we found [the organism], we had standing orders to give them medication ... They'd have to be in the throws of a chill. And if you can't find it in one chill ... then you'd have to wait until the next chill."[64]

The dressing of wounds consumed another major portion of nurses' time regardless of the theatre of war. The hospital survey of 1940-41 indicated that ordinary dressings were not necessarily a standard component of civilian nursing roles. Graduate nurses did dressings in only four of the six largest hospitals while only a limited number of nurses with extra training did dressings in 42 percent of the middle-sized hospitals and 62 percent of the small-sized hospitals. The popular nursing textbooks written by Bertha Harmer corroborate nurses' prewar roles with wound dressings as primarily those of assisting the physician, preparing the patient and the equipment, and cleaning up following the procedure. According to the 1939 edition, physicians prescribed the nature of the dressing for the wound and applied it while the nurse helped "provide the conditions that prevent discomfort and infection and promote healing." The nurse, however, had complete charge of the dressing carriage that contained the equipment.[65]

Most nursing sisters had completed additional courses after their basic training, particularly in operating room technique, that prepared them well for added responsibilities related to dressings, assessment of the healing process, and identification of infections. But no amount of prior experience prepared them for the number, complexity, or type of wounds encountered during war. NS Margaret Roe called them "more invasive wounds, exploding wounds, inside [of which] there would still be shrapnel,"[66] and NS Lamont described the difference as follows:

> It was just a totally different feeling, and they were all so wounded. A lot of civilian nursing is medical and long term. These were all terrible wounds that we had never seen in civilian nursing. So we did different dressings and different things that we would have never had to do in civilian nursing ... Shrapnel, abdominal wounds, terrible tank burns, amputations ... chests ... The MO [medical officer] would write the first order and then after that you used your common sense. You would just decide the thing to do or maybe they should have some more morphine or something. You sort of judged the condition and passed that on to the MO. And they were very good about taking your word.

The primary purpose of dressings shifted from one of limiting blood loss in the field to one of preventing infection and accelerating healing along the evacuation routes – while also shifting the level of knowledge and expertise required to perform dressing changes and treat the underlying wounds. Battle injuries typically required initial field dressings to be applied immediately, without cleaning the site, in order to staunch excessive blood loss. These initial dressings were followed by numerous reapplications during the evacuation process, which may or may not have included cleaning and/or surgical debridement with the dressing changes. Surgical and burn patients required extensive surgical dressings after remedial and/or reconstructive procedures. The vast majority of military surgical procedures involved serial operations on wounds in which repairs were done in gradual stages based either on need or time. Only essential work was done at each stage, as soldiers moved further back the chain of evacuation towards base general hospitals in England. Rather than suturing wounds shut while in the field and risking the formation of gas gangrene as well as other infections during transport, the medical units adopted Trueta's method of excision, drainage, and immobilization of open wounds within plaster casts. This method was used so widely that the Second World War became known popularly among the medical staff as the "Plaster War."[67] NS Cox was an operating room nurse in a field surgical unit in Sicily and the Italian mainland, where she described this process debriding wounds:

> We had two doctors, one surgeon, and one anaesthetist, and another nurse – two nurses with myself. And we had a couple of the boys with us. And the place we were in was a hotel ... The big lobby area was the recovery area (where they would prepare people for operations) and they would have these various rooms on either side ... Wounds were not being cleaned up quickly enough after injury. And they figured that they would improve (and certainly survive a lot better) if this was done more quickly ... so, we did a lot of debriding ... And they were in bad shape, an awful lot of maggots and ooze, and that sort of thing ... And or course, they leave some of the maggots in, because naturally, they were going to clean [the wound] and put it in a cast. So we were putting casts on, too. And then they would go back into that recovery area. Then somebody else would come in ... And everything [information and instructions] was written on the cast. And "maggots" was written in big letters. So that wherever they went, the first hospital they went to, that they would know ... We didn't attempt to clean it up completely. No, I mean we cleaned the wound but we'd leave some maggots there.

Abdominal wounds were another major type of injury that presented particular challenges for nursing sisters. At Falaise (France), in Belgium, and in the Liri Valley, there were whole wards of postoperative colostomy patients with abdominal injuries that required extensive surgical repair. These patients remained in a CCS for ten to twelve days to stabilize them prior to evacuation back to base hospitals for a long recovery. NS Mary Bray's ward was "full of the sickest people I have ever seen ... They'd be five days on intravenous and stomach lavages and then all we had to feed them was stew which they couldn't have ... It was very confusing if you looked down one of these wards with all those bottles hanging and to be sure what bottle was what."[68] NS Barbara Ross recalled that "I had a whole row of colostomies (the belly wounds) which had to be dressed frequently ... and after we'd done our stint, we'd go out and walk up and down the beach to get the smell out of the nose because it was so bad."[69] NS Fletcher questioned the long-term implications of such extensive technological interventions: "There is the lad from the Seaforths who got a bullet through the intestine and bladder. He has both a colostomy & suprapubic drainage. The third lad got a bullet in the groin, & now has osteomyelitis of the pelvic girdle, & lower spine. A cable telling of a loss would be much preferable to either of these." Several months later, Fletcher reported that one FSU did fifty-seven colostomies in the first one hundred cases.[70]

Abdominal surgery had other complications. Medical Officer W.R. Feasby pointed out that surgeons in the forward units quickly learned that resuscitation and surgery "were frequently of no avail if not followed by adequate post-operative care and nursing." He cited the notes of two surgeons who worked in the forward surgical units, in which they are explicit that orderlies "do a grand job but the patients seem to do better both practically and psychologically when sisters were there." When Feasby listed the twelve essential technologies required for successful abdominal surgeries, he included professional nursing care in the list along with morphine, oxygen, gastric suction, sulphadiazine, and penicillin – the nurse again became an embodied technology. His description of "nests of abdominal cases" in the Liri Valley, where patients "lay in reasonably comfortable beds, gastric suction tubes in place, intravenous fluids running, and carefully tended by skilled orderlies with one or two nursing sisters in each centre of 12 to 20 beds" obscures the nature of the embedded nursing care involved with gastric suction.[71]

Continuous gastric suction was also known as Wangensteen Suction, and it employed a closed system of glass bottles and tubing based on a principle that water flowing from one level to a lower level could be used to produce a partial vacuum and thereby drain the stomach or duodenal area following surgery to permit healing and prevent postoperative distension. Patients were connected to the system, consisting of a metal pole, two large glass bottles, various tubing, connectors, and clamps, by way of a nasogastric tube, and the entire system had to be maintained airtight – no simple task during wartime evacuations.[72] Although gastric suction had been used in civilian hospitals, nurses had to adapt the equipment to wartime conditions by improvising basic components. As NS Sloan said, "They had gastric suctions that they made up themselves with tubing that they had. You know – any old tubing and a stomach tube, and using intravenous bottles, and hanging them from the tents. And they had another bottle down beside the bed and they improvised all their gastric suctions because they didn't have gastric suctions."

Although military nurses were well prepared in terms of civilian nursing skills and experience, they were relatively unprepared for wartime working conditions, which contrasted with the ideal conditions described in textbooks, classrooms, and hospital procedure manuals. One nurse wrote to her alumnae association that "all our ideas of good nursing technique shattered completely. Every drop of water is as precious as gold, and has to be carried."[73] As NS Cole said, "You didn't fuss with a lot of things that we had been trained to do (the way you did it in civilian practice)." NS LaBonté agreed: "There was so very little in the way of technique. You did what you could with what you had. And it wasn't always the right thing but it produced often the same result." Matron Grace Paterson put it more positively: "In the Army we found out that we could do things just as well and a lot more quickly. The rituals we thought had to be followed weren't necessarily giving better nursing care."[74]

Nurses not only improvised techniques and equipment, but they also had to deal with dust, dirt, bombs, and flies, among other challenges. NS Kellough recalled the challenge of maintaining a sterile field in the operating room: "I can remember one day we were operating ... on stretchers and this bomb fell outside the window and the dust flew and the surgeons just calmly covered the incision with a towel and carried the stretcher to another room and carried on with their surgery." At No. 1 Field Dressing Station, NS Patricia Moll said, "We didn't remove the clothes ... Their tag would say what was wrong with them and we would operate on the parts. We would cut the uniform open and off then we would [send] them back to the follow up tents."[75] NS Cox describes the "filthy" conditions of rain and mud in Italy. Similarly, NS Roe, who was with No. 4 CGH receiving casualties from the Normandy invasion at Aldershot, remembers: "They were just full of the dust and the dirt and everything else on them ... First, I liked to get them a little bit cleaned up, as well as you could. You worked on them in stages, and then drawing blood and stuff ... They were very grateful to get cleaned up and freshened up. They went through a lot of hell for a few days." NS Pense had to recruit recovering patients to help her with dressings in North Africa, where flies swarmed over the wounds at No. 15 CGH, the base hospital for the Sicily invasion. She commented on the difficulties of admitting a thousand casualties from Cassino, who "just poured in":

> With the heat, the condition of their wounds when they got back, it was the first time I ever saw maggots. And the flies! When I was doing dressings, I used to get the patient with the strongest stomach to stand by with a fly swatter to shoo the flies away. And none of them could stand it for more than about ten minutes and I'd get somebody to take over the system ... I know in my own ward I was doing dressings on a ninety-six bed ward ... At the time of Cassino, I went on duty at eight in the morning, stopped for lunch and for dinner, and worked until ten o'clock at night doing dressings.

When it was not possible to resterilize instruments in makeshift autoclaves, nurses used "cold sterilization" (a method of soaking equipment in disinfecting solutions) between operations. Instead of individual sterile instrument sets for each surgery, as was the practice within civilian hospitals, they used a common instrument table for several surgeries taking place in the same tent. As NS Van Scoyoc described it, "We would have them on a table – all

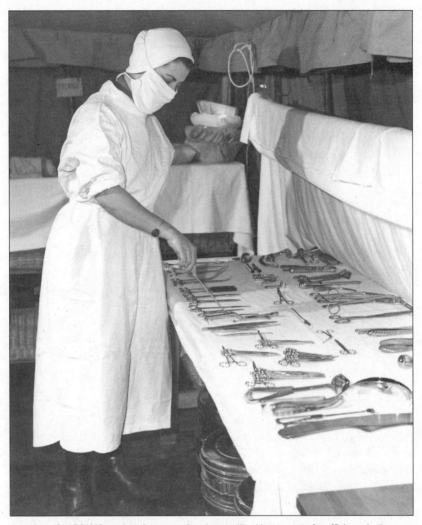

An unidentified RCAMC nursing sister organizes her sterilized instruments for efficiency in the operating room of No. 6 CCS in England, October 1943, anticipating the changes that might be required once the unit became mobile. *LAC/DND fonds/PA-213781*

different types of instruments would be on a table because we were so short. And the doctor would just take the one he wanted, or he'd ask you for the one he wanted. And so, that way you didn't have a set up [a tray] for a certain operation."[76]

Still another aspect of military nursing required a change in thinking for the nursing sisters – decisions about priority for resources and treatment among the sick and wounded soldiers. The origins of medical triage have been attributed to the Napoleonic Wars, when field surgeons sorted and treated the most seriously injured casualties first. Thus, grouping patients for attention was not a new concept, but the criteria used and the resulting decisions shifted during the Second World War. Triage determined not only the priority for immediate care but where that care would take place, and how much care would be given prior to the next level of evacuation. Those who were most seriously injured did not necessarily receive top priority. In situations where human and non-human resources had to be stretched and used efficiently for the greatest number of casualties, decisions were based on which casualties could reasonably expect to recover and return to combat within a reasonable time period. This approach differed from civilian practice, where the sickest patients and those who could most afford medical treatment typically received the most expert and time-consuming care.[77] As NS Roe explained,

> When triage came into being ... it was hard to grasp that at first. Then you could see the necessity in wartime for it ... There would be some terribly injured people but they wouldn't go to the top of your list; the doctors decided this because they needed people to fight – bodies, to put it in terms like that. And those that were recoverable – get them going. Get them up and going, and prepared. The ones in gradation – there is no use in spending all your time on the top few. I'm not saying you don't spend your time, but don't concentrate on them first. But you are going to give just as much care as you possible can. It's the logical approach in the military. People couldn't get that through their heads at first, you know.

Casualties arrived at each medical unit along the chain of evacuation with field medical cards attached to their uniforms, indicating their triage category and what procedure(s) were to be done next.[78] But as NS Nicolson said, "The very serious went right to hospital ships ... And we got the ones that we could do something for, and look after, and [could] send back [to the front]." Of the different types of units in the chain, CCSs had more resources than the forward mobile units, and patients could remain in a CCS for slightly longer recovery periods. The exceptions to this order of priority were those cases requiring immediate life-saving surgery or transfusions in order to survive evacuation back to rear units where more extensive repairs could be performed. Casualties in the lowest priority category (without reasonable hope of recovery) were not abandoned. As NS Sloan explained, "Everybody wanted everybody to get better or to at least be comfortable before they died ... It was a simple palliative care but that was one of the things that was important ... They were separated out in the triage tent." Some nurses reported giving morphine to the most seriously injured, hoping they would sleep through the evacuation process to their destination.

Casualties did not have a formal medical record until they reached a CCS or CGH. Key information was added to the field medical card or even written on their bodies in a manner that was highly visible and quickly accessible. NS Roe explained that, "on the stretcher cases, if they had been given morphine, it [the letter M] was in red on the forehead and also on the paper with the time [given]. And then, we had any information stuffed inside this envelope and a survival package." In a similar manner, the letter T on a forehead indicated there was a tourniquet in place, and it would need to be assessed frequently.[79] Plaster casts also made good communication devices, because they were not likely to be lost in transit. When the details of the injury were recorded on the plaster, the technology became known popularly as a "plasto-gram."[80] Ultimately, triage was a utilitarian strategy to selectively salvage men for quicker return to the frontlines. It also resulted in work "speed up" and fragmentation of care as casualties received only the essential care at each stage of evacuation, explaining how a hospital unit could admit and discharge a thousand or more patients within a 24-48 hour period.

Triage and rapid evacuation was inconsistent with nurses' prior training and experience. While they understood the rationale, they also sought, where possible, to mediate the effects of triage for individual soldiers. Nurses had been taught to treat patients individually and comprehensively in civilian practice, where they typically remained with their patients throughout the whole course of an illness or surgery – getting to know them and their families well, and seeing the results of their care. In the military, casualties arrived en masse, and the chain of evacuation called for rapid assessment, treatment, and evacuation. In addition, as CCS surgical NS Clegg explained, "We weren't able to make friends with them, because nobody was conscious most of the time we had them." NS Van Scoyoc recalled:

> You would just see the patient and then they would go ... We had six tables when I was in Bruges ... When the patients came in, one of the most skilful medical doctors would prioritize them. And you know, they had the field card, and it had [the procedure] on the card ... So we had nothing to worry about that. We just went from one table to the next table – the next patient, I should say ... Because you know, when we had a lot of casualties, we never even had a chance to clean up the floor! Until there was a lull, and then you'd do it. So you know there wasn't great technique. And that's why penicillin was so important.

Many of the interviewed nurses spoke about these differences in care, and what it meant not to have follow-up or closure with their patients. They were uncomfortable with assembly-line techniques, although they recognized the utility for managing mass casualties. As NS Cox said, "it was just a matter of operating and this is it. So it is not a very satisfying type of experience." NS Sloan described her ward of casualties in Holland, called the "walking wounded," this way:

Now these people came in, in droves, in ambulances and it meant that they were not so badly hurt that they couldn't move around. So when they came in, all we did for these people ... they just filed in and lay down. And essentially what you had to do in this sort of situation was check their dressings to see if they needed reinforcement, check their medical evacuation cards to see that they had the appropriate anti-gas gangrene shots ... We checked to see if they needed another penicillin shot before they left ... So that knowing a patient as an individual was almost impractical; they were coming and going so quickly ... There were so many. Those sorts of things were very hard ... You wouldn't know them. And they wouldn't remember where they were ... There weren't any signs that said, "This is No. 8 Canadian General Hospital." They never knew where they'd been.

But once the rush ended, as NS Lamont recalls, "You know, you wouldn't bother to straighten the castors or clean the bedside tables ... You had your priorities. And when the time was there, you made them comfortable – chat and have fun ... They wanted to talk. The boys wanted to talk."

Many nursing sisters achieved a new level of confidence with a variety of medical technologies, as they rose to the challenge of expanded roles. They learned to innovate, improvise, and adapt in different settings. According to one medical unit's war diary, "Except for a few difficult cases requiring assistance by an M.O., sisters were starting all blood, plasma, and saline infusions, taking blood pressures, and giving all serum and penicillin injections."[81] According to NS Lamont, "I think because these responsibilities were thrust on us, you learned how to improvise, make good judgments, and make do with what we had ... We suddenly became self-confident."

Reshaping Medical Technologies

Nursing sisters used their abilities to easily assume new roles associated with medical technologies to legitimate their presence in the armed forces. In the process, they partially reshaped these technologies. Even relatively straightforward medical therapeutics such as the administration of drugs required additional nursing surveillance and attention to prevent negative side effects. For example, NS Dorothy Surgenor pointed out the importance of fluids and monitoring the intake of patients taking sulfa drugs when she said, "the sulfathiazole drug was first initiated and that caused a lot of joy. But we had to drink, and drink, and drink because as I guess as people know today, sulfa was a terrific drug but it affected the kidneys and made crystals in the kidneys."[82] The provision of adequate fluids for individual patients was only one challenge, as thousands of casualties could be admitted and evacuated within a twenty-four-hour period, and water supplies could be uncertain due to enemy sabotage as well as mobility issues. Just giving tablets of sulfathiazole to a casualty with a tracheotomy tube required a great deal of skill, monitoring, and time, as NS Sloan explained:

A lot of them had tracheotomies, of course, so that was very heavy work. In contrast to civilian hospitals, who might have one tracheotomy or two tracheotomies in six months, we would have maybe six or seven on a ward ... You had to be fast and very observant ... The back of the tongue would flip back and cut off their windpipe (their trachea). You had to flip them over fast and give them oxygen and you just had to be on your toes all the time ... I think the exceptional cases were the ones that we had with the maxillo-facial teams (and very, very challenging). They were on sulfa too, most of them, and it takes an awful long time to grind up one sulfathiazole tablet in water and then put sips on the end of a spoon and hope they would be able to swallow – because of face wounds and tongue wounds, jaws shot away. Talk about challenging. Very, very challenging. That sort of thing. Or trying to get some food into them. Long, long time.[83]

In reality, most medical care involved the sharing of technologies among multiple personnel. Historians of nursing history have argued that civilian nurses shared equipment with both non-nursing women and physicians, noting that nurses did not typically have technologies reserved exclusively for their use.[84] In a similar manner, military nurses shared medical technologies with both physicians and orderlies. At times, nurses became the mediators or buffers between the technology and patients – interpreting and adapting procedures for individuals while assuring compliance to medical treatment regimes. In addition to the shared practices previously identified, two other situations in which nurses made substantial contributions to shared medical technologies were the care of burn patients and the care of psychiatric patients.

Prior to the war, nurses' experiences with burns in civilian populations were relatively limited. Hospitals rarely handled large numbers of burn victims, and students received minimal training in their care. But in the army, incendiary bombs and tanks produced horrific burns to large proportions of the body. In the air force, men who survived air crashes typically sustained major burns. And in the navy, destroyed ships spread fuel and flames across the surface of the water, burning any who survived the direct hit. The burns encountered during the Second World War challenged medical and nursing care both in immediate treatment and long-term recovery, provided the patient survived during the initial period, especially prior to antibiotics and extensive use of plasma and intravenous fluids in burn cases.

Although the medical treatment of burns changed greatly during the war, a major portion of treatment depended on basic nursing care for wounds, nutrition, comfort measures, and pain management in addition to the psychological support required for months and years of rehabilitation. Two excellent and detailed accounts of burn treatments appeared in the *Canadian Nurse* during 1943 – one written by NS Dorothy Macham while serving overseas and the other by two Montreal General Hospital civilian nurses, who

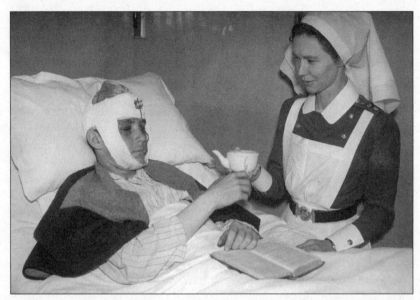

RCAMC NS Dorothy A. Macham based her published description of the care for burn patients on her many experiences with patients such as Harry Lord at No. 1 Neurological and Plastic Surgery Hospital in May 1943, while it was still located at Park Prewett, England. *Courtesy Eva Wannop*

emphasized that "the treatment of burns has always been in large measure a nursing problem."[85] Tannic acid sprays and dressings constituted the most common treatment for burns at the beginning of the war, but that changed rapidly as emulsions of sulfa drugs (and later, penicillin) became available.

Nurses had major roles and responsibilities in the care of these patients. The formation of specialized units and mobile teams to treat burns facilitated early standardization of treatment, which included morphine for analgesia; fluids, blood, and plasma for resuscitation; saline compresses and baths; surgical cleaning and debridement of dead tissue under anaesthesia; tulle gras dressings; skin grafting to cover large areas and to reconstruct missing body parts such as eyelids, ears, and noses; and close monitoring of blood work for haemoglobin, plasma protein, and blood urea nitrogen levels. During the invasion of northwestern Europe, so many patients had burns of both hands, and became totally dependent on nurses or orderlies to replace their fluid losses, that stomach tubes were used to supply a slow but continuous source of drinking water for them.[86] NS Wannop recalled the need to monitor blood work and to observe the patient carefully for signs of drug toxicity in relation to the sulfa medications.

Two main centres were established especially for the treatment of Canadian burn casualties – where the military clustered these patients together with specialized medical and nursing staff. They were the RCAMC wards

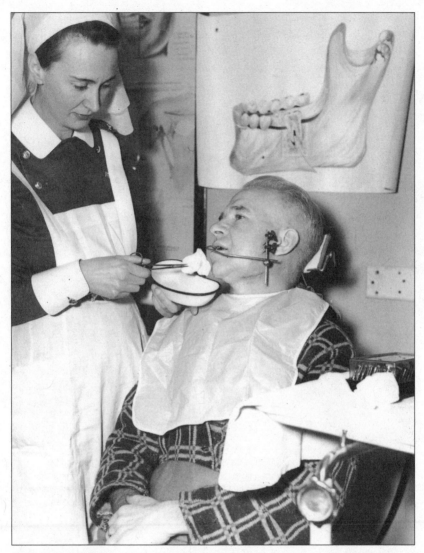

An unidentified RCAMC nursing sister provides wound and mouth care for a patient undergoing reconstructive jaw repair at No. 15 CGH unit, posted to North Africa during 1943. *LAC/DND fonds/PA-213778*

at No. 1 Neurological and Plastic Surgery Hospital at Basingstoke, and the RCAF Canadian wing at East Grinstead's Queen Victoria Hospital.

Basingstoke had two burn units with forty beds each, and nurses were responsible for all the dressings. NS Doree found that "the stench of forty severely burned people lying in two long rows in a Nissan [hut] hit like a blow every morning." Basingstoke never seemed to have enough staff, equipment,

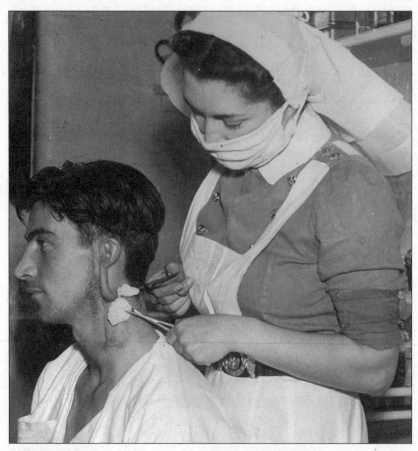

An RCAMC nursing sister at No. 1 CGH in Basingstoke, England, performs the delicate task of dressing a pedicle graft: the result of a surgical technique that uses live tissue from a nearby healthy body part to re-create body parts that have been destroyed by trauma. The new graft was left attached at the point of origin until the grafted tissue re-established a viable blood supply at the transplanted site. Skilled care was the key to preventing infection and promoting healing of the newly reconstructed part. *Courtesy Eva Wannop*

or supplies. Doree recalled, "Most of our patients received intravenous injections of four-times concentrated plasma to counteract the colossal loss of body fluid through their burns. This dried, life-saving plasma ... came in bottles to which we added 100cc's of fluid instead of the usual 400cc's. Then, as the bottle had to be shaken vigorously for some time to dissolve the plasma, it was not uncommon to see a nurse shaking the bottle with one hand and carrying out another procedure with the other hand."[87]

The East Grinstead wing began as a small unit within a British hospital. But as burn casualties increased, a special Canadian wing for fifty patients was built, opening in July 1944. It became well known for novel approaches to burn treatment, both psychologically and physically. The emphasis was on restoring normality by integrating patients into local community activities (particularly the pub life), relaxing discipline on the medical wards (with regular clothes and beer permitted), and including patients in decisions regarding reconstructive surgeries. Patients had the opportunity to go into operating rooms and watch surgical procedures prior to consenting for their own surgeries, especially for innovative grafts such as reconstructive pedicle grafts. As an anonymous author noted, "Much work was done in repairing and rebuilding distorted hands and faces, but fully as important was the restoration of personal morale and self-assurance which, almost inevitably, were burned away simultaneously with the normal features ... It required both the most highly specialized surgical skill and psychological ability."[88]

RCAF nurses became an embodiment of burn treatment technology at East Grinstead, becoming therapeutic measures themselves. Rita Donovan, in her account of the East Grinstead unit, claimed that chief plastic surgeon Dr. Archibald McIndoe "recruited the best-looking nurses he could find" for the unit: "Not only were they able to alleviate discomfort, but their female presence, their interest and concern in a patient, validated his ego and assisted his recovery ... Their role was clearly larger than that of medical support for they were also to assist in rebuilding the confidence of these damaged men."[89] NS Fran Oakes was responsible for organizing the original burn unit, and she recalled being "detailed" to accompany her patients to the local pubs after working twelve hours, in addition to walking the four miles to work and back to their billets: "This is the only place I ever knew ... where there was beer kept [on the ward]. And Mr. McIndoe would say, 'Go and get yourself a drink now ... Get down to the pub tonight. Get the girls to take you to the pub. And don't be sitting thinking to yourself. There's people worse off than you.'"[90]

But not all burn patients received treatment in these specialty units, at least not for their initial care. NS Ferguson was with No. 6 CCS near Caen, France, where "the burn cases and the tank injuries that came out of there were horrendous." There, burn care became highly routinized:

> They were sedated [with morphine] and then the clothing and the horrible burned skin would peel off them like a banana ... You couldn't touch them until you could sedate them. They were in shock. And then you could handle them quickly because we had to be able to remove their clothing and remove the burn as much as we could. And clean them up and put some sterile dressings and towels, and some clothes on them, and then get them over to Britain. That was our aim. We filled about six stretchers and as soon as the stretchers were ready (we had our landing strip near the hospital or near the casualty clearing station), they filled [the rest of the plane] up with walking-wounded, and they were over in Britain in just a few hours ... But the teamwork was excellent. You

could almost go ahead and do the job – boy, after boy, after boy without talking very much. You knew the routine. You knew what was going on. As long as they were labelled properly and you entered all the information about the sedation and everything onto the cards, why, they were cleaned up and ready to go.

At the HMCS *Niobe* in Scotland, one of NS Amy White's patients had third degree burns to his arms, thighs, perineum, face, and back. She wrote to her father, who was a physician, explaining that she thought he would be interested in the new ways of treating burns and describing two different methods used on this patient as an experiment: one arm and hand were treated with a sulfa emulsion dressing inside of a plaster cast while the other was enclosed in a plastic bag device filled with oxygen and irrigated with hydrogen peroxide three times a day. In addition, "the rest of him is done up in sulpha [sic] emulsion & elastoplast. He had four bottles of blood plasma."[91] NS Surgenor served at the HMCS *Stadacona* in Halifax, where burn patients were debrided in surgery and wrapped with penicillin emulsion and "cotton waste" as "one of the first improvements for burns that I can remember."

NS Wannop spent most of her military service at Basingstoke, working with burn patients, and developed such expertise that the RCAMC avoided posting her elsewhere. She was particularly articulate regarding her practice there, describing many aspects of patient care and the relative autonomy she experienced:

> When the big push would come on and patients would be brought in, you were pretty much on your own. But by this time, you knew pretty well what to do. We would start the intravenouses and that. We'd get them ready and put them in the saline bath and that was routine ... And if they were too sick to go in the bath, then we would treat them in their bed ... We would lower them in the bathtub of the normal saline. And when they were in that, then we would clean off all the dead debris underneath the water because it was easier for them. Cause most of these were about three-quarter burns, and then lift them out on a sterile sheet and then "dress" them [i.e., apply sterile dressings].

NS Wannop also talked about treating her patients for shock and pain, doing their blood tests, and monitoring the results as well as participating in decisions regarding patient readiness for surgical grafting.

Despite the innovations, medical technology had its limits. NS Roe recalled being on night duty in a surgical ward and making rounds with her flashlight when she noticed a burn patient with "these little 'rings of fire' around his eyes. He was all bandaged up to the face ... I called the medical officer, but there was not much he could do. But I kept [the dressings] moist [with boracic acid solution]. Pretty well all I could do ... I think I got his address to write to his mother after he was gone."

NS Wannop also described the need for psychological support for these burn casualties, as young as sixteen to twenty years old, whose lives had been "ruined." As she recalled, "They'd come in and talk to you about it, and I guess the talking would be part of the treatment too ... besides physical treatment ... They had a hard time and they needed a lot of nurturing." Some patients were "very bad physically and mentally," some were very angry, and others "swore like a trooper." Although official records deny any suicides among burn patients, NS Wannop, who maintained contact with some of her patients after the war, knew of several men who "ended their lives."

In addition to the psychological component of caring for burn patients, nursing sisters were also an essential part of the treatment for soldiers who developed psychiatric symptoms, especially on the frontlines. During the First World War, the term "shell shock" came to represent "a variety of conditions ranging from cowardice to maniacal insanity" including psychoneurosis, hysteria and neurasthenia. A diagnosis of shell shock risked being associated with or attributed to cowardice, which was perceived as a discipline problem and punishable by execution. As a result, Army regulations required medical officers to report all cases of shell shock and to certify a man's fitness for court martial and punishment, as well as to witness his execution if that were the sentence. Some soldiers with questionable mental status inflicted non-life-threatening wounds upon themselves to avoid combat. The medical services referred to these casualties as SIWs (self-inflicted wounds).[92] Later, the term shell shock fell into disfavour, replaced during the Second World War with "battle exhaustion" or "battle fatigue," which suggested a mild and recoverable condition and avoided the stigma of a psychiatric diagnosis. Soldiers with mental disorders were subsequently treated more as medical patients than as disciplinary problems. Labels might change, but consequences were still serious. Although the men didn't face execution, an SIW could result in a sentence of two to five years' hard labour and loss of postwar benefits – the latter a strong deterrent, especially so soon after the poverty and uncertainty of the Great Depression.[93]

As it had been during the First World War, psychiatry continued to be a contested field, as different practitioners sought professional recognition and the field began to emerge as a distinct medical specialty. On one side, key medical men from McGill and the University of Toronto who saw themselves as "neuropsychiatrists" were instrumental in the establishment of a psychiatric branch within the RCAMC by 1941. On the other side, psychologists, through the Canadian Psychological Association, argued for a greater emphasis on intelligence testing, personnel selection, and screening of recruits for mental stability prior to enlistment rather than relying on active treatment of disorders identified after enlistment.[94] Psychologists argued that screening was more cost effective, eliminating men from the military who might subsequently become eligible for pensions based on mental disabilities. During the early phase of the war, when recruitment was still relatively easy, the prevailing policy was to discharge problematic personnel rather than treat them within the military or initiate extensive screening processes during recruitment.

As the war continued, however, the number of soldiers discharged as medically unfit for psychiatric reasons due to this policy created a substantial manpower problem that increasingly worried the Department of Pensions and National Health, which was indeed responsible for their rehabilitation to civilian society as well as their pensions.[95] One postwar publication on the principal lessons learned during the war claimed that psychiatric disabilities accounted for approximately 30 percent of all medical discharges, and that less than 25 percent of those diagnosed with psychiatric problems and retained in the military had been rehabilitated to the point where they became "useful forward area soldiers."[96]

In comparison to wartime medicine and surgery, however, "the advances made by psychiatry during the war were not spectacular." The main RCAMC psychiatric unit was located at Basingstoke as part of the No. 1 Neurological Hospital, in addition to the burn units there. NS Doree wrote that the word "psychiatric" had been intentionally omitted from the hospital name to avoid stigma, but soldiers popularly referred to it as "No. 1 Nuts" anyway.[97] Initially, twelve nurses from the Montreal Neurological Institute and eight nurses from the Toronto General Hospital staffed the unit. Little treatment was available until 1943, other than electric shock and the creation of a special ward for psychotic patients.[98] But the movement of troops to the Mediterranean theatre, an impending invasion of northwestern Europe, and a full-blown conscription crisis at home lent mounting importance to the treatment of psychiatric disorders as efforts to salvage manpower.[99] When the Canadian forces landed in Sicily in July 1943, they were the first Canadian field formation to go into battle with a psychiatrist on strength. As well, No. 15 CGH in North Africa attached a base psychiatric centre for the evacuation of casualties from Sicily and mainland Italy. This unit increased in size to 200 beds prior to moving to Caserta, Italy, at the end of 1943. Over a twenty-one-month period (July 1943-April 1945), it treated 2,326 in-patients and 989 out-patients, with 22.7 percent returning to active duty, 62.8 percent medically boarded (i.e., examined) and reallocated to special work units, and 14.5 percent evacuated back to England.[100] NS Verna White, a graduate of the joint training program at the Provincial Mental Hospital of Ponoka (Alberta) and Calgary General Hospital, served with psychiatric units in Italy, where she recalled caring for patients receiving "deep sleep" treatments with sodium amytal sedation.[101] NS Marjorie MacLean, who also nursed in an Italian psychiatric unit, described narcosis therapy as follows:

> The doctor would say, "Wake him up for meals. He doesn't have to get out of bed. He doesn't have to do a thing." Because, well, some of the walk-in patients on

another ward – they would be given little jobs. And these weren't given any jobs at all. We were just told to let them sleep but wake them up for meals. Make them have meals. And after a week of this, [the doctor] would say, "Now come down to my office whenever you feel like it." And by the end of the week, they probably would. And then he would talk with them and keep them for another day or so, and then they'd go back to the lines. Well, the Americans couldn't get over this. They had never tried this. If somebody refuses to go ahead in the line, they're apt to be shot or something. I mean they did that in a lot of armies.[102]

The RCAMC created special work units (known as Pioneer Companies) to stretch manpower resources by using for heavy labour men who were illiterate or who had low mental abilities, thus releasing other men for active combat duty. In Italy (as Special Employment Companies or SECs), these units also included men with disciplinary problems, stress-related and psychiatric problems, and mild physical disabilities.[103] Three such SEC units absorbed a high proportion of the neuropsychiatric casualties who were unable to return to regular duty, ostensibly as a form of work therapy. Overall, at least 5,020 casualties received treatment for psychiatric disorders during the Mediterranean campaign.[104]

In both Italy and the rest of Europe, the main treatment for battle exhaustion and psychiatric problems consisted "simply of rest with sedation, if necessary; good bath facilities; clean clothing, new equipment, and psychotherapy in the form of explanation and reassurance." It was recognized that "the resolution of many of these cases depend[ed] in large part on Nursing Sisters who have had neuropsychiatric experience."[105] But psychiatric or mental nursing was a relatively new field of study and practice for nurses during the 1930s and 1940s. Between 1912 and the mid-1930s, only a few schools of nursing included several classes on psychiatry in their curricula, accompanied by a very brief period of service in a mental hospital.[106] One psychiatrist bemoaned the lack of student training, characterizing the average experience as a few lectures and "a single Cook's tour through the nearest mental hospital."[107] Two large teaching hospitals, the Montreal General Hospital and the Ottawa Civic Hospital, did not introduce psychiatric nursing into their curricula until the 1950s.[108] Thirty-four percent of the military nurses in my sample graduated in or before 1936 and may or may not have had courses or lectures on the topic because it was not recommended in the CNA curriculum guidelines until that year. Only 1.7 percent reported having had psychiatric or mental nursing experience as a graduate nurse prior to enlisting in the armed forces.

Eight nursing sisters from the main hospital at Basingstoke staffed the No. 1 Canadian Neuropsychiatric Wing that became attached to No. 10 CGH when it moved to Europe after D-Day. Some of the medical technological treatments available in this unit included two to four days of continuous narcosis with the drugs medinal and paraldehyde; induced suggestible states under the drug sodium amytal; psychotherapy; and an occupational therapy program wherein patients produced surgical dressings and cleaned medical equipment under supervision of the matron for No. 10 CGH. This psychiatric unit carried a convulsive therapy machine but, perhaps fortunately for the patients, lacked the electrical power to use it during the invasion.

NS Jean Ciceri recalled being "completely green" on arrival at Basingstoke. Mental nursing was not part of her basic training, but psychiatrists taught nurses about psychoses, neuroses, battle fatigue, and stress as well as treatments such as shock therapy; drug treatment with chloral hydrate, paraldehyde, phenobarbital, nembutal, and seconal; occupational therapy; diversion therapy such as sports, recreation, and gardening; exercise; fresh air; and enhanced diets for rapid weight gain and a sense of improved well-being. According to Ciceri, therapeutic narcosis therapy consisted of six days of sedation, which was supposed to get rid of anxieties. Noting that it didn't often work, she said nurses tried to make the psychiatric unit a "fun" ward, urging patients to join various groups as a form of therapy. It took her a long time to feel that this was nursing "work" because it was so different from the busy skills-oriented, physical work that she had always associated with nursing.[109]

Nurses were often the only treatment available for battle-stressed patients. As NS Anne Farries concluded, sometimes "the best nurses could do for men driven temporarily insane ... was to provide some sense of normalcy."[110] It was military policy to keep battle fatigue patients near the frontlines to discourage malingering rather than to evacuate them away from the action (unless they were severe cases and not expected to recover within nine days). In Sicily, NS Nicolson's battle fatigue patients lay on stretchers outside in the open, during a night assault on nearby Catania: "They could hear the bombs dropping. They could see the flares ... the whole ward would light up with the lights." She made sure her patients could also see and hear *her* throughout the bombardment, making herself visible as a nurse and a woman, to calm them and create a perception of safety: "I just got up and walked back and forth – just so that they could see me ... But that's all I could do at the time ... psychologically. They'd had it really ... and were anxious to get away." In a similar manner, NS Ferguson described SIW casualties with compassion and understanding. The military policy also kept these patients near the frontlines, where nurses such as Ferguson used therapeutic interpersonal skills: "We never called them S.I.W. Somebody else diagnosed them. ... I felt sorry for those fellows. Most times, they liked to bring out pictures of family, and talk about family, and that kind of thing. You had to let them do the talking. You became a good listener."

It is difficult to counterbalance these relatively positive experiences with less positive accounts of stress, anxiety, and psychiatric disorders, given the paucity of sources and the limited number of nurses involved in these units. NS Louise Jamieson provides one such example. She was with the SAMNS when she was posted to No. 84 British General Hospital in Barletta, Italy, in 1943. Jamieson was on night duty with four female civilian psychiatric patients without psychiatrists on staff or psychiatric treatment available to the patients. According to her, nurses focused on preventing patients from hurting themselves, one another, or the staff. She described how one nurse had to sit on a patient suffering from acute hysteria, another patient required constant observation because she "would chew everything in sight" including the handkerchief from your pocket, and a third patient had to be force fed.[111]

Doing "Real Nursing Things"

Nursing care has traditionally involved activities that provide comfort, relieve pain, provide nutrition, and support patients through illness and death. When NS Bayly was asked to describe her work at a CCS in Europe, she explained that, "All I was doing, was trying to make them comfortable: bathing them and doing all the real nursing things." Real nursing often involved invisible work like skilled observation and assessment of changes in a patient's condition, and decisions to use alternative techniques instead of relying on drugs. NS Roe explained that troops carried small, pre-prepared ampoules of morphine packaged with their field dressings that they could self-administer after being wounded and while waiting for stretcher bearers to pick them up. As a nurse, however, she was concerned with making soldiers comfortable without overloading them with narcotics that could mask important diagnostic signs and symptoms or impair respiratory and neurological functions. RCN Matron Rae Fellowes pointed out how important constant nursing vigilance and attention to detail were in restoring circulation to the feet of North Atlantic sailors who survived long periods with wet feet and developed "immersion foot," which could lead to amputation.[112] NS Cole described the importance of human touch for the care of a patient almost completely enclosed in a plaster cast:

> I had gone all around this 45-bed-ward doing the various things that had to be done, trying to get the bed patients comfortable, giving medications, and this sort of thing. And I was just about at the end and I came to this bed where this fellow was encased in a plaster cast from his toes up to his arm pits. And I always tried to say something to them rather that just go ahead and do the treatment or whatever – and ask them what unit they were with, where they had been, where they were from. And so I stopped at this bed and started doing whatever I had to do. He was all in plaster so I was trying to rub [to touch] whatever was available – you know, at the cut out area near the back.

Real nursing also included compassion extended to young single mothers and patients in internment camps. NS Cole decided to break the rules for a woman serving in the Women's Division who had just delivered a baby.

Recognizing the need for closure to a difficult experience, she said: "We weren't supposed to let them see their babies. [The mother] said, 'It's the hardest thing in the world for me to have to give him up ... For his sake, I have to do it.' And I've always remembered her crying while I was bathing the baby [in her presence]."

In the backwaters of Hong Kong, where NS May Waters and Kay Christie served as prisoners of war, nursing encompassed still different challenges.[113] During the eighteen days of fighting that preceded the British surrender, nurses' first concerns were for safety of their patients in the midst of bombing, shelling, and snipers as they moved patients continuously to lower floors and then to bomb shelters wherever possible. When patients could not be moved, nurses placed a folded mattress across the top bar of metal traction frames as protection; they also got under the beds of the sickest patients in order to remain available for assistance during air raids.

After surrender, the Japanese army declared the Bowen Road Military Hospital to be "Prisoner of War Camp A," put barbed wire all around the building and grounds, and patrolled the wards with armed guards. Medical supplies became increasingly scarce, and could not be replaced when they were used up. The nurses' own survival and the survival of their patients depended more and more on basic nursing knowledge and skills related to dietary deficiencies, dysenteries, basic sanitation and cleanliness, and the reuse of gauze bandages. Christie was appalled by the conditions. The nurses stretched dwindling supplies of medications by giving them only once a day, instead of the usual three or four doses per day, until the drugs were gone. They stretched dressing supplies by infrequent changes and by washing the used ones for reapplication. Christie wrote, "Before long we were not only re-using bandages that normally would be discarded, but were washing out and boiling gauze dressings, then re-using them. Ingenuity and the ability to improvise, yet preserve some semblance of surgical technique, became a constant challenge."[114] Although the drainage from wounds leaked through plaster casts and they were "high" – that is, smelled horrible – there was no material with which to make new casts, so they had to be left in place indefinitely.

Two particular examples serve well to illustrate the nature of nursing care, women's work, and medical technology in the Hong Kong POW and internee camps – the cases of Bud Sweet and Telegrapher Quinn. Bud Sweet was, according to NS Christie, a "young kid – freckles across his nose, a lock of hair down over his forehead. He should have been out in the streets playing marbles, not away over there. He looked about 14." Bud had been injured and was a patient at the Bowen Road facility with a compound fracture of the scapula. When the Japanese soldiers attacked the hospital, they bayoneted him as he tried to escape death a second time. He survived by "playing dead," but ultimately his left arm had to amputated. Christie focused on healing both his old and new wounds. Knowing the importance of adequate nutrition for the healing process, she "scrounged" extra food for him. Bud refused to accept the extra rations in the sight of other patients who were also hungry. As Christie wrote, "To give extra nourishment to one particular patient I had to hide him behind an opened cupboard door while he guiltily, but ravenously, ate whatever I had been able to scrounge from any source; however, he still had to be assured that these extras were a form of required medication."[115]

The left leg of eighteen-year-old Telegrapher Quinn had been amputated. He subsequently developed a "horrible pressure sore at the base of his spine" through which "you could get a [gauze] wipe on a forceps, put it in through the pressure sore, [and] bring it out through the amputation site."[116] He required a bed with a Balkan frame from which his leg could be suspended to relieve the pressure, at least two hours of nursing care each morning, and was addicted to morphine. Christie described his care as follows:

I strung him up in a hammock (which I thought was quite appropriate for a Navy boy to be strung up) ... to try and keep his back off the mattress. Oh, it used to take me an hour and a half, two hours, every morning for his basic care and he would scream and swear. I didn't blame the kid, you know, I wasn't too sure how I would act if I were in the same state he was in. But it did bother two young Navy boys – they were called Able-bodied Seamen, which I believe is the lowest form in which the Navy walks. Gray and Ward, (kids again, you know, skinny) and it bothered them the way he would speak to Sisters. And so anyway one morning he'd been particularly abusive, and when I finished with him and I went out to the bunk to get rid of the bath and dressing materials, these two followed after me and they stood very strictly at attention, saluted me and said, "Sister, on behalf of the Royal Navy, we wish to apologize for Quinn." Well, really, I could have cried ... Some weeks after, early one morning, Quinn mercifully died.[117]

Waters and Christie had little medical technology at their disposal, according to conventional understandings, but they relied on nursing knowledge and expertise for the benefit of patients even under extreme adversity. Their ability and opportunities to provide nursing care benefited patients while also providing purpose and meaning for the nurses. It is not surprising, therefore, that NS Christie found it extremely difficult when their Japanese captors removed the nursing sisters from hospital work. She explained: "Well this was bad enough for nurses (not to be able to care for your patients properly) but to leave them without any nurses, well, we thought this was the lowest thing they could do to us."[118]

Military medical technology included a wide variety of equipment, skills, procedures, roles, and knowledge during the Second World War. Nursing practice was contingent on not only the specific technology, where it was used, who was available with the necessary skills and knowledge to perform the roles, and whether the technology was perceived to be men's or women's work, but also what was at stake militarily, professionally, and socially.

"Civvy Street" and the Postwar Legacy

Through expanded technological roles and opportunities, nurses became essential to the military-medical system. But the postwar military nursing quota allowed for only eighty nurses in the permanent forces nursing service, distributed across the three branches. Outside the military, however, there were far more postwar nursing positions than nurses who wanted them. Nursing sisters were under pressure from the postwar profession, but the majority of them avoided "Civvy Street," as they called the civilian practice world. As NS Dorothy Grainger wrote, "civilian nursing had little appeal."[119] NS Tritt further explained that her friends "wanted something different ... They would not have been happy at a civilian hospital – having the doctors try to order them around."

There are two dominant discourses about postwar military nurses and civilian nursing practice. One claims that nurses used their considerable experience as a "leg up" in the profession, assisted by veterans' credits and educational opportunities. Another asserts that military nurses' success with technological changes during the war resulted in substantial postwar changes to hospital nursing practice.[120] With some exceptions, there has been little examination of postwar practice directly related to Canadian nursing sisters.[121] My research clearly indicates that very few military nurses engaged in hospital practice after the war, in spite of a shift from students to graduate nurses as the primary workforce in hospitals, and that the nursing sisters influenced postwar civilian practice mainly by their refusal to resume previous traditional nursing roles, forcing hospitals to consider changes to attract and retain graduate nurses. Public health and community nursing were the primary beneficiaries of the postwar educational opportunities granted to nursing sisters as part of their veterans' benefits.

As the civilian nursing shortage began to emerge during the early 1940s, Canada's nursing leadership became concerned about the pressure to enrol more student nurses and graduate them in less time to meet the short-term need. They expected that many military nurses would return to hospital work after the war and were wary that this might lead to an oversupply of nurses and an unemployment situation reminiscent of the 1930s. Nursing leaders exercised caution, participating in federal postwar planning endeavours while initiating strategies of their own.[122] As the nursing shortage deepened through the war years, the profession looked increasingly to demobilized nursing sisters as the solution. The focus shifted from protection of civilian jobs to recruitment of military nurses. The Registered Nurses Association of Ontario (RNAO), for example, established a Placement Service Advisory Committee, partially to match discharged nursing sisters with existing civilian vacancies. The Canadian Nurses Association (CNA) appointed a Committee on Reconstruction for postwar planning within the profession.[123] This committee surveyed overseas nurses regarding their discharge plans, and the CNA developed brochures to steer returning nurses towards "opportunities" and gaps in the civilian system. But nursing sisters did not necessarily conform to professional, societal, and military agendas designed for them: the vast majority of military nurses in this study left nursing, and those who remained in the profession avoided the resumption of traditional practice roles, preferring jobs in public health, teaching, supervision, or administration.

Several groups of military nurses left the profession immediately upon discharge, according to analysis of my sample. Department of Veterans Affairs (DVA) counsellors indicated on 29 percent of the discharge interview forms that the "nurse" would be "establishing a home for her husband" or "having a family." Included in this group were nurses who married prior to, or during, enlistment; nurses who planned to marry in the immediate future; and unmarried nurses who were pregnant. As one counsellor wrote of a married nurse, she was already "happily rehabilitated" – assuming heterosexual marriage as the ideal state. A second group consisted of nurses who planned to remain connected to the military or to the nursing care of veterans. They accepted positions with one of the armed forces branches (2.0 percent) or with DVA hospitals (12.0 percent). Nurses who planned to work outside the profession constituted a third group (5.1 percent).

Other nurses planned to work as supervisors, teachers, and administrators in either hospitals, community agencies, or international settings, including relief organizations and private enterprises (20 percent of the sample). According to their discharge interviews, many of these nurses were looking for non-traditional practice settings or to replace their wartime experiences with work that would offer similar challenges – such as outpost nursing, northern nursing, work with the United Nations Rehabilitation and Relief Administration (UNRRA),[124] nursing in other countries (China, South Africa, Persia, or Ceylon) or industrial nursing (with South American oil companies, insurance companies, or on steamships). A note on one nurse's file reads: "Hesitates to return to civilian nursing, not through lack of interest or qualifications, but due to civilian patients' failure to appreciate her efforts ... now realizes her capabilities from a professional point of view and more fully understands the opportunities open to her." After her POW experience, NS May Waters went as a missionary nurse to work in a leper colony on the island of Molokai, Hawaii. She remained single and eventually retired to Florida, where she died.[125]

Some nurses left the military as patients themselves with health problems such as tuberculosis, brucellosis, arthritis, psychoneurosis, fractured spines, burns requiring plastic surgery and rehabilitation, haemolytic anaemia, deafness, and cancer. Others accepted responsibility for the care of sick family members (1.6 percent). Some nurses had not yet decided on their plans when they spoke to DVA counsellors, while some planned to take a holiday before deciding, or simply did not indicate their plans (5.8 percent). Ultimately, only a meagre proportion of the nursing sisters (8.9 percent) planned to return to hospital nursing practice, although it is plausible that at least some of those without definite plans at discharge also remained in nursing or returned to the profession later in their lives.

Nursing sisters who used their credits for university enrolled in public health, supervision, teaching, and hospital administration courses – the primary courses available to nurses in Canada.[126] Many of these nurses subsequently married and left the profession after completing such courses. NS Tritt went to the McGill University School for Graduate Nurses for one year, taking courses in teaching and supervision, after which she taught briefly at a hospital school of nursing until she married. She explained that she took only the one-year course and received a diploma because she didn't have the qualifications for regular university admission (Grade 12) – like many nurses who were educated during the Depression. Taking into account those who planned to marry, transfer to the permanent forces, or work in DVA hospitals, private duty nursing, non-hospital nursing, X-ray or lab technician employment, and non-nursing employment – at least 69 percent of the nursing sisters in this study either left or planned not to return to civilian hospital nursing at the end of the war.

In their discharge interviews (from confidential DND files), some nursing sisters referred to military nursing as a patriotic, not a professional, endeavour. As one counsellor wrote, "Miss ____ is in the fortunate position of not having to work for a living. She studied nursing as a war duty and does not intend to continue to practise her profession." Another counsellor noted that the interviewed nurse was "definitely giving up nursing. She was not nursing before enlistment [she was a typist] and only came back to this profession because of the war."

Nursing sisters who did not want to continue in the profession proposed a wide variety of plans. Some were starting small businesses (either alone or with a partner): grocery stores, a hardware store, a tea room or a bar, a ski lodge, a leather goods store, a beauty shop, a restaurant, hotel management, or a tourist camp. Others wanted to go into advertising, farming, interior decorating, or handicrafts. Several planned to study art. One planned to become a musical accompanist. Other nurses remained in nursing out of necessity rather than by choice, as one file clearly explains: "This nursing sister appears to be a restless rather unhappy girl. She is 'fed to the teeth' with nursing and unable to break away from it. She has financial responsibilities which include the maintenance of a house and care of an aunt who is dependent on her. Miss —— is an orphan and the care of this relative devolves mostly on her shoulders ... [She] is hopeful that in taking public health training she may be able to obtain employment more congenial than general duty nursing."

The Second World War military nurses whom I interviewed made similar decisions. However, a small portion of these who married and left the profession returned (at least on a part-time basis) during the 1960s and 1970s after their children were grown. Two of the twenty-five nurses I interviewed married overseas, five married on discharge, and six more within the first year – for a total of thirteen (54.2 percent) who left nursing, although five of them worked part time at a later date. Only two nurses (8 percent) returned to bedside nursing at discharge. One worked while her husband attended university to become a pharmacist, resigning when he obtained his degree. The second had a baby, but her veteran husband, who was an amputee, cared for their baby while she worked part time for several years because the hospital "pursued" her as a result of the severe nursing shortage. Two nurses (8 percent) went to work in DVA hospitals but, after a brief period, retired to marry. Eight nurses (32 percent) used their veterans' benefits to go to university – five of these for public health courses or degrees. Two eventually completed doctorates and had careers in teaching and supervision, moving away from direct patient care. Four nurses (16 percent) joined the permanent force nursing service (two in the RCAMC and two in the RCAF), while another nursing sister re-enlisted within a year but stayed only briefly prior to her marriage. She found the postwar military situation changed, no longer offering the challenges and opportunities she had experienced during the war. The interviewed nurses were unsettled and restless when the war ended. NS Roe considered going to California or Costa Rica but said, "I wasn't ready at that time, mentally ... I had a chance to go back to university but I just wasn't ready for it." NS Cox recalls that "it took us awhile to adjust to civilian [settings] ... In the Army, you have your meals, you have your work, and everything is pretty much uniform and taken care of. And you were suddenly out doing it all on your own when you come back. It's an entirely different scene. And the very thought of working in a civilian hospital didn't attract me at that point."

If these nurses were restless, the profession was getting desperate. Dr. C.B. Parker, assistant-superintendent (medical) wrote to Air Commodore (RCAF) J.W. Tice in a series of letters in mid-1945 concerning the shortage of nurses at the Toronto General Hospital, suggesting the secondment of armed forces nurses to civilian hospitals "where the need is urgent." He argued that it would not only relieve the situation but also benefit the nursing sisters by providing them with civilian practice experience. Tice replied that the RCAF did not second nurses; although he anticipated the release of a considerable number of nurses in the near future, he could not control where they went or the work they chose once they left the RCAF.[127]

In 1945, the Canadian Nurses Association's Post-war Planning Committee attributed the need for more bedside nurses to the extension of DVA hospitals, increased delegation from physicians to nurses, unfilled positions in tuberculosis and psychiatry, and new practice areas such as industrial nursing.[128] The committee projected a need for more nurses and nursing instructors related to plans for postwar hospital expansion and the implementation of hospital insurance programs.[129] Initially, the professional literature exuded an understanding attitude towards demobilizing nursing sisters and their need to take some time and make their own decisions about future employment. Later messages became more urgent and more critical. Evelyn Mallory, the president of the Registered Nurses Association of British Columbia, for one, expressed her frustration bluntly in a 1946 editorial:

> We tell ourselves that we have worked hard during the last few years trying to keep civilian services going and to meet the nursing needs of war; but the war is over and the danger is passed ... The Canadian people have been very patient with us. We have been unable to meet their needs for nursing service, either in quantity or quality. But there was always the answer, "There is a war on!" ... We went to the Dominion Government and we said: "It is because of the needs of war that we have not enough nurses' ... We can no longer say that military needs are depleting the civilian service. Yet the shortage of nurses seems more acute than ever! ... There will be no glamour, and no awareness of a common danger to unite us."[130]

Some hospitals were downright deceptive in "trapping" nurses for their communities. NS Cole had just been discharged when a small, rural hospital begged her to come for just a few days of relief for their one and only nurse. Once Cole arrived, she realized there wasn't another train out for a week – and the nurse she replaced did not come back on it. She had to do everything: admit patients, "pour anaesthetics" during operations, and prepare baby formula. "I had to wash the damn diapers because they had no laundry service and I can remember washing the diapers on a scrubbing board, and crying into the tub: How did I get myself into this?" Cole remained six months because they were telling her how desperately they needed staff. But she finally decided, "I've got to get out of this."

As the military discharged nurses, the CNA and provincial organizations sought to match civilian needs to nurses' availability. A two-page spread in the *Canadian Nurse* classified available opportunities into two categories: positions open to newly graduated nurses and positions open to nurses with experience or advanced preparation.[131] It classified the employment opportunities as institutional nursing, public health nursing, nursing education, and private duty, with accompanying salary grids. The RNAO Placement Service reported only 54 inquiries for a total of 672 nursing vacancies in Ontario in March 1946, of which 18 were recently discharged nursing sisters. Of the 18, the service referred 5 nurses to interim placements while they waited for university courses. Another nurse never showed up for her placement. Two more went to the Toronto General Hospital as general duty nurses but "proved very unsatisfactory as they resigned after two days duty." Two nurses were placed successfully, two nurses placed themselves, and two more presented "definite problems related to handicaps."[132] By September 1946, the placement service report was even more disparaging. It noted a declining interest in bedside nursing and an "alarming" number of nurses seeking work in industry, clinics, and doctors' offices, but "unwilling to accept individual responsibility for hospital needs."[133]

Because so few discharged nursing sisters remained in nursing, it is important to examine the experiences of those who did. Returning military nurses made it clear, for the most part, that they were not interested in resuming previous practice roles, and the profession acknowledged to some extent that change was necessary. As one writer put it,

> War nursing ... has its own techniques, practices, methods and discipline ... A sudden change-over to duty in a civilian hospital after five years' absence will test the tolerance, understanding and patience of all concerned ... Many of the overseas nurses on discharge will feel the need for at least some re-orientation, and others will find satisfaction in taking a post-graduate course. As there is such urgent need for nurses in the administrative and teaching specialties every encouragement should be given the returned nurses with the necessary qualifications to take training along these lines. Their recent experience, so rich in providing an opportunity for a broader outlook and greater understanding, should be the best possible foundation on which to build future leaders in the nursing field.[134]

For the most part, nurses made choices that were consistent with their prewar career patterns. Many had held previous leadership, public health, industrial nursing, education, or supervisory positions. DVA counsellors typically described the nursing sisters as ambitious. One said, "Like many of these nurses she is very disappointed at not having had the opportunity of serving overseas. She is anxious to improve her value as a nurse now and take a post-graduate course in Lab work." Another counsellor described a nurse as a "small wiry girl of 29. She has worked hard for her opportunities to take advanced schooling and hospital training. In the process her outlook has become cautious, and she has learned to drive a good bargain." A francophone nurse planned to use her credits to enhance her English-language skills in order to increase her opportunities in home nursing, according to the counsellor who explained that she was "très désireuse de suivre un cours afin de devenir aussi bilingue que possible car elle considère, et avec raison, que la connaissance des deux langues pourrait lui être d'un précieux appui dans l'exercice de ses functions comme infirmière-visiteuse."

During the 1945-46 academic year, some 160 nursing sisters registered in universities across Canada, and there were more applicants than student places. The CNA successfully lobbied the federal government to extend the time limit for nurses to use their credits, arguing that returning nurses were also needed to help with the shortage.[135] As NS Mussallem recalled, "You even had to sit on the steps ... [Classes] were just overflowing, and a lot of them went back [to school]. That was a tremendous boost for Canada, wasn't it – all those nurses? ... It should have ultimately ended in better health care. Some of them were going for certificates and diplomas ... Others were completing their baccalaureate degrees." Mussallem took courses at the School for Graduate Nurses at McGill University, ultimately completing a baccalaureate degree there and taking both a masters and a PhD at Columbia University in New York.

The nursing profession and two university schools of nursing in particular, at McGill and the University of Toronto, benefited from the war and nursing shortage through special grants to expand their nursing education programs. In the *Canadian Nurse*, Ethel Johns urged nurses to "seize the priceless opportunity" to push for university education for nurses in 1941, arguing, "The community will accept financial responsibility for educating nurses if we prove that we are indispensable to health and welfare."[136] Recruitment efforts for civilian nurses had already begun in 1942 when the CNA lobbied for funding to prepare educators and supervisors to increase the enrolment of students in the schools of nursing. In that year, the W.K. Kellogg Foundation announced grants for nursing education to a maximum of $4,000 per school of nursing for 115 institutions in the United States and Canada. In the same year, the Canadian government provided the CNA with $115,000 for recruitment, teaching facilities, and the preparation of graduate nurses in teaching, supervision, and administration. Additional federal grants amounted to $250,000 for 1944-45 and to $159,970 for 1945-46.[137] While these sources of funding were very important, they were inadequate for long-term support, especially for nursing programs that had not been able to secure firm positions within universities to that point. Nonetheless, the great influx of nurses under the Veterans Charter of benefits was instrumental in placing these two university nursing programs on solid economic footing – regardless if nurses took certificate courses, diploma courses, or completed a degree.

Comparing the pre- and postwar situation at the School for Graduate Nurses at McGill University, NS Tritt concluded:

During the Depression, McGill wanted to close the school. They finally agreed if nurses could raise enough money to keep it going, they could keep it going.

So Miss Lindeburgh and all her staff had rummage sales, had card parties, had everything and anything to raise money plus many of the girls who couldn't afford it, handed in money. And they gave extra classes and they gave anything and everything ... Well then I guess about [1942], the Kellogg Foundation gave them a grant. So that put them on a better footing. Then, with all the girls coming back from overseas who took post-graduate – that really set them up. So from then on, it was a going concern.

Approximately one-third of the nursing sisters in this study used their educational benefits, but few returned to hospital nursing, where the greatest shortage of nurses existed. Almost 20 percent took certificate or diploma courses, and 12.9 percent completed degrees.

Some nursing sisters found themselves in contradictory positions related to postwar medical technology, fearing that they had been away from civilian hospitals too long and medical technology had changed too much during their absence from civilian practice settings. On one hand, they were more familiar with penicillin, transfusions, intravenous therapies, triage, burns, and wound care. But on the other hand, their expertise lay in a narrow domain associated primarily with trauma to young men. Civilian hospitals did not typically have a large proportion of young male patients, mass casualties, or wounds caused by bombs, shells, and artillery. NS Jean Wheeler said, "I felt I needed to be re-trained ... I was afraid to go into a general hospital" because of all the changes that had taken place during the war and because she lacked broader general experience.[138] NS Taylor avoided telling anyone she had been a military nurse: "I don't think I ever told anybody that I was an overseas nurse because they might think I didn't know anything ... People have different ideas. They just thought we went over there to have a fun time."

Other nursing sisters described a milieu within the military that did not exist in civilian hospitals. They referred to working as a team, being united by a common goal, and experiencing less competitiveness compared to prewar training school rivalries. NS Van Scoyoc, noting that "the spirit was so different" in the military, worked as a DVA hospital supervisor for seventeen years because her comfort level was greater there than in civilian nursing:

I think we felt when you'd been over almost for [over four] years, things had changed. And even if there hadn't been a war, things would have changed. And you felt ... curtailed in what you had done. But in some other ways you weren't as well-educated as the nurses that were [in civilian hospitals]. It was an odd feeling ... Eventually, I went into civilian nursing ... And I always thought I was fortunate when I went to the Montreal Children's [Hospital], that they would keep me as a supervisor because most of the supervisors there were well-educated ... I don't think that many nurses ... really got back into the act in the civilian field ... There wasn't really much room for these nurses who had been in the very senior [military] positions.

Many nursing sisters mentioned that they were used to more independence and autonomy. NS Cole said, "We were underemployed [regarding] what we were allowed to do [after the war]," while NS Oakes said, "I would think it would be difficult to go back to your own hospital and get back into the routine you left ... I didn't do that."

Civilian hospitals were unable to use the skills, knowledge, and autonomy acquired by the nursing sisters because the institutions still relied predominantly on a student workforce for direct patient care. NS MacLean worked for a brief period at the Ottawa Civic Hospital to support her husband, who was studying pharmacy under his veterans' benefits. She recalled the difficult workload and numerous patient complaints about care, noting that the conditions led to a judicial inquiry into the state of patient care in 1949. The final report fixed blame for the conditions on severe understaffing, an increased use of medical technologies, and a student workforce too novice to provide appropriate care.[139] Over the next decades, most Canadian hospitals continued to struggle with nurse shortages as nurses moved away from restrictive practice environments. Dr. Lorne Gilday of the Western Division of the Montreal General Hospital summed up the situation in 1948: "Nurses come and nurses go, and more seem to go than come."[140]

Although the majority of nursing sisters did not return to hospitals, many medical technologies that evolved during the war became part of hospital practice – for example, penicillin, transfusions, and intravenous therapy. As some of the first nurses to work with these technologies, those who did stay in practice helped to shape postwar uses and nursing roles based on their experiences with mass casualties. Various nurses claimed that their military experience influenced the development of nursing assistant programs, team nursing, specialty units, and early patient ambulation instead of prolonged bed rest for many conditions.

Nursing sisters had experienced both the advantages and the limitations of working with medical assistants, in the form of other ranks, throughout the war. After NS Ferguson returned to the civilian workplace and became involved in finding solutions to the shortage she found there, she spent a major part of her postwar career working to establish standardized training for nursing assistants in Alberta, based on her experience in the military, where medical orderlies served in this capacity. She said, "I came home convinced that we in nursing needed a second level of nursing to help us ... because the responsibilities were becoming so heavy ... Doctors were getting so many more complicated things to do ... Nurses were being trained as specialists ... So we needed a second level of nursing to help with the basics." Although there are references to trained attendants or aides in Manitoba and Quebec as early as the 1920s, and the Weir Report includes a brief analysis of the extent to which the public hired "practical nurses," it is not clear what level of training these assistants received.[141] Programs such as Ferguson suggested for training assistants began in Ontario in September 1946. The Montreal General Hospital listed nursing assistants, practical nurses, and trained attendants in its 1945 annual report, and by 1948 the hospital participated in an experimental, jointly sponsored Montreal School for Nursing Aides.[142]

In many ways, medical technology and the war complicated the situation on both ends of the nursing spectrum by adding another level of nursing assistant with less training and by adding nurses with more education at the university or postgraduate level. The technical skills and expertise that military nurses had used to become nursing sisters provided access to university education and professional advancement through veterans' credits. But professional advancement moved most of them away from direct patient care in hospitals, where medical technology was proliferating.

Some nursing sisters attributed changes in the *delivery* of hospital nursing care to their wartime experiences. For example, Navy NS Ruby Hull wrote in 1945 about the benefits of creating a "special department known as the post-anesthetic Recovery Room" where patients could be held overnight if necessary. She outlined a plan for oxygen therapy, duodenal tubes and Wangensteen suction, the use of sedatives and stimulants, and nursing observation required for cases of haemorrhage, shock, plaster casts, and surgical dressings. This was a change from the usual civilian practice of recovering patients on regular nursing wards.[143] Several nursing sisters mentioned a dramatic increase in the use of drugs during the war (compared to previous civilian practice). One hospital created a special unit in 1947, the Penicillin Treatment Centre, where a graduate nurse was responsible for administering all the penicillin throughout the hospital.[144] Specialty teams and units such as burn units, psychiatric wards, and maxillo-facial plastics team, where patients, equipment, and nurses were clustered for more efficient care under wartime conditions, were forerunners of the intensive care units, coronary care units, and dialysis units that emerged during the 1950s and 1960s.

Wages were another aspect of civilian nursing that benefited from the precedents set by nursing sisters during the war. Equally ranked Canadian female and male officers in the medical services earned equal pay, and this increased nurses' prewar earnings by two to three times their annual salaries and benefits. A 1944-45 Canadian Nurses Association recruitment brochure compared civilian nurses' monthly salaries by categories: $50-125 plus maintenance for staff nurses; $125 for a head nurse; $125-150 for an industrial nurse; $100-125 plus maintenance for operating room nurses; $125 for public health nurses; $150-175 for supervisors; and $125-150 for instructors.[145] These rates represented a substantial increase over those of the late 1930s and were more in line with military nursing salaries, as the civilian sector competed for the same pool of graduate nurses during the war. And when there was no relief to nursing shortages after the war, salary increases continued to be a primary recruitment strategy.

This generation of military personnel was also the first in Canada to experience the benefits of comprehensive health care programs, initiated partially to meet manpower commitments overseas by assuring healthy soldiers, and partially to avoid postwar pension liabilities due to health issues attributable to wartime military service. Many Canadians had gone through the Depression without medical or dental care, and on enlistment they got their teeth fixed or had minor surgical repairs done because these procedures made them fit for active duty. But as NS Tritt said, "During the Army, you got everything. Once we got home, we got nothing." Physicians were also aware of changing expectations for postwar medical care, and as the chairman of the general council of the Canadian Medical Association wrote, "Three quarters of a million young men and women in the Armed Forces are being educated to a new form of health care."[146] Although universal hospital insurance was widely contested, the first provincial program was in place in Saskatchewan by 1948.

American historians have argued that – among other claims to wartime nursing legacies – the Second World War led to the acceptance of black, male, part-time, and married nurses.[147] But it is likely that nursing shortages influenced change more than wartime experiences did – at least in Canada, where the eradication of racial and ethnic barriers in the profession was extremely slow.[148] The CNA definitely targeted men as one potential solution to the nursing shortage, surveying provincial requirements and legislation for nurse registration and reporting in 1948 that all provincial acts, except that in Quebec, were flexible enough to enable registration of male nurses. But the only provincial associations that accepted men into training programs at the time of the survey were Nova Scotia and Ontario. Other provinces trained men as attendants, mainly in mental hospitals.[149]

Thus, nursing sisters shaped postwar nursing practice by their refusal to accept prewar practice conditions as well as by their limited participation in the civilian workforce. Substantial changes were already beginning by 1940, and the nursing shortage that developed by the mid-1940s was not significantly exacerbated by the small percentage of nurses who enlisted in the military, or alleviated by those who returned. Student enrolment actually increased each year, and the profession implemented a variety of changes to retain nurses in practice. But when demobilized nurses moved away from the bedside and from nursing, it became clear that there were major underlying issues related to hospital working conditions, and that the shortage was not a temporary condition of the war.

Nursing sisters constituted an essential but temporary and contingent feminine workforce "for the duration" of the war. They embraced technological roles and responsibilities, enabled the movement of surgical care forward to the frontlines, and used newly acquired technological skills to legitimate their presence at the front. In return, military nurses gained access to expanded roles, increased autonomy, enhanced social status as officers, and decently paid stable employment. The work environment often placed medical officers and nurses in close proximity, where skills and knowledge were readily shared and developed. Nurses found, however, that gender continued to constrain what they could do, when they could do it, and where.

Military nursing experiences had a limited impact on the postwar nursing profession, as the majority of nursing sisters left the profession and those who returned to civilian nursing found it difficult to fit into the system again. Their decisions compounded an emerging nursing shortage, providing an impetus for reform of hospital working conditions over the subsequent decades. Several universities benefited from stable funding for nursing programs as military nurses capitalized on their benefits for further education. At the same time, public health nursing, psychiatry, and industrial nursing (occupational health) benefited greatly from an influx of military nurses, who brought advanced education and autonomy to these practice specialties. When the war ended, nursing sisters lost their legitimacy as officers, soldiers, and women in the military world. The camaraderie and collegiality forged through wartime experiences had contrasted greatly with the isolation and privation of private duty nursing during the Depression years. Although many nurses were eager to leave war and military duties behind for more ordinary lives, there were many others left to deal with personal losses and professional dissonances that remained long after peace had been declared.

"The Strain of Peace": Community and Social Memory

Nursing sisters had lived and worked in small, relatively isolated and strictly regimented residences during their student training days. Those experiences resembled military medical settings to some extent, although the exigencies of war intensified relationships, patriotism, and loyalty to the military system. As we have seen, war brought nursing sisters together from diverse regions and schools of nursing, but they were military nurses only "for the duration." They developed shared identities as Canadians, women, soldiers, and members of specific military medical units. The return of "peace," however, disrupted their newly created military identities almost as much as war had disrupted their prior civilian identities. While serving in Italy, NS Marguerite McLimont wrote a poem about the need to rebuild war-torn relationships as well as war-torn structures. In "Prayer on Hearing V-E Day Proclamation," she summarized her angst and uncertainty in the line "Lord, give us strength to stand the strain of peace."[1] In some ways, the postwar world was another "no-man's land" where many nursing sisters struggled to find a sense of belonging and purpose. Some found themselves suddenly isolated from both the professional and the military worlds, feeling that they no longer had a place in either after the armistice. They were no longer soldiers, and some doubted their identity as nurses, questioning their ability to, fit back into civilian practice.

For many nursing sisters, wartime experiences shaped an enduring postwar military nurse identity as members of an "imagined community" who engaged in constructing a collective social memory, including commemoration of their participation in this major world event. Their physical and social proximity intersected with gender to create a community of military nurses based on shared spaces and shared experiences. But it was remarkable that many of those whom I interviewed for this research continued to identify so strongly as an imagined or symbolic community despite postwar physical and social distance – even when they might never have known one another during the war. Almost sixty years after the war ended, NS Betty Nicolson still declared,

"I'm Army! ... You have a loyalty."[2] This symbolic community distinguished them from other women and from other nurses, while providing a place of acceptance, a social network, and a powerful gendered social memory with associated symbols, rituals, and stories.

Since the 1980s, our understanding of community has evolved from a spatial concept based on shared physical place to a structural concept based on shared social networks, to recent literature that considers community as a mental construct based on shared values, norms, and moral codes that provide a sense of identity. Sociologist and anthropologist A.P. Cohen points out that there are over ninety definitions of community in use, but, ultimately, it is the meaning (or importance) attributed to a community that constitutes its symbolism for the member. Thus, a symbolic community is one in which "members make, or believe they make, a similar sense of things ... with respect to specific and significant interests."[3] Community is always relational, with both similarity and difference implied, as some things are held in common and other things set a community apart. Benedict Anderson applies the term "imagined community" to nations, referring to a capacity for community even though most of the membership "will never know most of their fellow-members, meet them, or even hear of them, yet in the minds of each lives the image of their communion." He suggested that community exists regardless of inequality and exploitation because it is conceived as a "deep, horizontal comradeship."[4] Other scholars consider community as a collection of personal relationships that move beyond kinship, friendship, and neighbouring ties while questioning the assumption that such ties are necessarily supportive.[5]

Social historians point to the potential of community as a concept for research that examines how communities emerged, how they worked, and what meanings they held inside and outside their boundaries. They consider community as a "social process," predicated on relationships and change over time, in which social and spatial aspects are dynamic and changing.[6] Community takes on different meanings in different contexts, and its members attribute less or more importance to identification with it. Nursing sister Brenda McBryde, who was a member of Queen Alexandra's Imperial Military Nursing Service, wrote that, after the war, many British military nurses retired from the profession and buried wartime memories in domesticity and motherhood.[7] Canadian nursing sisters also indicated that they were busy "getting on with life" during the immediate postwar period. Some did not renew their associations with other nursing sisters until much later in life. Some never spoke of their experiences, publicly or privately, until the mid-1990s. As they entered their ninth and tenth decades, however, many expressed an urgency to re-establish community and to reconstruct meaning from their war experiences.

A collective social memory, defined as "the shared narratives of a community's past," is one important strategy to ensure a community's identity and survival. But *how* memories are selected, agreed upon, and transmitted is often more important than *what* memories are selected.[8] Gender plays a significant role in shaping social memory, particularly in relation to women and war. As Cynthia Enloe writes, "Postwar years in all countries are a time of continued gendered war waging. But now the battle is not to take the next hill. It is to capture the collective memory."[9] The literature and social memory related to the Second World War have been dominated by male perspectives; military women have almost disappeared from the accounts, relegated to margins and footnotes, if present at all. The nursing sisters created their own "memory on the margins" that served to sustain identity and meaning for them.[10]

Various social movements of the 1960s and 1970s, such as the New Left, anti-militarism, and second-wave feminism, rendered both military history and nursing history less and less popular among the populace and academics alike. Long-standing contested relations existed between feminists and nurses in general, and between feminists and military nurses in particular. Feminists were divided, however, and took stances that reflected "both a negation of militarism and an affirmation of the rights of women in the military."[11] Both anti-militarists and feminists contributed to nursing sisters' invisibility and silence by representing nurses as stereotypically female and subordinated while aligning them with male oppressors within a militaristic system. Postwar military nurses Nina Rumen and June Parker referred to the influence of these social movements as contributing to a morale problem among military nurses during the 1960s and 1970s.[12] It is hardly surprising, then, that many nursing sisters chose not talk about their experiences outside of their safe community. NS Betty Nicolson explained that, although all but two of her nursing sister friends remained in contact with one another over the years, "we never talked about our wartime experience." The paucity of commemorative material memory such as artifacts, texts, monuments, public heritage places, art, and photography also limited the transmission of military nursing social memory.[13]

To understand the nursing sister community as a "social and spatial process," we need to ask how it emerged, how it worked, how it re-created itself in postwar civilian settings, and what meanings it has held for its members.[14] The community had roots in at least three common sets of experiences: hospital training school culture, military culture, and the fledgling Overseas Nursing Sisters Clubs that convened locally from the 1920s and biennially as a national organization from 1932. The community reproduced prevailing gender- and class-based discourses related to military nursing, for the most part shaping a social memory that conformed to the dominant Canadian military social memory. Although there were diverse subgroups within the larger nursing sisters community that were not always cohesive and supportive, internal dissensions remained hidden from public view, and the dissenters were marginalized.

Although many nursing sisters married and left nursing careers behind, others never fit into the dominant socially prescribed roles for women. They left highly structured military settings where there were few individual decisions to make and privacy was rare, dispersing throughout Canada, where they often found themselves to be the only ex-military nurse in an area. Some "just got on with life" and never spoke of their experiences to family, friends, or co-workers, like NS Pauline Cox, who decided not to reveal her military service to co-workers in case they questioned her professional qualifications, or NS Pauline Lamont, who raised a family and followed her husband's career with no further involvement in the community for almost fifty years.[15] It is not clear what community may have meant for those military nurses who did not initially stay connected, either by choice or circumstances. But a substantial number of nursing sisters sought out and either maintained or rebuilt close relationships that endured over the rest of their lives. According to a 1958 Nursing Sisters' Association of Canada membership list, some 670 of them were still "members in good standing" at least a decade after the end of the war, and the organization continued to meet every two years until the year 2000.[16] The nursing sister community and its social memory have been constructed primarily by those military nurses who needed and found meaning in it.

The Emerging Community

Nursing sisters formed a distinct homosocial group that was isolated geographically, socially, and professionally from prewar relationships and identities. They frequently referred to a special camaraderie and closeness that lasted a lifetime and was both similar to and different from civilian nursing experiences. NS Van Scoyoc explained that it was hard to compare these relationships to anything they experienced before or after the war "because the spirit was so different ... We just seemed to be like one big family ... That was one thing that we missed so much when we came back to civilian life ... Right from the time you went in as a recruit, you had that until the very end ... All these friendships have lasted over the years which is a great plus for us ... Comradeship – it was the most wonderful thing."[17]

Camaraderie was not unique to nursing sisters. Other veterans shared war experiences in common, joined veterans' associations, and referred to themselves as "war buddies," including other women who served in various armed forces Women's Divisions or voluntary associations.[18] As well, the Australian nursing sisters joined the Returned Army Sisters' Association after the First World War and the Returned Sailors, Soldiers, and Airmen's Imperial League of Australia after the Second World War. British and American nurses may have established parallel communities, but we know little concerning their associations and reunions or what they ultimately meant to their members.[19]

One root of the enduring relationships among Canadian nursing sisters arose from nurse training schools. Early Canadian schools of nursing, like most North American training schools, were established during the mid- to late nineteenth century as a source of inexpensive labour. Student nurses exchanged their labour for marketable skills and enhanced occupational status. The number and size of schools increased rapidly over the first half of the twentieth century. In such schools, student nurse work culture focused on shaping both character and nursing practice. The students were effectively removed from their families, and often from their home communities as well, because of the requirement to live in residence with very little time off duty. This policy ensured plenty of opportunity for the inculcation of feminine values, norms, and moral codes during the three years of training, fostering the students' first homosocial professional community.[20]

After graduation, nurses often continued to maintain close relations with their training schools via membership in their respective alumnae associations. These associations provided a measure of job security for nurses as well as opportunities for social, educational, political, and economic activities. Private duty nurses depended on these associations with their training hospitals and physicians for referrals to patients. Moreover, most hospitals and alumnae associations maintained employment registries, and when there were requests for nurses, they recommended their own graduates first. Alumnae associations also provided limited economic assistance when work was scarce or when a nurse was unable to work as a result of illness.[21]

Thus, civilian nurses were already socialized as members of local nursing communities, with a strong sense of identification and pride in their training schools. Students who trained together often remained lifelong friends. NS Lois Bayly attended the sixty-fifth reunion of her class at Montreal General Hospital in 2002, for example, explaining that "Ida Johnson and I are the two oldest ones that attend. We graduated in 1937 and we've gone back every five years pretty well."[22] NS Betty Nicolson attended the sixtieth reunion of her Winnipeg General Hospital class of 1940, saying, "I think the nursing profession is more bonded than any other profession." It is not clear if nurses actually did bond more strongly than other professionals such as physicians, who also trained together and shared patient-related "life-and-death" events, but many of the interviewed nursing sisters perceived training school relationships as particularly significant and enduring.

The military further shaped nursing sisters as an all-women's community uniquely embedded within a much larger and dominant community of military men. Gendered boundaries shifted within military settings to accommodate nursing sisters, but, as we have seen, changes were understood as temporary and contingent on distance from usual civilian settings. There was far more flexibility within communal spaces that were socially and geographically isolated from mainstream civilian practice settings.

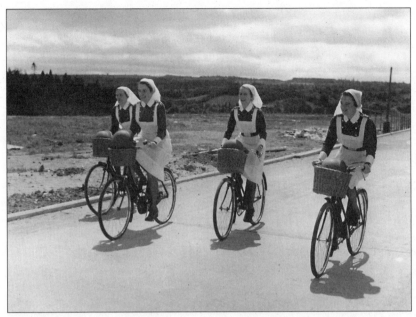

Close working conditions and the distance from families back home often meant that nursing sisters built close relationships within their assigned hospital units. Here, RCAMC nursing sisters Margaret Porter, Marg Walt, "Freddie" Hendricks, and an unidentified colleague bike to work in Bramshott, England. *Courtesy Nancy Mohan*

Isolation and mutual dependency facilitated development of this symbolic nursing sister community. On enlistment, nursing sisters moved into an environment that isolated them professionally and socially while inculcating values, beliefs, and norms specific to the military. Military service disrupted previous relationships, controlled all their activities, and intentionally fostered camaraderie – much as it did for other soldiers, whose survival under adverse conditions might depend on mutual trust and loyalty. NS Jean MacBain described military nursing as an "unnatural way of life away from home and families and old friends [that] resulted in strong friendships which have lasted through the years. Something which we as nursing sisters learned was that we always had to be optimistic and cheerful. The patients had many problems so it was up to us to make them as comfortable as possible in as cheerful a manner as possible."[23] On the positive side, NS Norma Fieldhouse called the military environment a "very, very pleasant social life," which was "a real contrast to civilian life because all the men you knew were overseas."[24]

Nursing sisters left families, friends, and work colleagues to travel further than most of them had ever been. They were totally dependent on the military, especially overseas in the midst of hostilities on the European continent or, as in the cases of NS Christie and Waters, in prisoner of war camps. In South

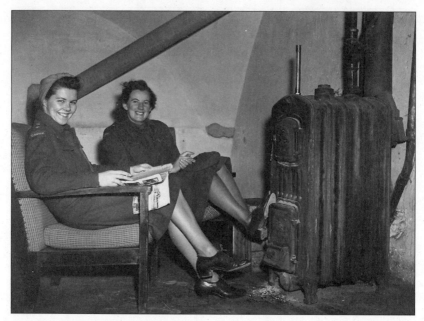

Two RCAMC nursing sisters took advantage of a break in the action in North Africa to relax. As many of them said, they became "as family" to one another. *LAC/DND fonds/PA-213777*

Africa, the small group of ten nursing sisters posted to Baragwaneth became a little "island of Canada" unto themselves.[25] NS Lettie Turner, referring to the nurses who served in Europe, said that they all formed a bond because "they were scared of the same things, facing the same things."[26] NS Lamont explained, "Anybody that was overseas never, ever, came back the same." NS Doris Carter wrote that, "Once I left England, I would have no civilian friends; they would all be from the fighting forces of various countries. It would take me three years to become socialized into my new way of life. And it would not be until I was on a troop ship leaving England for Canada in 1945 that I would realize how much I had changed during the preceding five years."[27]

Many nursing sisters referred to the military as their family. As NS Nicolson explained, "We were devoid of family connections. We were there with these people. So of course, they became our family at the time ... We would have done anything for each other ... Our whole attitude had changed. It was different altogether, military nurses." And they did look after one another, as RCN NS Elizabeth Dean illustrated. She was a dietician stationed at Sydney, Nova Scotia, where she roomed with a nurse who found ways to slip away from the barracks at night. Dean covered for her: in one situation, she "was called in ... to 'tell on her' because they figured she was going down to the ships and spending her night on the ships. I lived right beside the fire escape and I used to let her in every morning, and so on. But they accused her of this. And I would say, 'Oh, no. Her home is Glace Bay so she's just gone home, and probably missed the train.' ... But my roommate wasn't going home to Glace Bay!"[28] NS Margaret Van Scoyoc described nurses in Normandy lying in the dark at night and telling personal stories like real-life sisters, because they had no radios, lights, or other forms of entertainment. Some were homesick, and delayed or lost mail made the loneliness worse. Some nurses, such as NS Gaëtane LaBonté, "grew up during the war," which was a "coming of age" experience.[29]

Closeness, or community, was not dependent on previous relationships among nurses who had trained or worked together prior to enlistment. Early changes in military policy mandated the integration of nursing personnel from at least 187 different training schools into all the medical units. Consequently, nursing sisters did not necessarily know the medical officers or other nurses prior to postings, although some nurses from the larger teaching hospitals claimed to have recognized nurses who had been affiliated with their hospitals for at least part of their training.[30] Despite initial strangeness, nursing sisters quickly developed relationships, many of which were as close or closer than those they had experienced within civilian nursing culture. NS Pauline Cox referred to one nursing sister as a "very, very fine girl. Like I say, we celebrated our 60th anniversary since the day we met in Halifax when we were going overseas! I never had met Ethel because she was at the Vic and I was at the General. And we've been in touch ever since. Now, we aren't able to visit. I am always in touch with her. I phone every week or she phones me." NS Frances Oakes became godmother to a fellow nursing sister's children after the war. Although this friend is now dead, her children still "call me every Saturday or Sunday. I miss her very much. We got along very well. We didn't know each other [previously]. We met on the boat going over. And we got along fine."[31]

When times were tough, as NS Harriet Sloan recalled, "we were very conscious of one another's losses. When someone's boyfriend was killed, some dear relative, when a husband died – it was awful. There was compassion for one another ... Everyone knew. Everyone would express their sympathy ... People tried to make it as easy for you as possible under the circumstances, and we all would get tired and grumpy."[32] But not everyone appreciated closeness all the time. NS Doris Carter found there was too little privacy, especially while living under canvas: "Your tent was never quiet. You could hear everybody talking and they could hear you. You never had any secrets. Everybody could hear."[33]

The development of community depended partially on when a nurse enlisted and where she was posted. The armed forces began to accept younger nurses during the last years of the war, creating a noticeable gap in terms of age and experience that influenced feelings of belonging and comradeship. NS Beatrice Cole explained that camaraderie was stronger

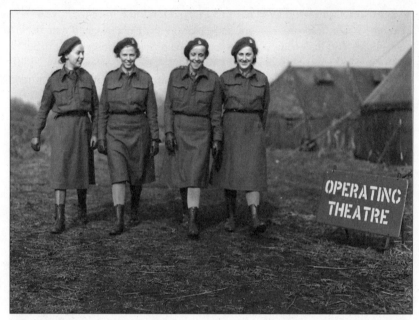

Wartime experiences forged bonds between nursing sisters, many of which lasted a lifetime. Here, four unidentified RCAMC nurses of No. 6 CCS in England, October 1943, join forces on the way to the operating theatre tent. *LAC/Lieutenant C.E. Nye/DND fonds/PA-213782*

among the older nurses and the physicians, while younger nurses were more easily intimidated by experience and rank.[34]

The case of NS Kay Christie and May Waters is unique: community became a physical and psychological tool of survival in the prisoner of war and internment camps of Hong Kong. On the one hand, POW camps were communities of fear, where members witnessed unspeakable torture, suffering, and death. Christie noted that the Japanese soldiers at these camps didn't discriminate between guilt and innocence among POWs. For example, when guards thought a mass escape was being planned, they identified the name of "Anderson" as one of the leaders. According to Christie, "They didn't know which Anderson so they took [killed] all six Andersons that were in the camp. That's the way things were done."[35] On the other hand, while the POW community faced constant danger and demoralization, it also called forth remarkable innovation and cooperation. Community became a necessary tool of survival as well as a mental construct that gave meaning to the situation. Christie's interviews and writings describe how adversity and deprivation forged bonds between nurses and patients, between nurses and civilian internees, and among nurses. POWs used whatever assets they could develop to endure the months and years of idleness. They taught one another bridge, new languages, and other skills. Bridge became a major obsession for Christie, who said that it helped her to forget about the surroundings, hunger, lack of privacy, uncertainty about the future, and what was going on around her.[36]

Community, as a POW survival strategy, sometimes elicited incredible commitments. Rumours of prisoner and internee exchanges circulated periodically within Stanley Camp. But in the fall of 1943, Christie and Waters learned that they were indeed going to be included in an American exchange. Because there had been almost no communication between their camp and the outside world, the other POWs were desperate to let their families know they were alive. Christie described a formidable process by which she delivered news of their survival to the outside world after she had been liberated:

> When word first got around the camp … every time you were out walking, you'd have somebody say, "When you get out, would you write to so and so?" And they would give me these great addresses in Britain, and Australia was just as bad, and when I'd go back to my room I'd write this down and who it was that had asked me. Then every time I would meet any of those people in the camp, I would repeat the name and address she or he had given me to write to when I got home. But I had quite a list. And I had the Brigade casualty list too, written but also memorized. So when we were down by the shore and were waiting, always in alphabetical order, to be searched before we went on ship, I suddenly remembered about these lists of names. You know, you were warned what would happen to you if you were caught with anything that you shouldn't have, and as I say, we had seen enough – that helped you to obey the rules. And so I took out the pages from that book and just ripped them into shreds and threw them. So when we finally got on the Teia Maru [the Japanese exchange ship] and were handed this roll of toilet paper, the first thing I did was, I went in and I sat down and wrote out all those names and addresses again on this orange toilet paper … When I got on the Grypsholm [a Swedish-American liner], then I began writing letters. I mailed some from South Africa when we stopped there; I mailed some more from Rio de Janeiro when we stopped there. And then the rest I mailed from home. Anybody I didn't hear from in a month or so, then I wrote again because I knew that mail was being lost.[37]

It was at least two decades before Christie spoke or wrote about her internment, but when she did, she balanced her memories with humour and accounts of "many friendships formed in those difficult days which not only have lasted but have become more firmly cemented as the years go by."[38] Although Christie remained in the military following repatriation, with postings to Chorley Park Military Hospital and a retraining centre in Canada, she claimed that after her experience as a POW, she never again quite fit in with the evolving military nursing community. She found military nurses in Canada during the last years of the war to be much younger in years and experience. Having less in common with them, Christie was less willing to accommodate a rigid military system after years as a POW.[39] She spent the rest of her long postwar life working in a physician's office and as an advocate for veterans. Indeed, she was a key witness at a Canadian Pension Commission compensation hearing in the case of Bud Sweet, who had been her patient at the Bowen Road Hospital. As an eyewitness to what he endured, Christie said, "I went to bat for Sweet."[40]

How Community Worked

The nursing sister community has portrayed itself publicly as one united, harmonious group. Yet closeness and camaraderie existed in tension with differences, conflicts, and fractures, whether perceived by community members or not. It is difficult to examine these conflicts because the nurses involved left few records of resistance or dissent, in contrast to conventional accounts of unified sisterhood. Reading against the grain of the existing sources and listening carefully to nurses' voices, however, it is possible to glimpse a community that was not always supportive, unified, or egalitarian, in spite of efforts to portray it as such.[41]

Only two Canadian Second World War nursing sisters have published memoirs, and both provide examples of differences and conflicts.[42] The community did not respond well to either publication, extending only limited recognition to Doris Carter's memoirs while considering Mary White's recollections atypical and best forgotten. Both memoirs refer to alcohol use and abuse, to sexuality, and to power struggles within military medical units, threatening a more desirable collective social memory. For the most part, interviewed nursing sisters denied having had similar experiences and distanced themselves from these accounts. Both Carter and White felt they were outsiders to the community, although both maintained their memberships in the postwar organization and regularly "paid their dues."[43] Their memoirs make an important contribution, however, that counterbalances more numerous narratives emphasizing camaraderie and harmonious relationships.

The first and most obvious commonality that shaped the nursing sisters community was Canadian identity. With few exceptions, Canadian military nurses served in Canadian forces' units – unlike nursing sisters of the First World War, who could be posted with British medical units as needed. Their written accounts and interviews are unanimously proud of this national identity, although many women denied that patriotism was a primary motivation for their serving in the military. Canadian identity could be problematic, however: Canada was still perceived as a colony in Great Britain, where Canadian nursing sisters sometimes encountered derogatory treatment and remarks from British nursing sisters and matrons. In many ways, the Canadian profession had achieved more control over nursing practice, and Canadian military nurses held officer rank long before the British nurses did.[44] These achievements served only to exacerbate friction between the regular British forces and the "territorial forces," as dominion military services were called. As the only Canadian nurses serving in Hong Kong, Christie and Waters encountered antagonism from British nursing sisters, and especially from the matron, who referred to them as "bloody colonials."[45] According to Christie, the matron's main objections stemmed from not understanding their language ("I can't make out a word they're saying"), their "nicer uniforms," their higher rate of pay and officer status, and the attention and "fuss" that they attracted wherever they went.

Canadian nursing sisters understood that their designation as colonials was pejorative and an attempt to position them as inferior to British nurses. Commenting on attitudes displayed by both patients and non-patients towards Canadian military nurses, NS Claire Murray wrote that the British "did not really expect to find us civilized ... [One patient] was very uneasy, though his injuries were not severe ... He was afraid of us, being 'colonials.'"[46] She concluded from her experiences that the British did not consider nursing a respectable occupation. NS Constance Bond was with No. 2 Casualty Clearing Station (CCS) when it landed along with a British medical unit at Courseulles, France, soon after the Normandy invasion. According to her account, "When we were landing we were on landing barges and one of our nurses started to step onto shore. There were British nurses with us. The British Matron prevented us from landing on the barge until all of her nurses landed first. She pulled the Canadian nurses back and said, 'We are the senior service.' So we joined No. 77 British General Hospital under canvas, just for one day, and the next day, July 12th, we rejoined our unit."[47] Although Canadian nurses did occasionally work in British military hospitals, it was only for brief periods and on an emergency basis. They clearly identified themselves as Canadians and typically exerted great effort to make sure their patients, of whatever nationality, understood that difference.

In spite of sharing a common Canadian identity, nursing sisters experienced contentious differences based on regional origins and language. Initially, military medical units recruited personnel accustomed to working together; for example, No. 15 Canadian General Hospital (CGH) was initially staffed from the Toronto General Hospital, and No. 5 CGH from the Winnipeg General Hospital in 1939. Attempts to create an all-French-speaking medical unit were unsuccessful, partially because the army had abandoned its plan for an all-French fighting brigade. But, in any case, it was not feasible to segregate casualties by language.[48] Whenever small work units were required for forward field units or on hospital ships, efforts were made to post "compatible" nurses together because of the limited working and social spaces. In general, however, the RCAMC followed a policy of mixing personnel from a variety of regions and training schools, and, as we have seen, that policy carried benefits for the armed forces. But it also exposed fractures within the community related to class, region, and language.

The civilian nursing workforce in general was dominated by the large teaching hospitals of central Canada, which were established well before those farther west. Graduates of these training schools dominated leadership positions within the profession, at least numerically, and also dominated the armed forces nursing services, leading to some resentment among westerners. NS Estelle Tritt, for example, herself a graduate of Reddy Memorial Hospital in Montreal, remembers the "intense rivalry and dislike" between two units with unusually distinct regional compositions: one dominated by nurses from Saskatchewan, the other by nurses from Nova Scotia.[49] NS Helen Mussallem enlisted at Vancouver, and, as she said, "Coming from the west (the far west in Vancouver), we thought that people in the East ... the Sisters were a little snobbish, you know. And they did things this way and that way."[50] NS Margaret Fletcher was also a westerner, serving in England with No. 7 CGH, which originated in Halifax. She wrote critically about the quality of care given by non-western nurses as well as tensions that resulted when the military posted nurses from disparate training backgrounds together: "I'm still taking a dim view of a lot of things – & the more I see of some people, the more respect I have for training schools in the west. Apparently people in the east get well in spite of the staff. All the ex #5 [referring to nurses who had served with No. 5 CGH prior to being transferred to No. 7 CGH] are very browned off [about their reassignment to the Halifax unit]." Later she referred to the antagonistic relations in the unit as "not conducive to good work."[51] In her effort to downplay regional differences, Matron Dorothy Macham decided to conceal her eastern origins when she arrived at No. 8 CGH, mobilized initially from Regina: "I began by saying I was from Corn Hill – this is actually the small community where I was born, near Barrie, but no one knew whether it was in Saskatchewan or Ontario."[52]

In addition to east-west rivalries, there were also rivalries between French- and English-Canadian nursing sisters within some units. As noted previously, over 99 percent of nursing sisters spoke English as either their first or second language; only 0.3 percent were unilingual francophones. With only a few exceptions, English dominated as the working language of the Canadian medical units, but cultural differences went beyond language, at times generating inequalities and precipitating prejudiced behaviour. NS Isabel Morrison completed a one-year contract with the South African Military Nursing Service and then joined the RCAMC for a posting to England, where she reunited with her twin sister, who was serving with a French-Canadian unit. Her sister felt very isolated in the unit because francophone nurses refused to speak English to her. The twins requested and received permission to room together at Leavesden Military Hospital, away from the rest of the unit. Winnipegger NS Margaret Roe recalled being "shocked" when Ontario nursing sisters used derogatory terms to refer to nurses from St. Boniface, a French community across the river from Winnipeg. Roe said, "Some of the French girls worked in our front office and at the telephone exchange; and we use to go to parties with them – in a group, you know ... They were just the French people from St. Boniface."[53]

Matron Suzanne Giroux of No. 17 CGH, initially designated as an all-French-speaking medical unit, illustrates the difficulty of maintaining a French-Canadian identity within overwhelmingly anglophone communities. Quite soon after the war began, her unit moved to England and spent a long time waiting there before Canadian forces began to move into northwestern Europe and Italy. According to her letter in the *Canadian Nurse*, the unit received much attention from a British organization whose mandate was to help "foreign groups" understand England: "We have been given very special attention and received a big box of books, all of them so interesting. They describe English life, English children, English schools, artists, musicians – a perfect choice. Beautiful original coloured prints (the kind you always want to buy and can never afford) were lent to us ... Now, if we can get a good piano, they will send us musicians and brilliant speakers. Well! It is very nice to be French-speaking in England."[54]

In addition to differences based on region, language, and culture, differing backgrounds sometimes generated tensions among the nursing sister community. Class differences played out in subtle ways, such as the use of personal and family privilege to gain entry to the military and coveted overseas postings, or to circumvent military policies. NS Carter's interview and memoir are full of anecdotes related to the myriad ways she used class privilege within the military – from modifying uniform regulations to suit her preferences for style to using family connections to obtain her discharge. Carter explained that she was unhappy with the way army-issued uniforms fit, but the matron had informed her, "'You will wear the same as everyone else whether it fits or not!' Traditionally there were only two sizes in the Army – too big and too small." So Carter waited until she got to England where she had her "greatcoat and walking out suit tailored, quietly and discreetly, as the Army seemed a place where things were done that way!" She also had special items made just for herself: a blazer for informal wear, a silk tie with the Medical Corps colours in stripes, and specially made uniform shirts to replace the "Boys Department" uniform shirts issued in Canada. Acknowledging that her new clothes were made from a darker fabric used for naval uniforms, she wrote, "The Matron was becoming more and more flexible about my uniforms being somewhat different from those of the others."[55] Carter used family influence to obtain her discharge when she was posted to a rehabilitation unit in Canada at the end of the war. Her sister's mother-in-law, Lady Kingsmill, was the widow of a Royal Canadian Navy first admiral from the First World War. Carter claimed that she used her influence to obtain an immediate discharge for her, writing: "It was a wonderful feeling to know I would be out of the Army soon, but I never dreamt it would happen the next day!"[56]

Class also manifested itself through long-standing training school rivalries, contentious relationships between matrons and nursing sisters, and differences in educational backgrounds that obscured class as a contested arena among nursing sisters. The three big nursing schools – the Montreal General Hospital, the Royal Victoria Hospital (also in Montreal), and the Toronto General Hospital – were among the oldest and most prestigious training schools. Because of their size and reputations, they received the largest number of applications and were selective with admissions.[57] Graduates of each of these schools insisted that their training and skills were the best, and in spite of shared class characteristics, they had a history of inter-school rivalry. In one of NS Carter's postings, for example, Montreal General Hospital graduates were running the unit according to their way of doing things and outnumbering the seven Royal Victoria Hospital graduates (including Carter). The Royal Victoria nurses wrangled a meeting with Matron-in-Chief Smellie during one of her visits to the unit and all requested transfers out of the unit.

Rank and postings were still other sources of rivalries and resentment that threatened to fracture the emerging perceptions of enduring community. Nursing sisters were subject to a military rank structure consisting of assistant matrons, matrons, principal matrons, and a matron-in-chief. Although most accounts portray these nursing leaders as well liked and admired, we can also glimpse less congenial situations in the nurses' accounts. NS Fletcher, for example, revealed her resentment of Matron Edna Rossiter's 1944 Royal Red Cross Award, apparently basing her criticism on a differentiation between nurses who served overseas and those who did not:

All the B.C. crowd are very amused at Rossiter's New Year's Honors R.R.C., & none of the girls who went to Italy or Africa even mentioned. Medals in this war are pretty phoney. The Boys who have to wear the 1939-43 medals call them the "spam" medal; obtained for slicing more tins of spam than anyone else – and they have been in action for years. This "stay at home" army who say they want to come over, but prefer crowns [the designations used for all ranks above nursing sister] to reverting to Nursing Sister [in order to obtain an overseas posting], amuse us all – & then they get medals for it!!![58]

Posted to England and eventually to the continent, NS Fletcher also resented the publicity paid to the "girls" who went to Sicily in 1943. She reprimanded her family for sympathizing with the nurses' hardships, revealing frontline jealousies in writing, "Glad you think that the girls in Sicily are having a hard time – they don't seem to think so – are working in palacial [sic] surroundings overlooking the straits of Messina, & are back in veils &

starched collars again. Don't bother feeling sorry for them – they are just gloating about it all. One of the #7 girls got tight the other night & informed us that if we had been any damn good they would have taken us too – so you see, life has its little difficulties."[59]

Educational backgrounds constituted yet another area of contention among nursing sisters. As the largest professional group within the nursing sister rank, nurses trained overwhelmingly in hospital apprenticeship programs, whereas most physiotherapy aides, occupational therapists, and some dieticians were university graduates.[60] NS Dean, who was a dietician, explained that relation-ships between nurses and dieticians were sometimes difficult:

> Back in those days, nurses did not go to university and they were very jealous. Let's face it. They really were. And consequently, I never talked about having been at university – ever. I mean, they might find out. But in order to be on friendly terms with them, I didn't tell them. Now is that naughty? I just felt it was important because after all I needed their assistance to make sure the food was properly served, or [that] I knew about a special diet immediately, or something like that … So when you say, did I run in to problems? I never did because I purposely never mentioned having been at university.

NS Mussallem also noticed friction between nurses and both physiotherapists and dieticians: "Some of the Sisters thought the physios and dieticians had greater respect … [T]hey were all graduates of universities and the nurses were not – or weren't at that time. And there was … not resentment, but friction shall I say. They were university graduates."

Clearly, the nursing sister community was not uniform, egalitarian, conforming, or universally supportive of its members. Based initially on shared spaces and shared experiences as women, nurses, and soldiers, it endured in spite of diversity and dissension within the rank, partially because it was embedded within the much larger and dominant male military community, and partially because of the isolation of nurses from previous relationships. Many nursing sisters transformed these temporary relationships into a postwar symbolic community within which they could maintain identities as military nurses, participate in meaningful public service activities, and create a social memory of nursing sisters – and others did not.

Postwar Disruptions and Community

The European war ended abruptly, following an intensive build-up of Allied troops for the Normandy invasion and a surprisingly rapid withdrawal of German troops. Demobilization, the process of closing units and releasing military personnel from the armed forces, proceeded cautiously for at least two reasons. First, there was still war in the Pacific theatre, with a request for Canadian volunteers to serve there, and one-third of the serving Canadian military nurses volunteered for this Pacific campaign. Some of them, such as NS Mussallem, were already in Vancouver for staging when, suddenly and unexpectedly, two atomic bombs brought about a swift end to the war. Second, the Canadian government was acutely aware of the potential for social, economic, and political unrest related to a rapid return of large numbers of demobilized soldiers, based on First World War experiences and unemployment crises during the Great Depression. Thus, the military developed a discharge priority system based on "points" accumulated in the service.[61] Soldiers were assigned to repatriation units located in England and underwent a variety of rehabilitation assessments while waiting to return to Canada. Medical units closed more slowly than combat units, as they still needed to care for recovering patients and their evacuations, first to England and then to Canada. The last Canadian medical units left Europe by 15 May 1946.[62]

Almost half of the nursing sisters served in the armed forces between three and six years. Many described their time in the armed forces as exciting, challenging, and rewarding. Without any hesitation, all of those interviewed for this research counted their military service as one of the highlights of their lives. Like Margaret Allemang, Frances Ferguson Sutherland, and Helen Mussallem, many said the experience changed their lives completely – providing educational and travel opportunities never before anticipated. NS Lamont felt "protected" in the RCAMC, with everyone "focused on one common goal." She also felt central to the main events of the war, being posted overseas. As she said, "You still were on that high roll of adventure ... Sure we had a hard life, but we were in the middle of it. It's better to be in the middle of things. It takes more courage to be on the outside and look in, and your imagination is far worse than the real thing." Although NS Carter took matters into her own hands to obtain her discharge, she still wrote, "You were leaving good friends you had been with for a long while ... It was like losing your family. Being sent out into civilian life, into a crowd of strangers, or even people you knew but hadn't seen in a long while, was frightening, as was the expectation of freedom. We hadn't made our own decisions since going into the Army!"[63]

With the war ended, nursing sisters lost both legitimacy as military nurses and status as military officers, along with the associated rights and privileges. After having their lives planned and orchestrated for years, they were supposed to "get on with their lives." But the civilian world was no longer familiar or desirable for many of them. They spoke and wrote about being restless or having a tough time personally and professionally after the war. NS Mabel Glew wrote, "I'd been four years over there – and it was a different life entirely. You came back here and you'd be amazed how hard it was to get back. They (the people at home) didn't know anything about war ... They didn't realize what we had been through. I was a nervous wreck when I got back."[64]

Similarly, few nurses knew or understood changes that had taken place in civilian contexts while they were away. As NS Van Scoyoc explained, "My family knows very little about my life experiences overseas, and I know not too much about what went on in Canada while I was away. Sort of a blank period."[65] NS Anne Gair wrote, "I felt lonely and found I missed my Army friends very much and I missed the active life I had had."[66] NS Margaret Mills "felt very flat. There was nothing more to see or do. The excitement had all gone."[67] NS Ruth Littlejohn was "scattered" and "at loose ends," with no sense of place.[68] Some, such as NS Louise Jamieson, returned to very different family circumstances: Jamieson's mother and grandparents had died, her brother was killed during the war, and her father had moved to a different house. In her search for a place to belong and perhaps a place to escape, she tried outpost nursing, considered joining the United Nations Relief and Rehabilitation Administration, applied to the World Health Organization, and then went to India for two years.[69]

Nurses talked frequently about being transformed personally by the war. As she approached her discharge, NS Fletcher tried to prepare her family for some of the changes they might notice in her. As she wrote,

You see we live in the midst of people who live high & sleep in slit trenches – & coming home to a family that is too prim & proper would be an awful shock. No – I haven't taken to "wine, men & song," but have learned to make the most of short opportunities. It will be difficult to settle down to an ordered life, where things are planned – & everyone in uniform doesn't accept you as a long lost friend at sight. It really will be a trifle lonesome for a while – no doubt."[70]

NS Van Scoyoc felt she had become too independent to fit into her former life again. Her family thought she was "ahead of her time" regarding the choice to remain single but, as she explained, "If I could have found someone that would have allowed me to do what I wanted to do, then probably I would have married. But I never met that individual."[71] Some nurses, such as NS Potts, expressed regrets about *not* getting married, saying, "I would probably have married, if I hadn't gone to the war ... I felt I had to go on and do more and more ... One man that I knew very well was killed in Israel ... He was a very fine person too. But, as you go on in years, it doesn't mean anything any more, you look back and say, 'Ah, I could have been married and had children by now.' I don't think of that any more at all."[72] Others, such as NS Bower, expressed regrets about *getting married* during the war. She suggested that if there had been adequate counselling, she might not have made poor choices, which led to a "marriage break up" and subsequent difficult life supporting three small children on her own: "I believe that at that time, I was just so homesick and the invasion had been on for quite some time. And the buzz bombs were going ... and all the frustrations of the war. I think that if I had had counselling, I would never have married."

The first troops to return to Canada received warm welcomes and much public attention. But nursing sisters were discharged later and under different circumstances from combat troops. They often worked during the homeward journey as well, caring for returning casualties or war brides and their children. NS Bond, along with many others, resented their inferior accommodations on these voyages: "We came back with a group of English war brides and their babies who were in first and second class and we were in steerage."[73] NS Lamont cared for a group of thirty war brides and twelve children under five years old, from England to Halifax, with the assistance of another nursing sister and a Red Cross worker. According to Lamont, the Red Cross worker went to bed for two weeks and "never lifted a finger" while the ship struggled through a severe North Atlantic storm. She said, "Those poor women and the babies! And somebody asked if I was seasick, and I said, 'I guess I must have been the first day, but we didn't have time. We were so busy all the time.' So we got to Halifax and I remember how tired I was." The war brides were welcomed warmly, but the nursing sisters were neither welcomed nor acknowledged: "Here was a big banner, Welcome to Canada, for the war brides. And there was hot coffee and donuts, and they got a wonderful welcome. We were left on the dock with our luggage there. Nobody said 'boo' to us. Until these two or three boys, soldiers, came and said, 'What can we do for you sisters?' And they helped us – took our luggage, took us to the train." NS Van Scoyoc had similar experiences, thinking it "very odd" that they didn't get the same kind of welcome earlier troops had received on their return and saying, "Maybe the public was tired of it."[74]

Some nursing sisters were reposted to military hospitals and rehabilitation centers across Canada to care for soldiers during the immediate postwar period until DVA hospitals could accommodate them. Others applied to the permanent forces, transferred to DVA hospitals as civil servants, or used this interim period to plan for the rest of their lives. While some nurses sought opportunities for travel, adventure, and autonomy similar to those experienced in the military, others wanted to leave the military life behind them. NS Elizabeth Pense was a member of the permanent forces prior to the war and ultimately served a total of twenty-one years. Even with permanent force status and years of service, she explained that the military took measures after the war to constrain her authority and privilege by posting her where she would pose little threat to the male hierarchy. She said, "They didn't quite know what to do with me, because I was the only overseas sister there. But they were going to make sure I wasn't throwing my weight around, so after the first few months, I was put in charge of the isolation hospital, and I loved that because I was all by myself and had the running of the place."[75] For NS Eileen MacGregor, postwar civilian work was "tedious and menial."[76] NS Roe wasn't ready to make decisions on her future at discharge but after a brief interval, she re-enlisted for one and a half years in the permanent

forces. The experience was not what she expected, however, and she soon
felt postwar military nursing was a "dead-end" for her. NS Allemang knew
right away that she was ready to get out of the air force: "I wasn't finding
it too much to my liking ... I think I was tired of the life and I decided if I
never went to another party, it would be too soon."[77] And NS Fletcher wrote
her family to "have the crystal pool all clear & a red evening dress ready. I'm
aiming to forget khaki."[78]

The Second World War nursing sisters had expected some form of
welcome, some recognition for their service, time to make the transition back
to civilian contexts, and a place where they might process the war experience,
possibly with some counselling. Instead, their community dispersed, and
they became invisible in the postwar world. According to NS Lamont, "I
don't think [the Canadian public] knew what to make of us, to tell you the
truth ... We didn't talk about it. Nobody was interested ... I'm not blaming
them – they just couldn't connect. So they really couldn't visualize what went
on over there ... I never opened my mouth until 1994 – literally ... But the
minute we got with war buddies, oh boy."

Shaping a Symbolic Community

The Nursing Sisters' Association of Canada was one of the logical places
where nursing sisters sought support from "war buddies." In April 1920, First
World War nursing sisters in Edmonton formed a club for military nurses
who had served overseas, in order to "continue a fellowship which was
peculiar to those who served overseas during the Great War, and to help one
another should the occasion arise."[79] Similar clubs emerged across Canada,
and by 1927 at the International Congress of Nurses at Montreal (1929) they
organized nationally as the All Canada Nursing Sisters Association. Renamed
the Overseas Nursing Sisters Association, this national body met biennially,
concurrent with the Canadian Nurses Association. Primary concerns at the
first national meeting in 1932 included nurses' employment, medical and
hospital care, and assistance to individual members – reflecting both the
dearth of nursing employment during the Depression and the absence of
social welfare programs for the unemployed.

During the Second World War, the Overseas Nursing Sisters Association
(ONSA), comprising veteran military nurses who had served outside of
Canada, was active in raising funds for the war effort and in continuing
support for serving military nurses, as well as relief support for British civilian
nurses who were suffering heavily during the war due to the bombing of
England as well as the rationing system and nursing personnel shortages.[80]
Sometime between 1944 and 1946, the organization dropped the requirement
for overseas service and changed its name to the Nursing Sisters' Association
of Canada (NSAC) while extending membership to "all Nursing Sisters
honourably discharged from the three military services." But dieticians,

physiotherapist aides, occupational therapists, and home sisters who had served as nursing sisters only became eligible for membership in 1960.[81] The NSAC affiliated officially with the Royal Canadian Legion in 1944, beginning a long association that proved instrumental in shaping the commemoration and social memory of military nurses. The thirty-fifth and final national biennial meeting was held in 2000 at Toronto, with eleven active units and 636 members, including military nurses who had served since the Second World War. Several local units continue to meet.

Many returning nursing sisters looked to this organization and the first generation of military nurses as a way to remain connected to one another. The NSAC held local "Welcome Home" parties and sent out letters of invitation to join the association. Several units extended free memberships for the first year and hosted returning nurses as speakers for their meetings. The Hamilton unit was eager for new leaders: "The present executive have carried on for many years, the unit having few members. With new and younger nurses joining the unit it is planned to pass the reins of office on to them at the annual meeting."[82] NS Jessie Morrison wrote that the Edmonton unit "opened ranks and received us warmly ... I believe ten of us joined that night."[83] Over the next six decades, the NSAC was instrumental in shaping the collective social memory of Canadian military nurses. It became the primary structure through which members communicated with one another and organized to represent the interests of military nursing to the public. In 1975, journalist Lotta Dempsey described the organization as a "sisterhood, forged in on-the-spot blood, sweat and tears," where "there's really no space for outsiders. Even husbands."[84]

For those nursing sisters who did not remain in active nursing practice, the association served to link them to both the ex-military and professional nursing communities through biennial meetings, newsletters, directories, and fundraising activities. They used these gatherings for social networking, as well as for activism in support of veterans' benefits, relief to countries affected by the war, political activism, and the advancement of military nursing. As NS Kay Poulton noted, "The friends I made are still my friends and even though we're scattered all over the country, we all try to keep in touch with each other [through the association's newsletters and directories]."[85] The NSAC network was so extensive that, according to NS Van Scoyoc, "There isn't a city or part of the country that I could visit, that I wouldn't know someone whom I could just phone and just say, 'I'm here. Let's get together.'" For some veteran military nurses, this nursing sister community provided an important social support network within a larger society where military nurses were no longer visible or needed. NS Nicolson explained: "We never talked about our wartime experience ... Just when we were together with veterans and our pals; and we would visit each other regularly, and we always had that close bond, that fellowship. Always. Still to this day." Members of the NSAC met regularly at the local and national levels; they frequently kept in contact via newsletters and telephone in-between meetings. In these ways, community worked not only to form a supportive and safe place in which to recall and reflect on experiences but also to shape a common memory of events as well as a public memory by which they wanted to be remembered.

Periodically, local units reported on their activities to the wider nursing body through the *Canadian Nurse*. They informed the broader nursing profession in Canada about individual members, their activities, and, ultimately, their members' deaths. Local units hosted returning military nurses; held bridge parties, teas, and picnics; visited veterans in DVA hospitals; sent relief packages overseas; met for annual vesper services in May and Remembrance Day dinners in November; volunteered together for Red Cross projects; collected and mailed uniforms to British and European nurses after the war; raised funds for the "rehabilitation of nurses in devastated countries"; participated in wreath-laying ceremonies at cenotaphs; and more. The Toronto unit organized as a group to join the Blue Cross Hospital Plan sponsored by the Ontario Hospital Service Association, thus assisting their membership to obtain hospital insurance.[86]

Local and national directories constituted another important link for members of the NSAC community. The 1958 membership directory includes the names of nursing sisters from sixteen units, with histories of each unit, a list of presidents, and important information for veterans regarding rights and benefits related to health care. At least 670 Second World War nurses were included in that edition. The directory listed each nurse's rank, decorations, address, service branch, and dates of service, as well as an unclear category called occupational code.[87] Later, a combined commemorative issue and national directory was published for the fiftieth anniversary of D-Day (June 1994). The final national directory was published in May 2000, commemorating the eightieth anniversary of the NSAC.

These organizational structures served to keep the community informed and connected. They also shaped a collective social memory by regulating what was included in and excluded from the organizational reports, newsletters, and directories – as well as whose voices were included or excluded. This collective social memory portrays the nursing sisters as a benevolent community whose members worked and socialized together on behalf of war's casualties, primarily for improvement in the care of and benefits for veterans as well as relief aid for nurses and nursing education in Europe. During the 1960s and 1970s, the association engaged in limited political activism, mounting a letter-writing campaign to protest "the change of the flag and proposed demotion of medals conferred for military service" and presenting a brief to the Parliamentary Committee on Veterans Affairs requesting that a nursing sister be appointed to the Pensions Commission.

Symbolic communities increase in importance as actual geo-social boundaries are undermined, blurred, or otherwise weakened – in this case, as nursing sisters dispersed after the war.[88] They no longer shared physical spaces; they seldom shared social spaces outside of commemorative occasions or biennial NSAC meetings. Their presence in the *Canadian Nurse* diminished with time, except for annual Remembrance Day features. Those who chose to maintain a military nursing identity found the NSAC a key resource. Through its official status as the voice of Canadian military nurses, the association and its leaders exerted substantial influence over the way in which the Second World War nursing sisters were commemorated and, thereby, the way in which social memory was created.

Commemoration and Social Memory

Historians Jay Winter and Jonathan Vance point out that the social construction of both commemoration and memory is as much about forgetting as it is about remembering.[89] Nursing sisters always existed in relation to groups of military men (medical officers, medical orderlies, and patients), and they all but disappeared from the armed forces and from Second World War social memory, especially mainstream histories and commemorations. Military nursing, like the armed forces in general, lost social approval during the 1960s and 1970s, when anti-war sentiments prevailed through much of North America. And as we have seen, military nurses were seldom considered by historians. In response, the NSAC collaborated with the Canadian Nurses Association to produce its own organizational history, and linked up with male veterans' groups to enhance the visibility of nursing sisters by way of participation in commemorative projects.

Commemoration, social memory, and the creation of a symbolic community are interrelated processes. Through commemoration, a group or society recalls an event or person(s) using specific images and discourse that have been consciously selected, usually to attribute respect or honour for that event or person(s). Commemoration can take the form of rituals such as celebrations, pilgrimages, or religious ceremonies. It includes symbols such as awards and medals, as well as the creation of material culture such as monuments, buildings, and architectural features, the naming of topographical features, and a variety of other artifacts. Commemoration both reflects and shapes the shared values, beliefs, meanings, and moral codes of a symbolic community. As nursing sisters' decisions about commemoration will illustrate, the shaping process may also be contested and negotiated.

Social memory, or "shared narrative," is constructed both within a community and outside it – that is, the symbolic community has both a private and a public face. There are particular images that a community desires to reinforce to the general public view, as well as shared private memories restricted exclusively to insiders of the community. The bonds of sisterhood have been relatively effective in protecting private memories from becoming public ones. Interaction among members, who contest, validate, and corroborate past events and interpretations of those events, shapes both the public and private narratives. Among the various documentaries, interviews, and written anecdotes provided by various nursing sisters, for example, there are surprisingly similar stories and themes. The language and portrayals are remarkably consistent regardless of settings, as if experiences have been well polished in the telling and retelling. One such story involves a nurse asleep in the lower bunk of a transport craft crossing the English Channel at night when it hit an object, causing a bucket of water on the floor to spill. The nurse is purported to have felt the water and yelled, "Girls, we will have to swim for it." Another example is NS Kay Christie's account of her experience in Hong Kong. Christie left several audiotaped interviews and written accounts of her POW experience. Although created from 1967 to 1992, these accounts are very consistent in terms of content and tone. Likewise, nursing sisters typically describe their patients as "very brave" and "wonderful boys," their medical orderlies as very helpful and supportive, and their medical officers as collegial, although as this study shows there was actually a range of behaviour among both soldiers and medical officers.

Jay Winter argues that the proliferation of images, metaphors, and discourses related to bereavement and commemoration after the First World War did not recur after the Second World War: "After Hiroshima and Auschwitz, the earlier commemorative effort simply could not be duplicated ... The Second World War helped to put an end to the rich set of traditional languages of commemoration and mourning which flourished after the Great War."[90] One of the ways to examine social memory is to consider what a community commemorates and how it does so, as well as what it chooses not to commemorate.[91] Although First World War nursing sisters were never subjects of commemoration or material memory to the extent that military men were, the social memory created around their experiences certainly exceeded that of Second World War military nurses: the women interviewed for this research confirmed that there was a profound silence after the Second World War.

The first generation of nursing sisters has been the primary focus of Canadian military nursing social memory. Ordinary women were not typically portrayed in public statues and monuments, partially because ordinary women did not die as a direct result of military involvement. But forty-six Canadian nursing sisters did die during the First World War, and the public was particularly enraged over the bombing of hospitals in France and the sinking of hospital ships that caused the deaths of twenty-one of them. It was their nursing colleagues, however, who raised the funds to commission the Canadian Nurses Association War Memorial and negotiated its location in the Hall of Honour of the Centre Block of Ottawa's Parliament Buildings in 1926.[92] This memorial has remained the only nursing symbol of its kind in Canada, and one of only two commemorations created for the Hall of Honour. The National War Memorial, unveiled at Ottawa in 1939, includes two nursing sisters among the twenty-two figures portrayed. Both memorials were subjects of further debate during the 1940s, related to decisions about the commemoration of the Second World War nurses.

First World War nursing sisters were commemorated in several other ways. Three individuals were honoured with the naming of a hospital wing, a hospital, and a mountain in their memories. There are at least four stained glass memorial windows in churches or chapels and a massive war art panel held (but not displayed) by the Canadian War Museum, titled *Third Canadian Stationary Hospital, France* by Gerald E. Moira, which depict nursing sisters.[93] The multi-volume set of Books of Remembrance kept within the Memorial Chamber of the Peace Tower on Parliament Hill, lists the names of Canadian nursing sisters who died in the line of duty. And the city of Saskatoon created living memorials in 1923, consecrating trees in memory of Canadians who had died during the war. One bears a simple plaque that reads "In Grateful Tribute to the memory of the 14 nursing Sisters who furished [sic] on the Llandovery Castle – A NURSE."[94]

By contrast, second-generation nursing sisters have remained relatively silent and invisible within social memory, whether it was because few people were interested in their experiences after the war, or because there were no adequate means to express their collective experience. There are no statues, hospital wings, or public buildings named in their honour, not even a memorial tree. Those who died during the war are included in the Books of Remembrance, and a recently erected Manitoulin Women's Memorial cenotaph includes one portion dedicated to Canadian nursing sisters. The Royal Canadian Military Institute at Toronto named a meeting room in honour of NS Kay Christie. On a far less public level, a Second World War nursing sister is represented in one panel of a memorial window at Hart House, at the University of Toronto, and in a song that none of the nursing sisters seem to have ever heard. Individually, some nursing sisters received recognition through various commemorative military awards and decorations.

Two little-known portrayals of nursing sisters appeared during and just after the war. In the spring of 1944, during the build up to D-Day, the *Canadian Nurse* published a small reproduction of a Victory Bond poster that bore the image of a nursing sister. It is difficult to know how this poster was distributed or just who the target audience might have been, but it is embedded with stereotypical messages about women, femininity, military service, and safety. It portrays the head and shoulders of an innocent-looking young military nurse wearing a billowing white veil and blue silk uniform, with an intense look of concern on her face. The caption simply read, "Now, more than ever … Buy Victory Bonds."

When the poster appeared in the *Canadian Nurse*, the accompanying text targeted nurses on several levels. Not only were nursing sisters portrayed as serving in danger "on land and sea and in the air," but civilian nurses were reminded that they worked at home in safety and, therefore, in debt to serving military nurses. Nurses were urged to invest in Victory Bonds, recalling their recent experiences during the Depression, now that there was "time to tuck away a dollar or two for a rainy day when jobs might be harder to find." They were admonished to sacrifice and invest towards a future home with "your own fireside." But most of all, they were to build up a savings account to furnish a home because, "when the war is over and *he* comes back from overseas, a new life will begin for many young Canadian nurses. There will be a house to build, gay curtains, cups and saucers, pots and pans to buy, all the things that go to make a home. It won't be as easy then to build up the savings account that every young couple ought to have. *Buy victory bonds!*"[95] There are at least three, interrelated messages apparent in the poster and accompanying text: a safety/danger discourse, a reminder of nurses' precarious economic situation, and a highly heterosexist discourse on femininity. It was assumed that a single woman would remain a burden to others and be unable to provide for her own needs. It was equally assumed that marriage would bring not only a man into her life but also material goods with which to create the "good life."

In a second portrayal of military nurses, John Murray Gibbon wrote lyrics for a song about nursing sisters, published in 1946.[96] Gibbon's image of the military nurse, however, bore little resemblance to reality. His nurse was a "Fairy Queen": ethereal, flitting around the tent of a casualty clearing station, or sitting by the soldier's bed. She relieved pain with soothing hands and drugs, and "wafted" care away. The Gibbon nurse did not wear heavy army boots or the same khaki shirt for days on end without an adequate water supply to launder it. Apparently, she did not evacuate hundreds of casualties while preparing to receive the next arrivals, for she had time to sit at the bedside. She was someone who flitted around rather than a competent, highly skilled professional. Her patients found her "irresistible," as she was, first and foremost, highly feminine.

The NSAC assumed that when official accounts of the war appeared, these histories would include nursing sisters. At its 1954 annual meeting, the association vetoed a proposal to commission a military nursing history, noting that "there would undoubtedly be historical material re the services of nursing sisters included in histories presently being compiled which would be adequate for all general purposes." The membership generally felt that the costs of publication and the subsequent purchasing cost for individuals would be prohibitive, if such an account were written exclusively for the nursing services.[97] By 1972, however, realizing that history was passing them by, the NSAC reconsidered their earlier decision and commissioned an organizational history by military historian Colonel G.W.L. Nicholson for $10,000. With four chapters on the Second World War nurses, Nicholson's history has been the main published account of Canadian nursing sisters. While many commend the book for its military aspects, individual nursing sisters suggest that it doesn't reflect their own experiences. NS Patricia Moll, for example, had collected "a great deal of material" from the Quebec units for Nicholson's research, including diaries, photos, and papers. But she claimed that Nicholson did not use the majority of this material, which represented rank-and-file nurses, saying "he only used incidentals from the lot we contributed." Everyday nursing practice and rank-and-file nurses are barely visible in this account. The situation is remarkably similar for Australian, British, and American military nurses.

Partially due to lack of interest from women's groups and feminist historians, nursing sisters, rather than pass into obscurity, aligned their quest for social memory more closely with men's wartime experiences. They adopted military portrayals and participated in veterans' activities. As members of the Veterans Association of Canada, nursing sisters participate in Remembrance Day activities at local and national cenotaphs in their regions; they still serve as ceremonial sentries, march in veterans' parades, attend vespers and church services as veteran representatives, and make presentations at local schools. More recently, they have served on a variety of veterans' committees.

Beginning with the thirtieth anniversaries of D-Day (1974) and the end of the Italian campaign (1975), nursing sisters participated in numerous commemoration trips, also referred to as "pilgrimages," to various battle sites. NS Jean MacAulay was an official delegate for the fifty-fifth anniversary of D-Day; NS Shirley Kelly went on the official pilgrimage to Hong Kong; NS Mary Hutton accompanied male veterans to France to repatriate the remains of Canada's unknown soldier; and NS Lois Bayly Tewsley represented Canadian nursing sisters at Juno Beach as part of the fundraising campaign to build a Canadian memorial there.[98] Interestingly, none of these women were involved in the events commemorated: they represent the perspectives of men who are veterans and the focus on "great battles" or watershed moments in the grand narratives of Canadian history. I found no commemoration of events that nurses might have perceived as significant, such as NS Christie and Water's prisoner of war experiences, or NS Wilkie's death in Newfoundland, or extraordinary services rendered in treating and evacuating thousands of soldiers within twelve to twenty-four hours, or thirty-two-hours stretches on duty in operating rooms, or nurses on the torpedoed *Santa Elena*, or the first-flight nurses to land in Normandy after D-Day.

Fiftieth anniversaries generated renewed public interest in Second World War commemoration during the 1990s. More recently, as sixtieth anniversaries approached and Second World War veterans continued to decrease in number, mainstream military historians demonstrated considerable urgency to enlarge museums and military collections. This urgency has resulted in the production of two documentaries on Canadian nursing sisters and one feature film with a supporting Canadian nursing sister character, as well as a perennial interest in nursing sisters during Remembrance Day, or Remembrance Week, activities.[99] This collective social memory, created in conjunction with veterans' associations, represents a sanitized universal narrative of war seen primarily through the experiences of men.

Social memory of Second World War nursing sisters within the nursing community has been shaped somewhat differently. Nursing sisters left relatively little material memory (such as public monuments) partially because they had fewer resources with which to create it, but also because they made different decisions regarding what to commemorate, and how to commemorate it. Public structures typically required large financial investments and considerable political influence – neither readily available within the nursing profession. Their first deliberations concerned modifications to the 1926 Canadian Nurses' Memorial to reflect the addition of a second generation of nursing sisters. The CNA appointed a War Memorial Committee in 1946 to consider how to commemorate nursing sisters who had died during the Second World War as well as "all Canadian nurses who had served in the armed forces." The committee initially felt that the existing Nurses' Memorial in the Hall of Honour would be appropriate and no further memorial necessary if they could add the names of nurses who died along with the total number of nurses who served in the armed forces during the Second World War.[100] The Minister of Public Works denied their request to add a carved plaque below the central figure of the Hall of Honour memorial, on the basis that any addition of that nature would "detract from its chaste dignity" and destroy its original intent. They then proposed simply engraving dates signifying each war period on either side of the central figure, but instability in world events caused the nurses to hesitate. As they reported in 1948, "in view of the present unsettled state of world affairs, this committee recommends that this project be abandoned ... and all moneys concentrated on the living memorial."[101] Perhaps the ominous uncertainty that accompanied the early days of the Cold War era left the committee pondering where the next set of dates could be engraved – and, indeed, the military called upon nurses again during the Korean War.

Through fundraising endeavours, donations, and bequests from members' estates, the NSAC did accumulate considerable assets over time. They chose, however, to invest these funds in less visible, non-material ways that did not necessarily leave traces in the form of a public social memory. After negotiations with the Minister of Public Works failed, the War Memorial Committee suggested a different type of tribute that would benefit members of the nursing profession in "war-torn countries" and have "lasting value." The NSAC then decided to establish a Rehabilitation Fund in support of nurses in "devastated countries," which they used for various overseas relief efforts including contributions to a Red Cross convalescent care facility for nurses in Geneva, Switzerland. Together with the CNA, they created education scholarships and loans that were available only to military nurses initially, but later to all Canadian nurses.[102]

The jointly sponsored NSAC-CNA "living memorial" project consisted of professional literature and educational material intended to provide nursing resources in countries disrupted during the war and to support re-establishment of nursing and the provision of health care. Each Canadian province had a quota for the fund based on membership in its professional nursing organization. By the fall of 1947, the committee had raised $22,701.58 for this living memorial. For its part, the *Canadian Nurse* donated fifty complimentary subscriptions for one year; the War Memorial Committee renewed those subscriptions for three additional years. The committee used the fund to purchase and ship libraries comprising fifty nursing textbooks to each of twenty countries: Austria, Belgium, Bulgaria, China, Czechoslovakia, Denmark, Finland, France, Germany, Greece, Hungary, Italy, Japan, Korea, the Netherlands, Norway, Philippines, Poland, Romania, and Yugoslavia.

In light of the substantial funds raised by nurses for these living memorials, lack of money does not appear to be a main barrier to more visible material commemorations. Instead, CNA and NSAC decisions were consistent with prevailing expectations among nurses and international nursing organizations regarding "service to others." A growing internationalism among women had emerged during the second half of the nineteenth century, taking root particularly within groups striving for the recognition of British nurses as professionals during the early 1900s. The leadership overlapped between groups associated with women's internationalism and nursing professionalization, partially as a result of a perception that they held common interests. Women's internationalism built on an understanding of gender as a unifying bond that superseded national and cultural boundaries. The overlap in interests and leadership is best exemplified through the International Council of Nurses (ICN), established in 1899. The ICN maintained a curious tension between "intense nationalism," with membership based on the principle of one professional organization per country, and nursing internationalism, wherein professional identity was supposed to transcend national identities. Indeed, Ethel Gordon Fenwick, founder of the British Nurses Association and key instigator for the International Council of Nurses, claimed that "there is no nationality in nursing."[103] This uneasy tension between nationalism and internationalism was particularly problematic during periods of war, when nurses responded to calls for military nursing service on national levels. Across Europe, national identities fractured professional unities, as did decisions regarding militarism versus pacifism.

Early ICN leaders, like those of other women's organizations of the period, often espoused pacifist ideologies, although, "officially, the ICN never advocated a pacifist position in relation to war," and pacifism was reportedly a minority perspective within the council.[104] When the CNA recommended in 1937 that the ICN "sponsor and support measures for the promotion of world peace and control of armaments," the suggestion was contested by the larger membership, and Canadian nurse Grace Fairley had to withdraw the recommendation. It was only after the Second World War that a new internationalism emerged that took a more activist stance in support of peace efforts and international relief work.[105]

A second way that the NSAC chose to commemorate their own contributions to the war was through education scholarships for military nurses, named after Matron-in-Chief Agnes Neill, the senior nursing sister officer at the end of the war.[106] Neill bequeathed $1,000 to the NSAC on her death in 1950, "to benefit nurses who have served or are serving in the RCAMS." Her two sisters matched that amount and individual NSAC units raised an additional $5,000, for a total of $7,000 to establish the Agnes C. Neill Memorial Fund. Initial terms stipulated that monies were for further education, hospital care for veteran nurses, and life membership grants. The CNA agreed to administer the fund. The first scholarship from the fund went to Second World War NS Janet Wallace at the June 1960 biennial meeting in Halifax. Criteria varied over the years, as fewer and fewer nursing sisters applied, and in 1970 it became a Canadian Nurses' Foundation bursary for which all Canadian nurses are eligible. The scholarship was a product of the nursing professional elite, donated by a well-known and respected leader and administered by other leaders through the CNA. Although many nursing sisters did take postgraduate courses after the war, most of them came from teaching, supervisory, or administrative positions and only a small proportion were rank-and-file (bedside) nurses.

Decisions regarding the CNA War Memorial, the living memorials, and the Agnes Neill award were initiatives taken by nurses to commemorate their colleagues. Public recognition was limited to the awarding of military medals, a type of commemoration associated primarily with military men. But nurses shared only in the campaign awards and stars, as well as length of service awards: the Canadian Volunteer Service Medal, the Defence Medal, the War Medal 1939-45, the 1939-45 Star, and the individual campaign stars for Italy, France, and Germany, and the Pacific – contingent on postings to those theatres. Instead of the decorations for valour that men received, nursing sisters were eligible for only two awards specially created for women. Queen Victoria had created the Royal Red Cross, First Class in 1883 and designated it as an award for fully trained nurses only. The Associate Royal Red Cross, also known as the Royal Red Cross, Second Class, was added in 1915 and designated for either trained or assistant nurses. These decorations were intended for demonstrated (and documented) "exceptional devotion and competency in the performance of actual nursing duties, over a continuous and long period" or "some very exceptional act of bravery and devotion at her post of duty."[107] During the Second World War, 71 Canadian nursing sisters received the Royal Red Cross, 4 received Bars to the Royal Red Cross, 311 received the Associate Royal Red Cross, and more than 100 nurses were "Mentioned in Despatches" – an internal military honour. One nursing sister, RCN Dietician Margaret Brooke, received the Order of the British Empire for heroism in trying to save the life of NS Agnes Wilkie when a German submarine sank the SS *Caribou* off the coast of Newfoundland.[108] But the nursing sisters themselves frequently indicated that they didn't know how or why nurses were selected to receive these awards. NS Dorothy Macham received the Associate Royal Red Cross decoration while in Italy and later claimed, "I had no idea what this was for. It must have come up in the rations that day ... I never knew why."[109] But in actual practice, overseas matrons typically received the Royal Red Cross and assistant matrons received the Associate Royal Red Cross because of responsibilities associated with supervising nursing care in medical units. The choices often failed to represent those whom the rank-and-file nursing sisters thought deserved the honour.

Beyond these official forms of commemoration and social memory, the Second World War nursing sisters do have personal private memories often supplemented by diaries or notes kept over the years. They also retained such mementos as entire uniforms, or pieces of the uniform such as a veil, their awards and commissions, poetry written by or about nursing sisters, playbills and luncheon menus, a few photographs, and occasionally a piece of equipment such as a canvas basin or field dressing. At least one nursing sister came home with a German sword, while another kept a piece of shrapnel from a patient. These items constitute the bulk of their personal material memory.

Material memory, social memory, and commemoration reflect a range of self-perceptions held by the nursing sisters community. During the immediate postwar period, the nursing profession portrayed nursing sisters as leaders, featuring them in the "Nurses to Know" section of the *Canadian Nurse* with descriptions of their military awards and decorations as well as their immediate civilian appointments or educational achievements. Within a few years, they disappeared into civilian life for the most part, except for occasional features in November issues associated with Remembrance Day. More interest developed during the late 1980s and 1990s within the profession and, to a very small extent, within women's history as feminists sought to recover some women from obscurity. These interests resulted in oral history collections and preservation efforts that included several nursing sisters, such as the Concordia University Oral History Project at Montreal in the mid-1980s and another oral history collection, "Nurses and Their Work," at the Provincial Archives of Manitoba.[110] Within the nursing discipline, renewed interests at the provincial level led to the creation of oral history projects in British Columbia and Ontario that included small cohorts of nursing sisters in the respective collections.[111]

More recently, the nursing sisters community has participated with journalists in the construction of another type of social memory, the portrayal of nursing sisters as agents of change, reluctant warriors, and heroines, and sometimes as feminists who broke gender barriers. This construction has sometimes represented military nursing as a calling, without acknowledging tensions or contradictions in caring for lives within the context of war, when innumerable lives will inevitably be lost. These journalistic accounts tend to avoid discussions of rivalries or dissensions among nursing sisters past or present, as well as the myriad forms of danger, risk, unpleasantness, and grief that were part of the war. They also avoid any hint of sexuality other than married, heterosexual relationships that were socially sanctioned at the time. For the most part, the community also downplays power inequalities – portraying military men and women, physicians and nurses, as equals. They speak of the military as breaking down gendered stereotypes and providing new opportunities for women, rather than as a system that reinforced gendered roles like military nursing.

During the Second World War, civilian nurses joined the Canadian armed forces and created a distinctly female community embedded within a large male military system. They legitimated the creation of this community by the need for nurses' skills in the military, and based it initially on shared physical and social spaces. But their community was temporary, gendered, and contingent on a state of war for its existence. Removed from their prewar social and professional networks, military nurses forged a different set of relationships that ultimately shifted their experience as a community from shared physical settings to a mental construct that endured across time and space.

With the cessation of war, this community dispersed, and nursing sisters sought to relocate themselves in civilian settings. Many of them also sought to re-create the nursing sisters community as a symbolic imagined community serving as a resource, a repository of meaning, and extended sisterhood. Through the community, they shaped a unified public image and social memory congruent with prevailing forms of male war commemoration. They continue to struggle for at least a small presence within veterans' groups, military museums, and historical records in spite of a paucity of material memory. As NS Jessie Morrison reminded a 1974 audience, however, "The branches of the tree are becoming bare. Hopefully there won't be a new crop of leaves. By the terms of our membership this necessitates war – and we don't want that ... We hope that when all the leaves have fallen there will be something of substance left behind for the enrichment of future generations. We hope they might read our records and learn from them that life's greatest rewards are found in giving service to others."[112] It was within this symbolic community that nursing sisters made, or believed they made, meaning out of their nursing experiences during times of war.

Conclusion

In order to fulfill society's expectation that sick and wounded soldiers during the Second World War would be well cared for, the Canadian armed forces looked to the civilian nursing profession to "fill the ranks" and serve alongside an almost non-existent, permanent force military nursing service. It was expedient to rely on the civilian profession to train nurses and provide them with the necessary professional credentials; the armed forces thus economized by avoiding the cost of that training and the expense of maintaining nurses during peace time. Civilian nurses "saved" the military by their overwhelming rush to enlist and by their willingness to deliver nursing care to the frontlines. Yet the military also "saved" hundreds of nurses who needed regular, full-time, decently paid work after almost a decade of underemployment associated with the Great Depression.

Gender shaped all aspects of military nursing during the Second World War. One cannot overlook the obvious construction of the nursing sister rank as a unique all-female military workforce, or the deliberate construction of nursing as women's work and combat as men's work. Gender was a pervasive, mediating variable that shaped who could serve as nurses, where they served and under what conditions, the duration of that service, what roles they could assume, and the expectations that both the military and Canadian society held with respect to nurses' postwar lives. The transformation of civilian nurses into military nurses required a series of careful negotiations regarding the number of nursing sisters and how to select the right kind of nurse, as well as how to balance military and civilian nursing needs. Without due consideration for civilian hospital staffing, the armed forces stood to lose public support and access to nurses for recruitment. It was important to select only the right kind of nurses: those who would conform to military discipline and could be shaped into "officers" and "ladies" – that is, respectable professional women to work within men's domain. But it was also necessary to conform to public perceptions that women needed the protection of men. The military had to reassure the Canadian public that military nurses served in safety, that they were always protected by men, and that they were soldiers only "for the duration."

. Once the nurses enlisted, gender continued to shape their social, professional, and technological boundaries. Nursing sisters were less afraid to "bend" gendered roles than were either civilian or military authorities. They learned to perform the soldier's role as "one of the boys" – wearing khaki battledress, enduring toughening up exercises and route marches, living and working under austere conditions, and scrambling up the side of battleships when their own ships sunk. They relished having "war buddies" but also used their femininity to advantage when either necessary or desirable. While the military recognized nurses' value in the care of soldiers, there was a great deal of ambivalence related to their presence in theatres of war. Prevailing social expectations related to masculinity and femininity meant that nursing sisters were to be protected at all costs from a variety of dangers and from death – even if that meant creating an official silence regarding their presence near and on frontlines or their exposure to dangers. Yet nursing sisters sought out opportunities to work ever closer to the frontlines of war and the frontiers of medical technology. They readily accepted adverse working conditions and military discipline.

The availability of men as medical officers and medical orderlies influenced nurses' work in the military. Nursing sisters capably assumed expanded roles and took on some of the responsibilities of both of these groups whenever physicians and orderlies were unavailable, or whenever those expanded roles reinforced their value to the larger military-medical system. Nurses' professional and social relationships were more flexible close to the frontlines, where patient acuity was higher, skilled personnel fewer, and risk taking more acceptable. But flexibility was temporary: once nurses left forward areas, they had to relinquish expanded roles and responsibilities. The degree to which boundaries were destabilized by wartime conditions was contingent on the relative closeness to military fronts and technological frontiers. Gender bend-ing was acceptable during the war because it was context-dependent, and those in power understood it as temporary. The contingent and temporary nature of war work was also acceptable to most nursing sisters, for whom a career was a relatively brief stage of life prior to marriage, as it was for most nurses of this period. For the most part, they were satisfied to assume traditionally gendered roles as wives and mothers after the war, although we don't know what choices they might have made if civilian nursing practice had been less constraining.

The Second World War was less of a technological watershed for nurses than assumed in existing literature. New medical technologies emerged during the war, and nursing sisters were heavily involved with some of the more dramatic innovations such as blood transfusions and penicillin. But civilian nurses were already experiencing a variety of technological role transitions during the 1930s, such as giving intramuscular injections and intravenous fluids, taking blood, removing sutures, pouring anaesthetics, taking blood pressure readings, and serving as first surgical assistants. Nursing sisters demonstrated that many additional newly developing technologies could be transferred readily to nurses. They also participated in shaping and reshaping these technologies from nursing perspectives. Furthermore, military nurses capitalized on their opportunities as essential personnel to gain additional technological skills and expanded nursing practice roles.

The military made key decisions to move medical personnel to the casualties rather than risk long evacuations of casualties to the personnel, as technological changes in transportation, communication, and weaponry influenced where the delivery of medical and nursing care took place. Although the military was ambivalent about nurses serving in active theatres of war and attempted to replace nurses by training medical orderlies for specific technological skills to be used on the frontlines, it found that nurses could not effectively be replaced by lesser-trained personnel. This need for nursing skills created occupational space for women in the military, while also creating a measure of tolerance for their occasional indiscretions, to which the military turned a "blind eye."

After the war, there was little opportunity to use these newly acquired skills, and many nursing sisters were reluctant to resume earlier roles and the practice constraints of hospital nursing. Conventional hospital nursing roles were no longer satisfying because hospitals were unable or unwilling to capitalize on nursing sisters' demonstrated abilities in expanded technological roles or their increased autonomy. Hospitals continued to rely heavily on student labour, with limited roles for "specially trained" graduate nurses. Thus, for many nursing sisters, the end of war also brought an abrupt end to meaningful work in direct patient care. They clearly resisted a return to prewar practice roles by using veterans' credits and benefits for advanced education, establishing small businesses, and retraining for career changes. For other nursing sisters, public health nursing as well as psychiatric and industrial (occupational health) nursing were popular choices, as they perceived these specialties to be more attractive than hospital nursing.

Contrary to what has been suggested in the literature, the enlistment of nursing sisters was not responsible for the Canadian nursing shortage that emerged during the early 1940s. Military nurses were only a very small proportion of the total civilian workforce at the time, although many of the teachers, supervisors, and more experienced nurses did have priority for enlistment, which placed an increased burden on training schools at a time when student enrolments needed to increase due to the developing nursing shortage. Nursing sisters' absence from the workforce merely exacerbated the underlying working conditions that made hospital nursing unsatisfying and unattractive. By the 1950s and 1960s, hospitals introduced a number of reforms to attract both women and men into the nursing workforce, removing barriers of race, ethnicity, gender, and marital status. Additional reforms during the 1970s shifted the delivery of nursing care from a student workforce to a graduate nurse workforce.[1]

Both during and after the war, several Canadian universities benefited greatly from more stable funding for nursing programs. During the war, funding came in the form of government grants and benevolent donations to train more nursing educators and increase the number of students in nursing programs. Following the war, funding came primarily in the form of veterans' benefits that nursing sisters used for further education. Universities were slow to develop nursing degree programs, however, and the nursing profession did not promote university education as basic preparation for practice until the late 1960s and 1970s.

The quest for professional status, the process of professionalization, and the class position of nursing occupy a good portion of nursing historiography. Class and professional status were reinforced in the military through deliberate decisions regarding officer rank as well as the manner in which the military intentionally shaped nurses as both officers and ladies according to embedded class and gender expectations of the period. The concept of professional status is historically situated and has to be understood within specific contexts. At least three separate sources contributed to the perception of Second World War nursing sisters as professionals: the Weir Report had studied and already concluded that nursing was as a profession according to sociological definitions of the 1930s;[2] the Canadian census classified registered nurses as one of a small group of professional classes in the 1941 census; and the armed forces reaffirmed nurses' professional status in granting them officer rank.

The full integration of nurses into the Canadian military eliminated many issues that had arisen during the First World War regarding untrained, partially trained, and volunteer nurses who provided auxiliary nursing services for the British, American, and French armies. Auxiliary services were not under the military's control, which led to problems with discipline and flexibility in postings. The Canadian armed forces exerted full control over the nursing sisters, with assurance of their availability and mobility as well as definite comportment expectations. Officer status also enhanced nurses' social and professional standings for the duration of the war. Their individual and collective activities appeared frequently in society columns and newspaper features. And among their peers, nursing sisters frequently carried an elite status, especially if they had served "at the front." While officer rank temporarily shifted traditional professional boundaries between nurses and physicians, war was understood to be an extraordinary set of conditions that justified the risks associated in shifting class and professional boundaries. The military could be flexible when there was little threat that equality would endure as permanent change.

Although nurses came into the military from a range of working- and middle-class backgrounds, the shared spaces and experiences of wartime practice were significant in creating an identity as a symbolic, imagined community. Nursing sisters came to perceive and portray themselves as comrades and patriotic citizens united to "win the war," downplaying differences, dissensions, and ambivalences regarding caring roles within the military system. Nonetheless language, culture, ethnicity, religion, regional origins, age, sexuality, class, and education differences did arise within the community, requiring us to rethink the categories "nurse" and "military nurse," and avoid any universal military nurse war narrative.

Nursing sisters lost their legitimacy and benefits as members of the armed forces at the end of the war. As they dispersed throughout Canada, many struggled to find a new identity and place of belonging within civilian settings. The nursing sisters community became a place of safety where they could negotiate shared meaning and a collective social memory. For the most part, they still maintain a code of silence about danger, risk, indiscretions, personal relationships, conflicts, and dissonances. Few military nurses were willing to talk about negative experiences or to criticize either the armed forces or the medical officers with whom they worked. But non-verbal language during the interviews and subtexts in their narratives and letters suggest that there were also less collegial and less congenial relationships within the community as well.

Demographic analyses of my sample from the Department of Defence personnel files have revealed some unexpected findings. For example, nurses were much older and much more experienced than the literature implied. They were overwhelmingly English speaking with strong British origins. They graduated from more than 180 schools of nursing, rather than only a few large teaching hospitals. And it is very doubtful that they caused a nursing shortage, given the small percentage they constituted of the total civilian nursing workforce in the 1940s. The oral histories provided glimpses of contention between British and Canadian military nurses, especially with respect to the colonial status attributed to Canadian nursing sisters, as well as contentions within and among the Canadian nurses themselves. The oral histories were also invaluable for rich descriptions of military nursing practice over a wide range of settings and wartime conditions.

Military nurses increasingly identified as soldiers and perceived war as nurses' work, but it is not clear to what degree they did or did not acknowledge complicity in military agendas. Both civilians and nursing sisters assumed (and were told) that military nurses went to war under the protection of the Geneva Convention, which guaranteed their status as non-combatants among nations that recognized the agreement and declared the neutrality of medical services. As such, they were not to be held as prisoners of war.[3] Yet, as fully integrated members of a national armed force, nursing sisters wore the same uniforms, carried the same rank and pay, and moved with the troops. It was increasingly difficult to maintain any neutral status. They considered their work to consist of "winning the war" through the salvage of damaged men. They increasingly accepted risks and dangers associated with soldiers, including becoming casualties or prisoners of war. Some of the nursing sisters expressed futility in repairing men for a return to the battlefield. Some nurses differentiated the collective "enemy" from individual prisoners of war whom they knew as their patients. Most nursing sisters viewed war as a terrific waste of human lives and resources on both sides of the conflict. But few of them chose to talk about the dissonance of saving lives in the midst of war and the taking of lives, or how they reconciled these contradictions – if indeed they ever did.

For some of the nursing sisters, participating in oral history interviews provided an opportunity to review memories and bring some closure to their wartime nursing experience. Several described "seeing the wards" exactly as they did during the war and "being there now" as they described patients. NS Norah Mallandaine had kept her army belt that patients had "autographed." She described it as "a precious mememto [sic] ... On occasion I take it out and try to put faces to those names."[4] Nursing sisters provide alternative perspectives for understanding the Second World War, to balance traditional accounts of war as political and military strategies.

Appendix: Biographical Profiles of Interviewed Nursing Sisters

Margaret M. Allemang

Margaret Allemang was born in Toronto of British and German parents. She graduated from the University of Toronto School of Nursing (1940). After one and a half years' experience as a general duty nurse and as an assistant head nurse at the Toronto General Hospital, she joined the RCAF in February 1942. She was posted to various RCAF stations within Canada over the next forty-four months (to December 1945). On discharge, she used veterans' credits to complete a Bachelor of Science in Nursing degree at the University of Toronto, followed some years later by master's and PhD degrees from the University of Washington. Margaret was a professor and researcher at the University of Toronto School of Nursing for the rest of her career. She was interviewed 26 April 2001 at Toronto, and died at in that city on 14 April 2005 at the age of ninety-one.

Lois Bayly

Lois Bayly was born in Ottawa, the only child of Canadian parents with British ancestry. She graduated from the Western division of the Montreal General Hospital School of Nursing (1937) and practised in general duty and private duty nursing for five years before enlisting in the RCAMC (January 1942). Her enlistment did not please her mother. Lois served in Canada, England, and continental Europe until January 1946 (twenty-one months in Canada and twenty-six months overseas) at No. 2, No. 8, and No. 22 CGH and No. 6 CCS. She married while overseas, and resigned her commission to return to Canada for the birth of her first child. Lois Bayly Tewsley was interviewed at Ottawa on 11 June 2001.

Mary Marguerite Bower

Mary Bower was born in Blairmore, Alberta, the third of five children of Irish-Canadian parents. Her father was a veteran of the Great War, who survived being gassed at Ypres. Mary graduated from the Holy Cross Hospital in

Calgary (1938) and completed further courses in operating room technique at the Mayo Clinic in Minnesota. With four years' experience in general duty and the operating room, Mary enlisted in the RCAMC in June 1942. She was posted in Canada for sixteen months and overseas in England for seventeen months, primarily with No. 11 CGH and No. 7 CGH. Married overseas, Mary was discharged in March 1945 to return to Canada for the birth of her first child. Ten years later, she took a refresher course and returned to work in nursing. Her memoir, published in 1992, is entitled *Hello War, Goodbye Sanity*. Mary Bower White was interviewed on 20 October 2001 in Surrey, British Columbia.

Doris V. Carter
Doris Carter was born in England, the second of seven children, and immigrated with her parents as a baby to Canada. Her father served with the Canadian Expeditionary Force during the Great War, and two of her brothers served in the Canadian forces (RCN and RCAF) during the Second World War. Doris completed normal school, earning her teaching certificate, before deciding that teaching was not for her. She then entered training to become a nurse. She graduated from the Royal Victoria Hospital (1935) and worked in private duty nursing until enlisting in the RCAMC in October 1940. She was posted in Canada (four months) and overseas (fifty-four months) in England, the Mediterranean, and Europe. Doris served with No. 1 CGH, No. 4 CCS, No. 8 CGH, No. 15 CGH, No. 5 CGH, and No. 5 CCS. On discharge, she used her veterans' credits to complete a public health diploma at McGill University and worked in public health the rest of her career, retiring in 1975. She published her memoir, *Never Leave Your Head Uncovered: A Canadian Nursing Sister in World War Two* in 1999. Doris was interviewed at Ottawa on 22 June 2001.

Beatrice Cole
Bea Cole was born in Wapella, Saskatchewan, to Canadian and English parents. She graduated from the Regina General Hospital (1943), working in general duty only briefly before, in contrast to most of the RCAMC nursing sisters, she received a call, asking her to enlist in March 1944. She was posted twelve months in Canada and twenty months overseas with No. 19 CGH and No. 22 CGH in England. After discharge in November 1946, she completed a Bachelor of Science in Nursing degree and taught at St. Paul's Hospital School of Nursing in Vancouver. She went to Edmonton as a clinical teacher and then as director at the Misericordia Hospital School of Nursing in that city (1974-82). In the late 1960s, she married an engineer who had been responsible for drilling the Leduc No. 1 oil well in 1947. Bea wrote a book based on oral histories of the experience from the workers' perspectives, entitled *Last Chance Well: Legends and Legacies of Leduc No. 1* (1997). Bea Cole Hunter was interviewed on 13 October 2001 in Edmonton.

Pauline Cox

Pauline Cox was born in Wolverhampton, England, and immigrated with her parents to Quebec. A 1937 graduate of the Montreal General Hospital School of Nursing, Pauline worked three and a half years as a general duty nurse, an operating room nurse, and an industrial nurse at Grand-Mère, Quebec. She enlisted in the RCAMC in May 1941, serving in Canada (three months), England and the Mediterranean (forty-seven months) with No. 14 CGH until July 1945. Pauline was on the *Santa Elena* when it was torpedoed near Gibraltar. She worked in a field surgical unit – one of at least four small mobile units that moved rapidly behind the troops and close to the frontlines. After discharge, Pauline went to university for a public health diploma and worked in public health until her marriage in 1947. Pauline Cox Walker was interviewed on 13 June 2001 in Kingston, Ontario.

Elizabeth Dean

Elizabeth Dean was born in Kingston, Ontario, and recalls her father's war injuries from being gassed at Ypres during the First World War. She graduated from the University of Toronto with a Bachelor of Household Science in 1940, and completed her dietician internship at the Toronto General Hospital in 1941. She worked as a dietician and teacher at Hamilton General Hospital for a year prior to enlisting in the RCN (1943) as a nursing sister (dietician). Elizabeth recalled teaching male student nurses in the area of dietetics – one of the first experimental programs to train men as nurses. She was posted in Canada (twelve months) and at the HMCS *Niobe* in Scotland (eighteen months). Elizabeth married a naval officer at the *Niobe* in 1944 and was discharged in October 1945. Her husband became an oceanographer for the Fisheries Department after the war, and they travelled widely in South America and Europe while raising a family. Elizabeth Dean Doe was interviewed in Ottawa on 30 June 2001.

Frances Ferguson

Frances Ferguson was born in Edmonton, Alberta, to Canadian and Scottish parents. Her father was a veteran of the First World War. Frances graduated from the Royal Alexandra Hospital in Edmonton in 1938. She completed postgraduate courses, and practised in both general duty and private duty for four and a half years prior to enlistment in the RCAMC as a nursing sister in January 1943. Her postings included nineteen months in Canada and nineteen months overseas in England and continental Europe with No. 12 CGH, No. 7 CGH, No. 6 CGH, No. 6 CCS, and No. 10 CGH. She was then a volunteer for the Pacific theatre of war. After discharge in September 1945, Frances was instrumental in establishing a school for nursing aides in Calgary, where she taught for ten years. She went to Ceylon for five years with the World Health Organization to establish nursing programs there.

Later, she served as president of the Alberta Association of Registered Nurses and on the Canadian Nurses Association executive committee. Married later in life, Frances Ferguson Sutherland was interviewed on 10 October 2001 in Edmonton.

Pauline Lamont

Pauline Murray Lamont was born in Denfield, Ontario, of Scottish parents. She enlisted with the RCAMC in Ontario on her twenty-third birthday in 1943 after graduating from the Toronto Western Hospital (1941). She had worked as a general duty nurse and industrial nurse in the Bren Gun factory in Toronto to gain the requisite nursing experience prior to military service. She served as a nursing sister from 1943 to 1946, with twenty-five months in Canada and twenty months overseas in England with No. 9 and No. 4 CGH, in Belgium with No. 2 CGH, and in Holland with No. 3 CCS. She was assigned to escort thirty war brides with their twelve children on her way home to Canada in 1946. Pauline's postwar career included DVA nursing at Sunnybrook Military Hospital and at Shaughnessy, British Columbia, prior to marriage and raising a family. Her husband was a member of the public service and the family spent considerable time in Washington, DC. Pauline Lamont Flynn was interviewed 3 April 2001 in Ottawa.

Marjorie MacLean

Marjorie MacLean was born in Campbelltown, New Brunswick, the fourth of eight children to Canadian parents of English and Scottish ancestry. She graduated from the Montreal General Hospital (1939). After working as a private duty nurse for one and a half years, she enlisted in the RCAMC in December 1940. Four of her brothers served with the RCAF during the war. She was posted in Canada (eleven months) and overseas in England and the Mediterranean (forty-eight months). Marjorie was on the *Santa Elena*, which was torpedoed in the Mediterranean while transporting hospital units to Italy and North Africa in 1943. After discharge, she nursed at St. Anne-de-Bellevue, Quebec, prior to her marriage in 1945 and at the Ottawa Civic Hospital until the birth of her first child while her husband studied pharmacy on his veterans' credits. Marjorie MacLean Root was interviewed 15 June 2001 in Ottawa.

Muriel Catherine McArthur

Muriel McArthur was born in Oro, Ontario. Her parents were English and Scottish. An aunt raised her after her parents died when she was seven years old. Two other aunts (Mary Christina McCuaig and Isabella Ann McCuaig) had been nursing sisters during the First World War. Muriel initially obtained a teacher's certificate and taught public school for one year before entering nurses' training at the Toronto General Hospital, where she graduated in

1937. She enlisted in the RCAF in December 1941 after working as a general duty nurse, a summer camp nurse, and a private duty nurse for three and a half years. She served in Canada (thirty-six months) and Yorkshire, England, at #6 Bomber Command (twenty-one months), and then transferred to the permanent forces in September 1946. Her postwar postings included NATO headquarters at Metz, France. Prior to her retirement from the military, she was the first matron-in-chief of the integrated Canadian Forces Medical Services, Nursing Service (1960-64). She worked briefly in Edmonton at the University of Alberta Hospital after her retirement from the military. Muriel was interviewed 14 May 2001 in Barrie, Ontario. She died in Barrie on 18 October 2006 at the age of ninety-three.

Isabel Morrison

Isabel Morrison was born in Halifax, Nova Scotia, to Scottish parents. Her grandmother and mother had both been nurses trained in Boston. Both Isabel and her twin sister became nurses and nursing sisters, but they graduated from different training schools. Isabel graduated from the Victoria General Hospital in Halifax (1940). She worked in private duty for one and a half years and then enlisted in the RCAMC (1942), immediately volunteering for the South African Military Nursing Service in a special draft of 300 Canadian nurses. She served her one-year contract there at Baragwanath and returned to Canada, rejoining the RCAMC in August 1943. With her combined service, Isabel served eleven months in Canada and thirty-five months overseas (in England and Europe with No. 23 CGH, and in South Africa). She also volunteered for the Pacific theatre. On discharge, she married a regimental medical officer and retired to raise a family. Isabel Morrison Fraser was interviewed on 27 November 2001 in Ottawa.

Helen K. Mussallem

Helen Mussallem was born in Prince Rupert, British Columbia. Her parents were Lebanese and immigrated to Canada in 1899. Helen graduated from the Vancouver General Hospital in 1937 with the highest award for operating room technique. She went on to complete courses in supervision and teaching, and worked primarily in the operating room for six years prior to her enlistment in the RCAMC in August 1943. Helen was posted fourteen months in Canada and fifteen months overseas (in England with No. 19 CGH at Marston Green). She volunteered for the Pacific theatre and was in preparation for embarkation when Japan surrendered and the war ended. After discharge in April 1946, she used her veterans' credits to complete a course in supervision, administration, and teaching at McGill University. She went on to complete a Bachelor of Science in Nursing at McGill University, as well as master's and PhD degrees at Columbia University in the New York (1962). She conducted a major study on the state of nursing in Canada for the Canadian Nurses Association, published as the *Royal Commission on Health Services: Nursing Education in Canada* (1965). Helen became executive director of the Canadian Nurses Association in 1963 and was actively involved in international nursing projects in more than forty countries. She was interviewed on 24 September 2001 in Ottawa.

Constance Betty Nicolson

Betty Nicolson was born in Scotland, the sixth of seven children. She immigrated with her parents to Winnipeg and graduated from the Winnipeg General Hospital School of Nursing (1940). She completed a postgraduate course in operating room technique and worked two years in the operating room prior to enlisting with RCAMC No. 5 CGH in January 1942. Betty was posted in Canada, in England at Taplow, in the Mediterranean at Sicily and mainland Italy, and returned to Canada on compassionate leave as result of family illness. She continued to serve at Fort Osbourne, Manitoba, and volunteered for the Pacific campaign. Betty served a total of fifty-two months – twenty-five in Canada and twenty-seven overseas. One of her older sisters was a nursing sister with the British forces during the First World War while another had been a voluntary aid detachment. On discharge, Betty married an RCN officer. Betty Nicolson Brown was interviewed 5 June 2001 in Ottawa.

Frances Marion Oakes

Frances Oakes was born in Fergus, Ontario. Her parents were Scottish and English; Lord Lister was one of her grandfather's nephews. She graduated from the Kitchener-Waterloo Hospital School of Nursing in 1930, after which she took several postgraduate courses in X-ray and operating room technique at both the Montreal General Hospital and the Toronto General Hospital. Fran worked as an operating room supervisor until October 1940, when she was one of the first nurses to join the RCAF after it became a separate branch of the Canadian armed forces. She served in Canada at the St. Thomas Technical Training School, a part of the British Commonwealth Air Training Plan, with a 700-bed hospital unit. She was one of the first two RCAF nurses posted overseas and was instrumental in setting up the specialized burn and surgical unit at East Grinstead in Sussex. She became an honorary member of the "Guinea Pig Club" based on her work with soldiers who underwent extensive reconstructive surgery following their burns. She served fifty-six months in Canada and twenty-four months overseas, for a total of eighty months (the longest-serving nursing sister interviewed for this research). At the end of the war, she transferred to the permanent forces as principal matron, RCAF, until her mandatory retirement in February 1958. In this role, she was responsible for nursing sisters who staffed medical facilities along the DEW Line in northern Canada and along the Alaskan highway. Many of the nurses who served under Fran credited her as the impetus for nurses' training in air evacuation and other educational opportunities. She was interviewed 15 May 2001 in Guelph, Ontario.

E. June Parker

June Parker was born in Regina, Saskatchewan. Her father was a British soldier and her mother was a Territorial Forces nursing sister during the Great War. June enlisted in the RCAF (WD) in 1943, working as a radar technician in British Columbia. With her veterans' benefits, she went to the University of Manitoba for a year of home economics, hoping to get into physiotherapy. On the death of her father and the family's move to England, June completed nurses' training at the Leed's Infirmary in 1954. She then enlisted in the RCAF as a nursing sister in 1959. She served in England, Labrador, Canada, and with NATO forces in France and Germany retiring in 1974. June completed the Air, Evac course at Brooks Air Force Base in the United States (1963). She was posted to the Operational Training Unit (OTU) at Trenton, Ontario, where she was involved in establishing the Canadian Air Evac course with Flight Lieutenant Ella Manix. Along with Peggy Corkum and Eve Gibbons, these four nurses became the first instructors with Sgt. Ballantyne in Air Evac (1963). June described this course as unique, as it was "all medical ranks, all services, French and English, men and women, three weeks course in class, pool, chamber, and five days flying (usually a Hercules or whatever aircrew were training on) to Vancouver, San Francisco, Colorado, New Jersey, or Trenton. Students reversed roles daily, applying their training and improving their skills. Some of the ranks were highly trained, and we nurses learned a lot from them!" June was interviewed on 23 November 2001 in Ottawa, on the topic of postwar military nursing in Canada.

Betty Young Ramage

Betty Ramage was born in Galston, Scotland, and immigrated with her parents to Canada when she was three. She graduated from the Misericordia Hospital in Edmonton (1939). She completed a postgraduate course and worked as a general duty nurse, an assistant head nurse, and a public health nurse for the Department of Social Hygiene for four and a half years prior to enlistment in the RCAMC, in May 1945. She was posted twelve months in Canada and volunteered for the Pacific theatre. On discharge in May 1946, Betty returned to the hospital while waiting for placement at university. She married in 1949 and worked part time in response to the severe nursing shortage while her disabled veteran husband took care of their baby. She returned to public health, becoming a supervisor of Alberta District Nurses and retiring in 1972. Betty Young Ramage Hamilton was interviewed on 12 October 2001 in Edmonton.

Betty Riddell

Betty Riddell was born in Winnipeg and had both Welsh and Scottish origins.

Her father was an RCAF veteran of the First World War and ultimately served in the Second World War as well. Betty graduated from the Misericordia Hospital School of Nursing in Winnipeg (1938) and completed postgraduate courses in the operating room. She worked in private duty briefly and decided to enlist with the U.S Army Nurse Corps because of the long waiting list in the Canadian forces. She enlisted at Detroit in May 1943 and was posted in the United States and Papua New Guinea, where she served a total of thirty-six months until April 1946. After discharge, she completed a public health degree at the University of Minnesota and was a school nurse in Los Angeles until returning to Canada to work in public health. Betty then entered the Canadian civil service and worked in nursing research until her retirement in 1980. Her experience offers a good comparison to the Canadian military nurses' experience, and she represents a large number of Canadian nurses who were unable to enlist with the Canadian forces due to the quota. Betty was interviewed on 26 November 2001 in Ottawa.

Margaret Roe

Margaret Roe was born in Neepawa, Manitoba, one of eight children of British parents. Margaret's mother was a nurse who trained in Minneapolis. Margaret graduated from the Winnipeg Children's Hospital (1941) and worked three years in general duty nursing until she enlisted in the RCAMC (1944). She was posted for six months in Canada and twenty-five months overseas (in England, the Mediterranean, and continental Europe) with No. 4 CGH, No. 17 CGH, No. 1 CGH, and No. 23 CGH. She was a volunteer for the Pacific theatre. After discharge in October 1946, Margaret re-enlisted in the permanent forces from April 1947 to November 1948, when she married. Margaret Roe Dewart was interviewed on 15 October 2001 in Edmonton.

Harriet J.T. (Hallie) Sloan

Hallie Sloan was born in Winnipeg but grew up in Saskatchewan and graduated from the Vancouver General Hospital School of Nursing (1940). Her parents were of Irish and British ancestry, and her father was a Great War veteran. She enlisted in the RCAMC on February 1942 at the age of twenty-five, serving in Canada for thirty-five months and overseas for nineteen months in England, France, Belgium, and Holland. Hallie transferred to the interim forces and then the permanent forces postwar. She was command matron of NATO forces in Germany (1953), command matron Canadian Western Command (1954-56) and Canadian Forces Medical Services Training Centre (1959), major principle matron (1960), and lieutenant-colonel matron-in-chief Canadian Forces Medical Services (1964-68). After her retirement in 1968, she worked for the Canadian Nurses Association until the early 1980s. She was interviewed on 14 March 2001 in Ottawa.

Dorothy Surgenor

Dorothy Surgenor was born in Cornwall, Ontario. Her father had been a Great War veteran and her mother a schoolteacher – both Canadians of the United Empire Loyalists line. Dorothy graduated from the Montreal General Hospital in 1943. After a half-year of experience in general duty and operating room nursing, she enlisted in the RCN the day before V-E Day in May 1945, as preparations were being made for the Pacific theatre of war. She was posted in Canada for eight months, resigning in April 1946 to marry. She worked part time briefly after marriage until her first child was born, and returned to nursing during the 1960s in renal dialysis, retiring in 1982. Dorothy Surgenor Maddock was interviewed on 26 June 2001 in Ottawa.

Doris Taylor

Doris Taylor was born in Little Harbour, Nova Scotia. Her parents were Canadian of British and German ancestry. She graduated from the Women's General Hospital School of Nursing in Montreal (also known as the Reddy Memorial Hospital) in 1940. She completed postgraduate courses and worked as a general duty nurse, an operating room nurse, a head nurse of the out-patient clinic, and an assistant-supervisor for two and a half years prior to enlistment in the RCAMC in October 1943. She was posted in Canada (seventeen months) and overseas in England and continental Europe (nineteen months). Her two brothers served with the army and navy while her sister served with the Canadian Army Women's Corps – thus, four of the five children in her family served during the Second World War. On discharge in August 1946, Doris worked at Queen Mary Veterans' Hospital under the DVA until her marriage to a veteran in 1951. She returned to nursing from 1962 to 1984 in out-patient clinics. Doris Taylor Rasberry was interviewed on 19 June 2001 in Pointe Claire, Quebec.

Estelle Tritt

Estelle Tritt was born in Montreal, one of seven children. Her parents immigrated from the Austro-Hungarian Empire between 1886 and 1890. She graduated from the Women's General Hospital (also known as the Reddy Memorial Hospital) in 1941 after an attempt at teaching public school. She worked as a general duty nurse for one and a half years prior to enlisting with the RCAMC as a nursing sister. Estelle was posted in Canada for seventeen months and overseas in England and Europe for twenty-seven months, serving with No. 18 CGH, No. 8 CGH, and No. 7 CGH. In addition, she volunteered for the Pacific theatre. Soon after her discharge in August 1946, she married a veteran and retired from nursing to raise a family. She returned to nursing briefly during the 1970s. Estelle Tritt Aspler was interviewed in Montreal, 13 August 2001. She died in May 2007 at the age of eighty-eight.

Margaret Van Scoyoc

Margaret Van Scoyoc was born in Montreal to English and Dutch parents. Her mother was a teacher who had graduated from Oberlin College in the United States. Margaret graduated from the Montreal General Hospital School of Nursing (1936). Her pre-enlistment experience included work in Bermuda and at a munitions factory in Quebec. With five years experience in general duty, public health, VON, and industrial nursing, she enlisted in the RCAMC in December 1941. She served in Canada (ten months) and overseas in England and continental Europe with No. 12 CGH (thirty months) prior to transferring to the permanent forces in October 1946. She retired from the military in February 1966 and worked at the Montreal Children's Hospital as a central supply nurse. She was interviewed on 13 June 2001 in Kingston, Ontario.

Eva Wannop

Eva Wannop was born in Carmangay, Alberta, to English and Canadian parents. She graduated from the Holy Cross Hospital School of Nursing in Calgary (1939). After a year of experience in private duty nursing, she had saved the funds for further study and was accepted by the University of Toronto for a course in nursing administration, supervision, and public health. Eva requested the university to hold her position, and she enlisted in the RCAMC in September 1940. Her mother was against her enlistment and refused to "see her off," but her father did. She was posted in Canada (twenty-two months) and England (thirty-eight months), serving at Basingstoke Neurological and Plastics Hospital, where she developed special skills with burns and plastic surgery patients. She was discharged in August 1945 after sixty months of service and returned to take up her public health course at the University of Toronto. She worked as a public health nurse and industrial nurse with the Manulife Insurance Company until her retirement in 1979. She was interviewed 25 April 2001 in Toronto. Eva died in Toronto on 21 April 2004 at the age of ninety-two.

Notes

Introduction

1 Roger Cooter, "Medicine and the Management of Modern Warfare: An Introduction," in *Medicine and Modern Warfare*, ed. Roger Cooter, Mark Harrison, and Steve Sturdy (Amsterdam: Rodopi, 1999), 4; Desmond Morton and Glenn Wright, *Winning the Second Battle: Canadian Veterans and the Return to Civilian Life, 1915-1930* (Toronto: University of Toronto Press, 1987).

2 Sue M. Goldie, ed., *Florence Nightingale: Letters from the Crimea, 1854-1856* (Manchester: Manchester University Press, 1997), 1-14; G.W.L. Nicholson, *Canada's Nursing Sisters* (Toronto: Samuel Stevens Hakkert, 1975), 52.

3 Janet S.K. Watson, *Fighting Different Wars: Experience, Memory, and the First World War in Britain* (Cambridge: Cambridge University Press, 2004), 59, 62-65, 69-70; Eileen Crofton, *The Women of Royaumont: A Scottish Women's Hospital on the Western Front* (East Lothian, Scotland: Tuckwell Press, 1997); Anne Summers, *Angels and Citizens: British Women as Military Nurses, 1854-1914* (New York: Routledge, 1988); Vera Brittain, *Testament of Youth* (New York: Seaview Books, 1980) and *Chronicle of Youth: War Diary, 1913-1917*, ed. Alan Bishop with Terry Smart (London: Gollancz, 1981); Linda Quiney, "Assistant Angels: Canadian Voluntary Aid Detachment Nurses in the Great War," *Canadian Bulletin of Medical History* 15, 1 (1998): 189-206.

4 In this context, *nursing sisters* are not to be confused with nuns who were members of religious orders that provided nursing services.

5 C.P. Stacey, *Official History of the Canadian Army in the Second World War*, vol. 1, *Six Years of War: The Army in Canada, Britain and the Pacific* (Ottawa: Queen's Printer, 1955), 3, 43, and 118-22; G.W.L Nicholson, *Seventy Years of Service: A History of the R.C.A.M.C.* (Ottawa: Borealis Press, 1977), 138; W.R. Feasby, ed. *Official History of the Canadian Medical Services, 1939-1945*, vol. 1, *Organization and Campaigns* (Ottawa: Queen's Printer, 1956), 311-12.

6 Stella Goostray, *Memoirs: Half a Century in Nursing* (Boston: Boston University Mugar Memorial Library, 1969), 126-27; Mary T. Sarnecky, *A History of the U.S. Army Nurse Corps* (Philadelphia: University of Pennsylvania Press, 1999); Phillip A. Kalisch and Beatrice J. Kalisch, "The Women's Draft: An Analysis of the Controversy over the Nurses' Selective Service Bill of 1945," *Nursing Research* 22, 5 (1973): 402-13; Darlene Clark Hine, *Black Women in White: Racial Conflict and Cooperation in the Nursing Profession, 1890-1950* (Bloomington and Indianapolis: Indiana University Press, 1989), 179-83.

7 *Rights and Duties of Nurses, Military and Civilian Medical Personnel under the Geneva Conventions of August 12, 1949: Red Cross Principles*, brochure (Geneva: International Committee of the Red Cross, 1970); "RCAMC Nursing Sisters on Duty in Hong Kong," *Canadian Nurse* 38, 1 (1942): 32.

8 Erich Maria Remarque, *All Quiet on the Western Front* (Toronto: Random House of Canada, 1958), 263.

9 Jan Bassett, *Guns and Brooches: Australian Army Nursing from the Boer War to the Gulf War* (New York: Oxford University Press, 1992), 1-2.

10 C.P. Stacey, *Official History of the Canadian Army in the Second World War*, vol. 1, *Six Years of War*, and vol. 3, *The Victory Campaign: The Operations in North-West Europe, 1944-1945* (Ottawa: Queen's Printer, 1960); G.W.L. Nicholson, *Official History of the Canadian Army in the Second World War*, vol. 2, *The Canadians in Italy, 1943-1945* (Ottawa: Queen's Printer, 1957); J.L. Granatstein, *Canada's Army: Waging*

War and Keeping the Peace (Toronto: University of Toronto Press, 2002) and *Canada's War: The Politics of the Mackenzie King Government, 1939-1945* (Toronto: Oxford University Press, 1975); Desmond Morton, *A Military History of Canada*, 3rd ed. (Toronto: McClelland and Stewart, 1992); J.L. Granatstein and J.M. Hitsman, *Broken Promises: A History of Conscription in Canada* (Toronto: Oxford University Press, 1977); Peter Neary and J.L. Granatstein, *The Veteran's Charter and Post-World War II Canada* (Montreal and Kingston: McGill-Queen's University Press, 1998); Norman Hillmer, Bohdan Kordan, and Lubomyr Luciuk, *On Guard for Thee: War, Ethnicity, and the Canadian State, 1939-1945* (Ottawa: Canadian Government Publishing Centre, 1988); Jeff Keshen, "Getting It Right the Second Time Around: The Reintegration of Canadian Veterans of World War II," in *The Veteran's Charter and Post-World War II Canada*, ed. Peter Neary and J.L. Granatstein, (Montreal and Kingston: McGill-Queen's University Press, 1998), 62-84; Jeffrey Keshen, "Revisiting Canada's Civilian Women during World War II," *Histoire sociale/Social History* 30, 60 (1997): 239-66; and Jeffrey A. Keshen, *Saints, Sinners, and Soldiers: Canada's Second World War* (Vancouver: UBC Press, 2004).
11 W.R. Feasby, ed., *Official History of the Canadian Medical Services, 1939-1945*, vol. 1, *Organization and Campaigns* and vol. 2, *Clinical Subjects* (Ottawa: Queen's Printer, 1953); Bill Rawling, *Death Their Enemy: Canadian Medical Practitioners and War* (Ottawa: author, 2001); Harold M. Wright, *Salute to the Air Force Medical Branch on the 75th Anniversary Royal Canadian Air Force* (Ottawa: author, 1999); Rita Donovan, *As for the Canadians: The Remarkable Story of the RCAF's "Guinea Pigs" of The Second World War* (Ottawa: Buschek Books, 2000); and Stanley T. Richards, *Operation Sick Bay* (West Vancouver: Cantaur Publishing, 1994).
12 Nicholson, *Canada's Nursing Sisters*. Despite an initial effort during the 1920s to collect records for the purpose of creating a history of the First World War Nursing Sisters, the project was never completed; see Susan Mann, *Margaret Macdonald: Imperial Daughter* (Montreal and Kingston: McGill-Queen's University Press, 2005), 165.
13 Jean Bruce, *Back the Attack: Canadian Women during the Second World War – At Home and Abroad* (Toronto: Macmillan, 1985), viii, 124-39; Carolyn Gossage, *Greatcoats and Glamour Boots: Canadian Women at War, 1939-1945* (Toronto: Dundurn Press, 1991); Lisa Bannister, producer, *Equal to the Challenge: An Anthology of Women's Experiences during World War II* (Ottawa: Department of National Defence, 2001); Barbara Dundas, *A History of Women in the Canadian Military* (Montreal: Art Global, 2000); Jean Portugal, *We Were There: The Navy, the Army, and the RCAF: A Record for Canada*, vols. 1-7 (Shelburne, ON: Battered Silicon Dispatch Box, 1998).
14 Susan R. Grayzel, *Women's Identities at War: Gender, Motherhood, and Politics in Britain and France during the First World War* (Chapel Hill: University of North Carolina Press, 1999), 244.
15 Angela K. Smith, *The Second Battlefield: Women, Modernism and the First World War* (Manchester: Manchester University Press, 2000), 7-8 and 75-77.
16 Margaret R. Higonnet, *Nurses at the Front: Writing the Wounds of the Great War* (Boston: Northeastern University Press, 2001).
17 Cynthia Enloe, *Does Khaki Become You? The Militarisation of Women's Lives* (Boston: South End Press, 1983).
18 Cynthia Enloe, *Maneuvers: The International Politics of Militarizing Women's Lives* (Berkeley and Los Angeles: University of California Press, 2000), 3, 199, 218. Emphasis in original.
19 Joan W. Scott, "Rewriting History," in *Behind the Lines: Gender and the Two World Wars*, ed. Margaret Randolph Higonnet, Jane Jenson, Sonya Michel, and Margaret Collins Weitz (New Haven: Yale University Press, 1987), 21-30.
20 Margaret R. Higonnet and Patrice L.-R. Higonnet, "The Double Helix," in Higonnet et al., *Behind the Lines*, 31-47.
21 Ruth Roach Pierson, "Beautiful Soul or Just Warrior: Gender and War," *Gender and History* 1, 1 (1989): 77-86.
22 Jean Bethke Elshtain, *Women and War* (New York: Basic Books, 1987), 184-85 and 10-11.
23 The University of Ottawa Research Ethics Board granted approval for this project. Each participant gave informed written consent as well as permission to be quoted in presentations and publications resulting from the research. Interviews ranged from 45 to 180 minutes in length with an average of 90 minutes per participant. Initial participants volunteered through the Nursing Sisters' Association of Canada; subsequent participants were referred to me, based on areas of military service such as posting to a specific theatre of war, type of medical unit, or branch of the armed forces.
24 Library and Archives Canada (hereafter LAC), RG 24 (Department of National Defence). To minimize sampling biases, individual records were selected randomly according to letter sampling techniques

developed in collaboration with the archivist responsible for the records. The data are reported in aggregate form to maintain the privacy and confidentiality of these records.

25 Only three files had to be rejected because the folder contained too little content, although many records have sustained extensive water damage due to flooded storage facilities.

26 Tim Cooke, "Clio's Soldiers: Charles Stacey and the Army Historical Section in the Second World War," *Canadian Historical Review* 83, 1 (2002): 52 and 55.

27 Ibid., 35-36, 39, 47, and 52.

28 Kathryn McPherson, "Science and Technique: Nurses' Work in a Canadian Hospital, 1920-1939," in *Caring and Curing: Historical Perspectives on Women and Healing in Canada*, ed. Dianne Dodd and Deborah Gorham (Ottawa: University of Ottawa Press, 1994), 71-101.

29 Wiebe E. Bijker, Thomas P. Hughes, and Trevor J. Pinch, *The Social Construction of Technological Systems: New Directions in the Social History of Technology* (Cambridge, MA: MIT Press, 1989); John Law and John Hassard, eds., *Actor Network Theory and After* (Oxford: Blackwell, 1999); Thomas P. Hughes, "The Evolution of Large Technological Systems," in *The Social Construction of Technological Systems*, ed. Wiebe E. Bijker, Thomas P. Hughes, and Trevor J. Pinch (Cambridge, MA: MIT Press, 1989), 51.

30 Hughes, "The Evolution of Large Technological Systems," 51.

31 Kathryn McPherson, Cecilia Morgan, and Nancy M. Forestell, eds., *Gendered Pasts: Historical Essays in Femininity and Masculinity in Canada* (Don Mills, ON: Oxford University Press, 1999), 4-5.

32 A.P. Cohen, *The Symbolic Construction of Community* (New York: Tavistock, 1985), 9, 12-15, and 118.

33 Ibid.; Charles Wetherell, Andrejs Plakans, and Barry Wellman, "Social Networks, Kinship, and Community in Eastern Europe," *Journal of Interdisciplinary History* 24, 4 (1994): 639-63; Benedict Anderson, *Imagined Communities: Reflections on the Origin and Spread of Nationalism*, rev. ed. (New York: Verso, 1991); John C. Walsh and Steven High, "Rethinking the Concept of Community," *Histoire sociale/Social History* 32, 64 (1999): 255-73; and Jenéa Tallentire, "Strategies of Memory: History, Social Memory, and the Community," *Histoire sociale/Social History* 34, 67 (2001): 197-212.

34 Cohen, *The Symbolic Construction of Community*, 7, 9, and 12.

35 Ruth Roach Pierson, "Wartime Jitters over Femininity," in *The Good Fight: Canadians and World War II*, ed. J.L. Granatstein and Peter Neary (Toronto: Copp Clark, 1995), 141-68, and *"They're Still Women after All": The Second World War and Canadian Womanhood* (Toronto: McClelland and Stewart, 1986).

Chapter 1: "Ready, Aye Ready"

1 Kathryn McPherson, "Science and Technique: Nurses' Work in a Canadian Hospital, 1920-1939," in *Caring and Curing: Historical Perspectives on Women and Healing in Canada*, ed. Dianne Dodd and Deborah Gorham (Ottawa: University of Ottawa Press, 1994).

2 George M. Weir, *Survey of Nursing Education in Canada* (Toronto: University of Toronto Press, 1932).

3 Kathryn McPherson, *Bedside Matters: The Transformation of Canadian Nursing, 1900-1990* (Toronto: Oxford University Press, 1996), 124.

4 Beth Light and Ruth Pierson, *No Easy Road: Women in Canada, 1920s to 1960s* (Toronto: New Hogtown Press, 1990), 16, 149-50; Paul Axelrod, *Making a Middle Class: Student Life in English Canada during the Thirties* (Montreal and Kingston: McGill-Queen's University Press, 1990), 156-57.

5 E.P. Scarlett, "Till the Barrage Lifts!" *Canadian Nurse* 36, 8 (1940): 479.

6 *"Fisher's Folly": A History of the Ottawa Civic Hospital, 1924-1984* (Ottawa: Banfield-Seguin, n.d.); Ottawa Civic Hospital School of Nursing Archives (hereafter OCHA), Hospital Annual Reports, 1924-44.

7 Gertrude LeRoy Miller, *Mustard Plasters and Handcars: Through the Eyes of a Red Cross Outpost Nurse* (Toronto: Natural Heritage Books, 2000).

8 Weir, *Survey of Nursing*, 498 and 15.

9 McPherson, *Bedside Matters*, 129-30, 137; Barbara A. Keddy, "Private Duty Nursing: Days of the 1920s and 1930s in Canada," *Canadian Woman Studies/Cahiers de la femme* 7, 3 (1986): 99-102; Weir, *Survey of Nursing*, 15, 498.

10 Eva Wannop, audiotaped interview with author, Toronto, 25 April 2001.

11 Muriel McArthur, audiotaped interview with author, Barrie, Ontario, 14 May 2001.

12 Keddy, "Private Duty Nursing," 100; Doris V. Carter, audiotaped interview with author, Ottawa, 22 June 2001; Valerie Knowles, *Leaving with a Red Rose: A History of the Ottawa Civic Hospital School of Nursing* (Ottawa: Ottawa Civic Hospital School of Nursing Alumnae Association, 1981), 41; McPherson, *Bedside Matters*, 134, 151-60.

13 Frances Ferguson Sutherland, audiotaped interview with author, Edmonton, Alberta, 10 October 2001; Lois Bayly Tewsley, audiotaped interview with author, Ottawa, 11 June 2001; Betty Riddell, audiotaped interview with author, Ottawa, 26 November 2001; Dorothy M. (Grainger) Anderson, in *Military Nurses of Canada: Recollections of Canadian Military Nurses*, vol. 1, ed. E.A. Landells (White Rock, BC: Co-Publishing, 1995), 411.

14 James Struthers, *No Fault of Their Own: Unemployment and the Canadian Welfare State, 1914-1941* (Toronto: University of Toronto Press, 1983), 81-83; Veronica Strong-Boag, *The New Day Recalled: Lives of Girls and Women in English Canada, 1919-1939* (Toronto: Copp Clark Pitman, 1988), 48.

15 McPherson, *Bedside Matters*, 151-2.

16 Charles E. Rosenberg, *The Care of Strangers: The Rise of America's Hospital System* (New York: Basic Books, 1987); Joel D. Howell, *Technology in the Hospital: Transforming Patient Care in the Early Twentieth Century* (Baltimore: Johns Hopkins University Press, 1995); Margarete Sandelowski, *Devices and Desires: Gender, Technology, and American Nursing* (Chapel Hill: University of North Carolina Press, 2000), 72-78.

17 Kathryn McPherson, "Science and Technique: Nurses' Work in a Canadian Hospital, 1920-1939," in *Caring and Curing: Historical Perspectives on Women and Healing in Canada*, ed. Dianne Dodd and Deborah Gorham (Ottawa: University of Ottawa Press, 1994), 76-77, 86-94.

18 Bill Rawling, *Death Their Enemy: Canadian Medical Practitioners and War* (Ottawa: author, 2001), 117-19.

19 G.W.L. Nicholson, *Canada's Nursing Sisters* (Toronto: Samuel Stevens Hakkert, 1975), 102-3; Rawling, *Death Their Enemy*, 117-18; Leslie Newell, "'Led by the Spirit of Humanity': Canadian Military Nursing, 1914-1929" (MA thesis, University of Ottawa, 1996); W.R. Feasby, ed., *Official History of the Medical Services, 1939-1945*, vol. 1, *Organizations and Campaigns* (Ottawa: Queen's Printer, 1956), 12, 37, appendix A.

20 Newell, "Led by the Spirit of Humanity"; Rawling, *Death Their Enemy*, 126.

21 Elizabeth B. Pense Neil, interview with Norma Fieldhouse, Kingston, Ontario, March 1987, from the Oral History Collection, Margaret M. Allemang Centre for the History of Nursing (MMA); G.W.L. Nicholson, *Seventy Years of Service: A History of the R.C.A.M.C.* (Ottawa: Borealis Press, 1977), 121-22; Rawling, *Death Their Enemy*, 119, 126.

22 During the First World War, according to Geneviève Allard, 37 percent of all active Canadian nurses had enlisted as Nursing Sisters. See "Des anges blanc sur le front: L'expérience de guerre des infirmières militaires Canadiennes pendant la première guerre mondiale," *Bulletin d'histoire politique* 8, 2-3 (2000): 120.

23 Rawling, *Death Their Enemy*, 117-18.

24 "Nursing Sisters: Royal Canadian Army Medical Corps," Library and Archives, Canadian Forces Base Borden; "Nursing Service, R.C.A.M.C., C.A.S.F.," *Canadian Nurse* 36, 2 (1940): 87-88.

25 Cynthia Enloe, *Does Khaki Become You? The Militarisation of Women's Lives* (Boston: South End Press, 1983), 77.

26 Jean S. Wilson, "Notes from the National Office," *Canadian Nurse* 35, 8 (1939): 453.

27 Robert Craig Brown and Ramsay Cook, *Canada, 1896-1921: A Nation Transformed* (Toronto: McClelland and Stewart, 1994), 271-72; Desmond Morton, *A Peculiar Kind of Politics: Canada's Overseas Ministry in the First World War* (Toronto: University of Toronto Press, 1982), 136; Cynthia Enloe, *Maneuvers: The International Politics of Militarizing Women's Lives* (Berkeley and Los Angeles: University of California Press, 2000), 213; John Herd Thompson with Allen Seager, *Canada, 1922-1939: Decades of Discord* (Toronto: McClelland and Stewart, 1985): 115-17, 325-29.

28 James Eayrs, *In Defence of Canada*, vol. 1, *From the Great War to the Great Depression* (Toronto: University of Toronto Press, 1964), and vol. 2, *Appeasement and Rearmament* (Toronto: University of Toronto Press, 1965); J.L. Granatstein, *Canada's War: The Politics of the Mackenzie King Government, 1939-1945* (Toronto: Oxford University Press, 1975); J.L. Granatstein and J.M. Hitsman, *Broken Promises: A History of Conscription in Canada* (Toronto: Oxford University Press, 1977).

29 Mary T. Sarnecky, *A History of the U.S. Army Nurse Corps* (Philadelphia: University of Pennsylvania Press, 1999), 269-70; Phillip A. Kalisch and Beatrice J. Kalisch, "The Women's Draft: An Analysis of the Controversy over the Nurses' Selective Service Bill of 1945," *Nursing Research* 22, 5 (1973): 402-3; Ann Graber Hershberger, "Mennonite Nurses in World War II: Maintaining the Thread of Pacifism in Nursing," *Nursing History Review* 11 (2003): 153-4.

30 *King's Regulations and Orders for the Canadian Militia, 1939* (Ottawa: King's Printer, 1939); Jean S. Wilson, "Military Service," *Canadian Nurse* 35, 10 (1939): 562.

31 See McPherson, *Bedside Matters*, 17, 118; Harriet J.T. Sloan, audiotaped interview with author, Ottawa, 14 March 2001; Alice Michiyo Uyede, "A Spotless Reputation," *Canadian Nurse* 35, 2 (1939): 93-94.

32 Frank Graham, audiotaped interview, Nursing History Digitization Project, Mount Saint Vincent University Archives, http://www.msvu.ca/library/archives/nhdp/history/malenurses.htm, accessed 14 February 2007.

33 Dean Care, David Gregory, John English, and Peri Venkatesh, "A Struggle for Equality: Resistance to Commissioning of Male Nurses in the Canadian Military, 1952-1967," *Canadian Journal of Nursing Research* 28, 1 (1996): 103-17.

34 These comments are taken from the military files of individual nurses who were discharged within the first six months after enlistment. Respecting confidentiality, I omit identifying details.

35 Nicholson, *Seventy Years of Service*, 137; "V.A.D. Training," *Canadian Nurse* 36, 2 (1940): 105.

36 Jean S. Wilson, "National Enrolment," *Canadian Nurse* 35, 1 (1939): 31.

37 Ethel Johns, "Guarding the Flame," *Canadian Nurse* 35, 10 (1939): 563.

38 Frances Oakes, audiotaped interview with author, Guelph, Ontario, 15 May 2001.

39 F.I. McEwen, "Report of the National Joint Committee on Enrolment of Nurses," *Canadian Nurse* 36, 9 (1940): 584.

40 E. Frances Upton, "Provincial Reports," *Canadian Nurse* 36, 9 (1940): 611.

41 "RNAO Reports to Annual Meetings, 1944-49," 2-3, RNAO, 96F-2-04, Archives of Ontario (hereafter AO); Rawling, *Death Their Enemy*, 117-18.

42 McEwen, "Report of the National Joint Committee," 584.

43 Helen Morton Rendall, interview with Margaret M. Allemang, Toronto, 14 and 21 March 1986, MMA.

44 Constance Betty Nicolson Brown, audiotaped interview with author, Ottawa, 5 June 2001.

45 Doris V. Carter, audiotaped interview with author at Ottawa on 22 June 2001.

46 Beatrice Cole Hunter, audiotaped interview with author, Edmonton, Alberta, 13 October 2001.

47 The Nursing Sisters Database (hereafter NSD) was constructed from Department of National Defence records held by Library and Archives Canada (hereafter LAC).

48 Harriet J.T. Sloan, audiotaped interview with author, Ottawa, 14 March 2001.

49 Lois Bayly Tewsley, audiotaped interview with author, Ottawa, 11 June 2001.

50 Mary M. Bower White, audiotaped interview with author, Surrey, British Columbia, 20 October 2001.

51 Isabel Morrison Fraser, audiotaped interview with author, Ottawa on 27 November 2001.

52 Letter from Elizabeth Smellie to the Department of National Defence, 17 February 1943, "Correspondence and Instructions regarding Nursing Sisters for British South African Nursing Service," 324.009 (D204), Department of National Defence Directorate of History and Heritage (hereafter DHH).

53 J.W. Tice, letters of 4 July 1941 and 24 April 1942, file 400-2-1, "Nursing Sisters, RCAF: Appointment of, Policy governing," RG 24, E-1-b, v. 3365, LAC.

54 Letter to C.G. Power, 31 March 1942, file 400-2-1, "Nursing Sisters, RCAF: Appointment of, Policy governing," RG 24, E-1-b, v. 3365, LAC.

55 Letter to C.G. Power, 5 October 1942, file 400-2-1, "Nursing Sisters, RCAF: Appointment of, Policy governing," RG 24, E-1-b, v. 3365, LAC.

56 "Report of the Committee on Nursing and Nurse Education in Canadian Hospitals," Bulletin #36 (1941), presented to the sixth biennial meeting of the Canadian Hospital Council, 96B-5-14, RNAO fonds, AO.

57 Ethel Johns, "The Home Front," *Canadian Nurse* 37, 9 (1941): 603-4; Marion Lindeburgh, "Our National Duty," *Canadian Nurse* 38, 10 (1942): 760; "A 'Practice' Raid," *Canadian Nurse* 37, 7 (1941): 478.

58 Jean S. Wilson, "Report of the Executive Secretary," *Canadian Nurse* 36, 9 (1940): 546; "Notes from the National Office," *Canadian Nurse* 38, 5 (1942): 310; "Notes from the National Office," *Canadian Nurse* 39, 4 (1943): 276; *Eighth Census of Canada, 1941*, vol. 7 (Ottawa: King's Printer, 1946), 32; *Report of the National Health Survey*, part 8, *Nurses* (Ottawa: King's Printer, 1945), 219.

59 Kathleen W. Ellis, "The Report of the Emergency Nursing Adviser," *Canadian Nurse* 38, 9 (1942): 636-45.

60 Marion Lindeburgh, "Important Emergency Measures," *Canadian Nurse* 38, 12 (1942): 925.

61 Kathleen W. Ellis, "Some Pertinent Questions," *Canadian Nurse* 39, 4 (1943): 269-71. The National Selective Service was a compulsory registration of all women between twenty and twenty-four years of age (single or married) except for members of religious orders, hospital patients, prison inmates, and women in insurable employment; see Ruth Pierson, "Women's Emancipation and the Recruitment of Women into the Labour Force in World War II," in *The Neglected Majority: Essays in Canadian Women's History*, ed. Susan Mann Trofimenkoff and Alison Prentice, 125-45 (Toronto: McClelland and Stewart, 1977), 126.

62 Jean S. Wilson, "Notes from the National Office: Registration of Nurses," *Canadian Nurse* 39, 6 (1943): 407; *The Leaf and the Lamp: The Canadian Nurses'Association and the Influences Which Shaped Its Origins and Outlook during Its First Sixty Years* (Ottawa: Canadian Nurses Association, 1968), 88.

63 Kathleen W. Ellis, "The Final Report," *Canadian Nurse* 39, 8 (1943): 531-33.

64 "Report of the Committee on Nursing and Nurse Education in Canadian Hospitals," 7, RNAO fonds, 96B-5-14, AO; Allard, "Des anges blanc sur le front," 120.

65 Kathleen W. Ellis, "An Interim Report," *Canadian Nurse* 39, 6 (1943): 398-400.

66 Ellis, "Final Report," 532-33.

67 Jean S. Wilson, "Notes from the National Office: Labour Exit Permits," *Canadian Nurse* 39, 5 (1943): 345.

68 Ibid.

69 There is a formidable body of Second World War Canadian military literature. I focus on the medical services and in particular, the nursing sisters and how events of the war influenced their practice. For an overview of major events, see Norman Hillmer, "World War II," *The Canadian Encyclopedia: Year 2000 Edition* (Toronto: McClelland and Stewart, 1999), 2551-53.

70 Stacey, *Six Years of War*, 27-34, 43-45, 60-61.

71 Morton, *Military History of Canada*, 194.

72 Stacey, *Six Years of War*, 82.

73 Morton, *Military History of Canada*, 188.

74 Charles G. Roland, *Long Night's Journey into Day: Prisoners of War in Hong Kong and Japan, 1941-1945* (Waterloo, ON: Wilfrid Laurier University Press, 2001).

75 Stacey, *Six Years of War*, 517.

76 Muriel McArthur, "52 RCAF Mobile Field Hospital," in *The Military Nurses of Canada: Recollections of Canadian Military Nurses*, vol. 3, ed. E.A. Landells, (White Rock, BC: Co-Publishing, 1999): 271.

77 "List of Canadians who Served with South African Nursing Service – Second World War (1939-1945)," and 325.009 (D575), "Correspondence, reports, instructions, etc. re. Nursing Sisters enrolling in South African Forces, August 41-November 45," 000.8 (D91), DHH.

78 Authors typically cite John Murray Gibbon and Mary S. Mathewson, *Three Centuries of Canadian Nursing* (Toronto: Macmillan, 1947), 456-58, or Nicholson, *Canada's Nursing Sisters*, 208. Much of the variation in statistics can be explained by three factors: who was included in the calculations (nurses only or all Nursing Sisters), what date was used as the end point (since the services were not completely coordinated for reporting purposes), and whether the reported figure is cumulative or date specific.

79 Three Nursing Sisters transferred from RCAMC to RCN, and twelve transferred from RCAMC to RCAF. At least sixty-nine Nursing Sisters served in both the SAMNS and RCAMC. Therefore, there were at least eighty-three or eighty-four fewer Nursing Sisters than commonly reported.

80 "Appointment Statistics – Nursing Sisters, Physiotherapy Aides, Occupational Therapists, Dieticians and Home Sisters," 000.8 (D93), DHH.

81 Letter, K.W. Ellis to J.E. Porteous, 9 December 1943, RG 24, file 400-2-1, vol. 3365, E-1-b, LAC.

82 Nicholson, *Canada's Nursing Sisters*, 199-200. A lack of full qualifications likely influenced decisions about RCAF physiotherapy aides. See "Memo on Physiotherapy Aides and Occupational Therapists," 2 December 1943, 400-2-1, in "Women Medical Officers, Nursing Sisters, Physios, Orthopists, and Opthalmical Assistants," 181.003 (D1467), DHH; and Feasby, *Official History of the Canadian Medical Services*, 1: 329-31, 202-7, 442.

83 Nicholson, *Canada's Nursing Sisters*, 202-3; and Stanley T. Richards, *Operation Sick Bay* (West Vancouver: Cantaur Publishing, 1994), 52.

84 Feasby, *Official History of the Canadian Medical Services*, 1: 315-23.

85 Elizabeth Dean Doe, audiotaped interview with author, Nepean, Ontario, 30 June 2001.

86 "List of Canadians who Served with South African Nursing Service," 000.8 (D91), DHH.

87 "The Royal Canadian Army Medical Corps," presented at the Victory Meeting of the Canadian Medical Association, Banff Springs Hotel, Banff, Alberta, June 1946, MG 31, G19, vol. 5, LAC.

88 Feasby, *Official History of the Canadian Medical Services*, 1: 325.

89 Pauline Lamont Flynn, audiotaped interview with author, Ottawa, 3 April 2001; Ella Beardmore, audiotaped interview with Joan Williams, 26 November 1975, ISN 196092, LAC.

90 McPherson, *Bedside Matters*, 117-18.

91 Axelrod, *Making a Middle Class*, 139, 149.

92 Strong-Boag, *The New Day Recalled*, 20-21.

93 McPherson, *Bedside Matters*, 39-40.
94 *What You Want to Know about Nursing* (Montreal: Canadian Nurses Association, n.d.), 14, in "Background/Supplemental Material for CNA Nurse Recruitment, 1944-45," RNAO, 96B-5-20, AO.
95 McPherson reported no male nurses in the 1931 census in *Bedside Matters*, 116, but they are present in the *Eighth Census of Canada, 1941*, 7: 328. See also Care et al., "A Struggle for Equality," 103-17.
96 "District #4 Report for March 1940," Nursing Education Section, Minutes and Reports (1928-41), and CNA annual report for 1940, RNAO, 96B1-1-09, AO.
97 Care et al., "A Struggle for Equality," 104.
98 Estelle Tritt Aspler, audiotaped interview with author, Westmount, Quebec, 13 August 2001.
99 Copies of "Undertaking" forms are in every Nursing Sister's personnel record. Regulations regarding marriage were set out in paragraphs 136 and 263 of *King's Regulations*.
100 Department of Defence letter regarding nursing sisters and marriage policy, 29 December 1942, confidential record, LAC.
101 Elizabeth Smellie, memo dated 6 January 1943, LAC.
102 "Appointment Statistics," 000.8 (D93), DHH.
103 RCAF Memo, DMS (Air), 16 November 1943, file HQ 400-1-1, RG24, E-1b, vol. 3365, LAC.
104 Elizabeth Smellie, "Minutes of the Matron's Conference," Ottawa, 27-29 May 1943, in "Correspondence and Minutes of Meetings regarding Nursing Sisters – July 43/October 45," 147.73 C 132009 (D2), DHH.
105 "Policy of NS marrying and requesting discharge," 28 July 1943, Department of Defence Memorandum, NSD files.
106 See Constance Backhouse, *Colour-coded: A Legal History of Racism in Canada, 1900-1950* (Toronto: University of Toronto Press, 1999), 1-6.
107 Thompson, *Canada, 1922-1939*, 6.
108 Darlene Clark Hine, *Black Women in White: Racial Conflict and Cooperation in the Nursing Profession, 1890-1950* (Bloomington and Indianapolis: Indiana University Press, 1989), 102-4, 151-53, and 162-84.
109 R. Scott Sheffield, "'Of Pure European Descent and of the White Race': Recruitment Policy and Aboriginal Canadians, 1939-1945," *Canadian Military History* 5, 1 (1996): 8-11.
110 Ibid., 12.
111 *Eighth Canadian Census*, 7: 334-35.
112 Ethel Johns, "This Heritage of Freedom," *Canadian Nurse* 36, 7 (1940): 401.
113 Lisa Bannister, producer, *Equal to the Challenge: An Anthology of Women's Experiences during World War II* (Ottawa: Department of National Defence, 2001), xiii-xv.
114 Gaëtane LaBonté Kerr, audiotaped interview with Lisa Weintraub, Montreal, 11 April 1985, Concordia Oral History Project, ISN 167796, LAC.
115 Gaëtane LaBonté Kerr in *Military Nurses of Canada*, 1: 338.
116 E. Frances Upton, "The A.R.N.P.Q. Meets in the City of Quebec," *Canadian Nurse* 38, 4 (1942): 266.
117 Thompson, *Canada, 1922-1939*, 325-29.
118 Neil Sutherland, *Growing Up: Children in English Canada from the Great War to the Age of Television* (Toronto: University of Toronto Press, 1997), 74-77; Strong-Boag, *The New Day Recalled*, 53; McPherson, *Bedside Matters*, 125; Axelrod, *Making a Middle Class*, 159.
119 John Porter, *The Vertical Mosaic: An Analysis of Social Class and Power in Canada* (Toronto: University of Toronto Press, 1965); Strong-Boag, *New Day Recalled*; and McPherson, *Bedside Matters*.
120 Porter, *Vertical Mosaic*, 9.
121 Andrew C. Holman, *A Sense of Their Duty: Middle-Class Formation in Victorian Ontario Towns* (Montreal and Kingston: McGill-Queen's University Press, 2000), 11-16, 98.
122 Porter, *Vertical Mosaic*, 9-10.
123 Strong-Boag, *New Day Recalled*, 3.
124 Ibid., 53; McPherson, *Bedside Matters*, 125.
125 McPherson, *Bedside Matters*, 117, 121, 125.
126 *Eighth Census of Canada, 1946*, vol. 6, *Earnings, Employment and Unemployment of Wage-Earners* (Ottawa: King's Printer, 1946), xiii-xvii.
127 Weir, *Survey of Nursing*, 70, 98, 119, 168; McPherson, *Bedside Matters*, 121, table 4.1.
128 Kathi Jackson, *They Called Them Angels: American Military Nurses of World War II* (Westport, CT: Praeger, 2000), xviii.
129 Sarnecky, *A History of the U.S. Army Nurse Corps*, 177, 231.

130 Ibid., 270.
131 Ibid., 277.
132 Elizabeth M. Norman, *We Band of Angels: The Untold Story of American Nurses Trapped on Bataan by the Japanese* (New York: Random House, 1999), 47.
133 Hine, *Black Women in White*, 102-4, 151-53, and 162-84.
134 Sarnecky, *History of the U.S. Army Nurse Corps*, 233-34; Enloe, *Maneuvers*, 215-17.
135 Jan Bassett, *Guns and Brooches: Australian Army Nursing from the Boer War to the Gulf War* (New York: Oxford University Press, 1992), 112-13, 172.
136 Juliet Piggott, *Queen Alexandra's Royal Army Nursing Corps* (London: Leo Cooper, 1975); Penny Starns, *March of the Matrons: Military Influence on the British Civilian Nursing Profession, 1939-1969* (Peterborough, UK: DSM, 2000) and *Nurses at War: Women on the Frontline, 1939-45* (Stroud, Gloucestershire: Sutton Publishing, 2000).

Chapter 2: Incorporating Nurses into the Military

· 1 T.S. Wilson, "Resuscitation in Battle Casualties," *Journal of the Canadian Medical Services* 2, 5 (1945): 520.
2 "Nursing Sisters' Association of Canada, 1920-1966," Agnes MacLeod papers, College and Association of Registered Nurses of Alberta Archives and Museum (hereafter CARNA); "Overseas Nursing Sisters Association," *Canadian Nurse* 36, 1 (1940): 32.
3 M.B. Clint, *Our Bit: Memories of War Service by a Canadian Nurse* (Montreal: Barwick, 1934); Ethel Johns, "A Valiant Heart," *Canadian Nurse* 35, 8 (1939): 459-62; Constance Bruce, *Humour in Tragedy: Hospital Life behind Three Fronts by a Canadian Nursing Sister* (London: Skeffington and Son, 1918).
4 Jessie Morrison, "Address to Royal Alexandra Hospital Nurses Alumnae – Edmonton, 9 December 1974," Record numbers 87.4, 91.30, and 92.10, CARNA.
5 "Nursing Service, RCAMC, CASF," *Canadian Nurse* 36, 7 (1940): 425-26; "The Matron-in-Chief in Canada," *Canadian Nurse* 36, 8 (1940): 497-98.
6 Elizabeth Smellie, "A Message from the Matron-in-Chief," *Canadian Nurse* 36, 9 (1940): 622-23.
7 Ruth Littlejohn McIlrath, audiotaped interview with Nina Rumen at Vancouver, 20 October 1987, and Burnaby, BC, 23 November 1988, Oral History Collection, College of Registered Nurses of British Columbia (hereafter CRNBC).
8 "Nursing Service, RCAMC, CASF," *Canadian Nurse* 36, 2 (1940): 87-88; Ethel Johns, "The Shape of Things to Come," *Canadian Nurse* 37, 2 (1941): 84.
9 C.P. Stacey, *Official History of the Canadian Army in the Second World War*, vol. 1, *Six Years of War: The Army in Canada, Britain and the Pacific* (Ottawa: Queen's Printer, 1955), 30-31, 43, 110-22.
10 E.L. Smellie, "Recommendations from Minutes of Matrons' Conference," in "Correspondence and Minutes of Meetings re. Nursing Sisters, July '43/Oct '45," 147.73-C-132009 (D2), Department of National Defence Directorate of History and Heritage, Ottawa (hereafter DHH).
11 G.W.L. Nicholson, *Canada's Nursing Sisters* (Toronto: Samuel Stevens Hakkert, 1975), 53.
12 *King's Regulations and Orders for the Canadian Militia, 1939* (Ottawa: King's Printer, 1939).
13 Estelle Tritt Aspler, audiotaped interview with author, Westmount, Quebec, 13 August 2001.
14 Evelyn Pepper, in *The Military Nurses of Canada: Recollections of Canadian Military Nurses*, vol. 1, ed. E.A. Landells (White Rock, BC: Co-Publishing, 1995), 45-6; Mary (Benwick) Baldwin, in *The Military Nurses of Canada: Recollections of Canadian Military Nurses*, vol. 2, ed. E.A. Landells (White Rock, BC: Co-Publishing, 1999), 131-32; Nicholson, *Canada's Nursing Sisters*, 125-26; Evelyn A. Pepper, Gaëtan (LaBonté) Kerr, Harriet J. T. Sloan, and Margaret D. McLean, "'Over There' in World War II," *Canadian Nurse* 62, 11 (1966): 32.
15 Frances Oakes, audiotaped interview with author, Guelph, Ontario, 15 May 2001; W.R. Feasby, ed., *Official History of the Canadian Medical Services, 1939-1945*, vol. 1, *Organization and Campaigns* (Ottawa: Queen's Printer, 1956), 439; Jean Ellen (Wheeler) Keays, audiotaped interview with Sheila Zerr, 16 August 1994, White Rock, BC, CRNBC; Betty Riddell, audiotaped interview with author, Ottawa, 26 November 2001.
16 Dorothy Surgenor Maddock, audiotaped interview with author, Ottawa, 26 June 2001.
17 Kay Christie, audiotaped interview with Joan Williams, 20 November 1975, ISN 196090, Library and Archives Canada (hereafter LAC).
18 "The Organization of the CWAC," *Canadian Nurse* 37, 8 (1941): 545.
19 Smellie, "A Message from the Matron-in-Chief," 623.
20 Anne A. (Gair) Evans, *Military Nurses of Canada*, 1: 345-46; Dorothy M. (Grainger) Anderson, ibid., 1: 412; Rossalea O. (Hughes) Crowe, ibid., 1: 250.

21 There were approximately twenty of these cars in service by the end of the war; the first ones were donated by the Canadian National Railway in 1940 and the Canadian Pacific Railway in 1941. See Nicholson, *Canada's Nursing Sisters*, 195-98; "Hospital Car for Canadian Casualties," *Canadian Nurse* 37, 10 (1941): 716; and Helen (Bright) Armstrong, in *Military Nurses of Canada*, 1: 184-85.

22 Kathleen G. Christie, "Experiences as a Prisoner-of-War, World War 2," interview with Charles G. Roland, 8 December 1982, HCM 28-82, Oral History Archives of the Hannah Chair for the History of Medicine, McMaster University (hereafter HCM 28-82).

23 Nicholson, *Canada's Nursing Sisters*, 192-94 and 213; Muriel McArthur, in *The Military Nurses of Canada: Recollections of Canadian Military Nurses*, vol. 3, ed. E.A. Landells (White Rock, BC: Co-Publishing, 1999), 271-76; Muriel McArthur, audiotaped interview with author, Barrie, Ontario, 14 May 2001; "The RCAF Nursing Service," *Canadian Nurse* 40, 3 (1944): 164-66; "History of the RCAF Plastic Surgery and Jaw Injury Unit," *Journal of the Canadian Medical Services* 4, 1 (1946): 90-4; Rita Donovan, *As for the Canadians: The Remarkable Story of the RCAF's "Guinea Pig"' of The Second World War* (Ottawa: Buschek Books, 2000).

24 Nicholson, *Canada's Nursing Sisters*, 182-85; Marjorie G. Russell, "The Royal Canadian Naval Nursing Service," in *Military Nurses of Canada*, 3: 230-35; "Royal Canadian Navy Nursing Service," *Canadian Nurse* 37, 12 (1941): 830; "Royal Canadian Naval Nursing Service," *Canadian Nurse* 40, 2 (1944): 96-98; Norman K. Harrison, "The Hospital Ship That Never Puts to Sea," *Nursing Mirror*, 15 January 1944, ii-iii.

25 Nicholson, *Canada's Nursing Sisters*, 187; Surgenor Maddock interview; "Last Post," *Canadian Nurse* 38, 12 (1942): 938-39; Marjorie (Cowan) Horton, *Military Nurses of Canada*, 1: 554-55.

26 Wheeler Keays interview, CRNBC.

27 "List of Canadians who Served with South African Nursing Service – Second World War (1939-1945)," 000.8 (D91) and "Correspondence, reports, instructions, etc. re. Nursing Sisters enrolling in South African Forces, August 41-November 45," 325.009 (D575), DHH; Isabel Morrison Fraser, audiotaped interview with author, Ottawa, 27 November 2001; Florence Louise Jamieson, interview with Margaret M. Allemang, Toronto, 24 April and 3 May 1987, Oral History Collection, Margaret M. Allemang Centre for the History of Nursing (hereafter MMA); Gladys Sharpe, "Our Canadian Nurses in South Africa," *Canadian Hospital* 20, 8 (1943): 20-22; "Canadian Nurses for South Africa," *Canadian Nurse* 37, 9 (1941): 623; "Canadian Nurses for South Africa," *Canadian Nurse* 37, 10 (1941): 698; "Canadian Nurses for South Africa," *Canadian Nurse* 37, 12 (1941): 830; "On Active Service at Home and Abroad," *Canadian Nurse* 38, 2 (1942): 95.

28 Marguerite McLimont, "Canada Goes to South Africa," *Canadian Nurse* 38, 12 (1942): 914-20.

29 Angela M. (La Croix) Smith, in *Military Nurses of Canada*, 1: 354.

30 Elizabeth Louise Clement, in *Military Nurses of Canada*, 1: 434.

31 Feasby, *Official History of the Canadian Medical Services*, 1: 17-20, 27-29, 56-58, 62-67, 83-87; Bill Rawling, *Death Their Enemy: Canadian Medical Practitioners and War* (Ottawa: author, 2001), 129-236 and 275-78.

32 "Advances in Military Medicine," *Journal of the Canadian Medical Services* 2, 1 (1944): 78.

33 Patricia Moll audiotaped interview with Lisa Weintraub, 5 July 1985, ISN 167813, LAC.

34 Wilson, "Resuscitation in Battle Casualties," 520; Feasby, *Official History of the Canadian Medical Services*, 1: 187-89, 200; "Front Line Surgery," *Canadian Nurse* 39, 2 (1943): 130; Wallace Reyburn, "Medicine Goes to War," *Maclean's Magazine*, 1 September 1943, 32; and Rawling, *Death Their Enemy*, 157-59.

35 Pepper et al., "Over There," 32; W.A. Scott, "Letter on Transfusion Service in Sicily and Italy," *Journal of the Canadian Medical Services* 1, 2 (1944): 108-9; "A Canadian F.T.U. – C.A. Overseas," *Journal of the Canadian Medical Services* 2, 2 (1945): 113-15; J.C. McC. Brown, "A Simple Method of Serum Transfusion in the Field," *Journal of the Canadian Medical Services* 3, 2 (1946): 144-46.

36 Elsie M. Clay (Barr), in *Nursing Sisters' Association of Canada: Commemorative Issue and Membership Directory*, June 1994, 18.

37 Feasby, *Official History of the Canadian Medical Services*, 1: 189.

38 F. Mills, "A Letter from a Field Surgical Unit C.M.F. (Overseas)," *Journal of the Canadian Medical Services* 1, 3 (1944): 187.

39 "A Canadian F.S.U.," 115.

40 Helen (Bright) Armstrong, in *Military Nurses of Canada*, 1: 181-83.

41 February 1944, No. 5 Casualty Clearing Station war diary, RG 24, series C-3, v. 15941, LAC.

42 A.M. MacPherson, "Camp Borden Military Hospital," *Journal of the Canadian Medical Services* 3, 5 (1946): 481; Rawling, *Death Their Enemy*, 196-98.

43 Jean Dorgan, in *Military Nurses of Canada*, 1: 128.
44 Agnes J. Macleod, "With a RCAMC Casualty Clearing Station," *Canadian Nurse* 37, 2 (1941): 95-6.
45 Evelyn Pepper, in *Nursing Sisters' Association of Canada: Commemorative Issue and Membership Directory*, June 1994, 34-35.
46 Eva Wannop, audiotaped interview with author, Toronto, 25 April 2001; and Donovan, *As for the Canadians*.
47 Margaret Roe Dewart, audiotaped interview with author, Edmonton, Alberta, 15 October 2001; Feasby, *Official History of the Canadian Medical Services*, 2: 109-14.
48 No. 1 Canadian General Hospital War Diary, 15-16 November 1940, RG 24, Series C-3, v. 15666, serial 282, LAC; "RCAMC Sisters to the Rescue," *Canadian Nurse* 37, 2 (1941): 115.
49 Letter from Margaret Fletcher to her family, 30 October 1944, Margaret Fletcher fonds, 1933-1945, SC042, University of Victoria Archives and Special Collections, BC Archives (hereafter Fletcher letters).
50 Constance Betty Nicolson Brown, audiotaped interview with author, Ottawa, 3 June 2001.
51 "The RCAF Nursing Service," *Canadian Nurse* 40, 3 (1944): 164-66; "Royal Canadian Naval Well Baby Health Service," *Canadian Nurse* 40, 7 (1944): 469-72.
52 Feasby, *Official History of the Canadian Medical Services*, 1: 99, 110.
53 Nicholson, *Canada's Nursing Sisters*, 122; Wannop interview; Joan Doree, audiotaped interview with Nina Rumen, 11 February 1987, CRNBC; Jean Ciceri, audiotaped interview with Nina Rumen, 13 January 1987, CRNBC.
54 Margaret Helena Kellough, interview with Margaret M. Allemang, Toronto, April and May 1987, MMA.
55 Memo, R.W. Ryan to Air Commodore, DMS (Air), 4 January 1943, file 400-2-1, vol. 3365, Series E-1-b, RG 24, LAC; Joan Doree, in *Military Nurses of Canada*, 2: 97-98.
56 Helen K. Mussallem, audiotaped interview with author, Ottawa, 24 September 2001.
57 Frances Ferguson Sutherland, audiotaped interview with author, Edmonton, Alberta, 10 October 2001.
58 Rawling, *Death Their Enemy*, 125-26.
59 Pepper et al., "Over There," 31.
60 Littlejohn McIlrath interview, CRNBC; Lois Bayly Tewsley, audiotaped interview with author, Ottawa, 11 June 2001.
61 Margaret H. Mills, interview with Margaret M. Allemang, 5 April 1991, MMA.
62 Doree interview, CRNBC.
63 Harriet J.T. Sloan, audiotaped interview with author, Ottawa, 14 March 2001; Evelyn Pepper, in *Military Nurses of Canada*, 1: 55. See also Brenda McBryde, *A Nurse's War* (London: Chatto and Windus, 1979), 146-47, 152.
64 Mary Bray Hutton, letter to Major Hayes at CFB Borden, 8 February 1994, inserted into a Camp Borden copy of Joyce Hibbert, *Fragments of War: Stories from Survivors of World War II* (Toronto: Dundurn Press, 1985).
65 Pepper et al., "Over There," 32. Emphasis in original.
66 Fletcher letters, 20 February 1945.
67 Margaret Van Scoyoc, audiotaped interview with the author, Kingston, Ontario, 13 June 2001.
68 Lotta Dempsey, "Canada's Blitz Sisters," *Maclean's Magazine*, 1 September 1943, 24.
69 Doris Carter, *Never Leave Your Head Uncovered: A Canadian Nursing Sister in World War Two* (Waterdown, ON: Potlatch Publications, 1999), 24.
70 Helen K. Mussallem, audiotaped interview with the author, Ottawa, 24 September 2001.
71 Ann Graber Hershberger, "Mennonite Nurses in World War II: Maintaining the Thread of Pacifism in Nursing," *Nursing History Review* 11 (2003): 154.
72 Littlejohn McIlrath interview, CRNBC; Mary M. White, *Hello War, Goodbye Sanity* (N.p.: New Leaf, 1992).
73 "On Active Service," *Canadian Nurse* 39, 10 (1943): 647-50.
74 Edith Dick, "Overseas Mail," *Canadian Nurse* 40, 5 (1944): 343.
75 "Tells of Death of Winnipeg Nursing Sister," undocumented news clipping, Winnipeg General Hospital Nurses Alumnae Archives (hereafter WGHA); "Last Post," *Canadian Nurse* 38, 12 (1942): 938-39; Marjorie (Cowan) Horton, in *Military Nurses of Canada*, 1: 554-55.
76 Canadian Nurses Association, *The Leaf and the Lamp* (Ottawa: CNA, 1968), 81; "Appointment Statistics – Nursing Sisters, Physiotherapy Aides, Occupational Therapists, Dieticians and Home Sisters," 000.8 (D93), DHH; "In the Service of Their Country," *Canadian Nurse* 39, 8 (1943): 511-12; *Journal of the Canadian Medical Services* 1, 1 (1943): 89; ibid. 2, 2 (1944): 203; ibid. 2, 6 (1945): 718; ibid. 3, 2 (1946): 169.

77 The deaths of Margaret McCullough Stirling Parkinson (apparently a SAMNS nursing sister), Margaret Agnes Briggs, and Marie Cecile Dussio do not appear in corroborating sources.

78 Confidential DND personnel files, LAC.

79 Pearl (Lundgren) Swift, in *Military Nurses of Canada*, 2: 159; Tritt Aspler interview.

80 Helen Morton Rendall, interview with Margaret M. Allemang, Toronto, 14 March 1986, MMA. See also Dorothy M. Dent, "Battles with Bicycles," *Canadian Nurse* 39, 6 (1943): 411-12; Carter, *Never Leave Your Head Uncovered*, 24; Tritt Aspler interview; Mussallem interview.

81 Pauline Cox Walker, audiotaped interview with author, Kingston, Ontario, 13 June 2001. See also "Courage and Discipline," *Canadian Nurse* 40, 1 (1944): 21; notices in the *Journal of the Canadian Medical Services* 1, 1 (1943): 89; 2, 2 (1944): 203; 2, 6 (1945): 718; "A Salute to Our Nursing Sisters," *Canadian Nurse* 39, 12 (1943): 795-99; Irene D. Courtenay, in *Nursing Sisters' Association of Canada: Commemorative Issue and Membership Directory*, June 1994, 19-22.

82 Margery MacLean Root, audiotaped interview with author, Ottawa, 15 June 2001.

83 Rendall interview, MMA.

84 Pepper et al., "Over There," 27-28.

85 "Appointment Statistics," 000.8 (D93), DHH.

86 Confidential DND personnel files, LAC.

87 Jean D. (Scrimgeour) Wilson, in *Military Nurses of Canada*, 1: 248.

88 Harriet J.T. Sloan, personal communication and in Jean E. Portugal, *We Were There: The Navy, the Army, and the RCAF: A Record for Canada*, vol. 5 (Shelburne, ON: Battered Silicon Dispatch Box, 1998), 2276.

89 Nicolson Brown interview; Nicholson, *Seventy Years*, 165-66; and *Canada's Nursing Sisters*, 136-37.

90 Kellough interview, MMA.

91 Marion C. (Story) McLeod, Scrapbook of the *Lady Nelson*, April 1943, CARNA archives.

92 Littlejohn McIlrath interview, CRNBC; and Ruth (Littlejohn) McIlrath, in *Military Nurses of Canada*, 3: 18.

93 Confidential DND personnel files, LAC.

94 Doris V. Carter, audiotaped interview with author, Ottawa, 22 June 2001; and "Jungle Weapon," *Canadian Nurse* 41, 10 (1945): 803.

95 Carter, *Never Leave Your Head Uncovered*, 79; "DDT Studied for Outdoor Use," *Canadian Nurse* 41, 9 (1945): 702.

96 Christie interview, HCM 28-82. Although the Japanese attack on Hong Kong is generally attributed as occurring on 7 December 1941, on the other side of the international date line, it was actually 8 December 1941, as Christie points out.

97 Christie interview, LAC; and Kay Christie, "Behind Japanese Barbed Wire: A Canadian Nursing Sister in Hong Kong," *Royal Canadian Military Institute Year Book* (Toronto: RCMI, 1979), 11-13.

98 The civilian nurse was Pearl Needham, a Vancouver General Hospital graduate who went to Shanghai in public health, married an Englishman, and settled in Hong Kong; see Christie interview, HCM 28-82.

99 Ibid.

100 Kathleen G. Christie, audiotaped interview with Margaret Allemang, 5 April 1992 and 3 June 1992, MMA; Kathleen G. Christie, "M. & V. for Christmas Dinner," *Canadian Nurse* 63, 12 (1967): 28-30; Kay Christie, audiotaped interview with Bill McNeil, January 1992, Kay Christie fonds, 94.41, CARNA; Jessie G. Morrison, "Kathleen Georgina Christie, 1911-1994: In Memoriam," 91.31, CARNA; Bill McNeil, *Voices of a War Remembered: An Oral History of Canadians in the Second World War* (Toronto: Doubleday, 1991), 96-104; Constance Murray, "A Repatriate from Hong Kong," *Canadian Nurse* 42, 3 (1946): 242-43.

101 Jean (MacBain) MacAulay, in *Military Nurses of Canada*, 2: 190; Rendell interview, MMA.

102 Margaret Van Scoyoc, audiotaped interview with Lisa Weintraub, Montreal, 4 June 1984, ISN 167825, LAC.

103 Rita (Murphy) Morin, in *Military Nurses of Canada*, 2: 176.

104 Barbara Ross in Jean E. Portugal, *We Were There*, 2250.

105 Elizabeth L. (Burnham) Lowe, in *Military Nurses of Canada*, 1: 154-58.

106 Christie interview, MMA.

107 Pepper, in *Military Nurses of Canada*, 1: 48-49, 53-54; Elizabeth B. Pense, interview with Norma Fieldhouse, Kingston, Ontario, March 1987, MMA.

108 Betty (Herringer) Campbell, in *Nursing Sisters' Association of Canada: Commemorative Issue and Membership Directory*, June 1994, 17.

109 Ross, in Portugal, *We Were There*, 2254.
110 Lettie Turner, video-interview, *Nurses on the Battlefield*, TV documentary, producers Lori Kuffner and Barbara Campbell (Cooper Rock Pictures, 2001).
111 Margaret Fletcher, in *Military Nurses of Canada*, 1: 87.
112 Nicolson Brown, Van Scoyoc, Mussallem, and Ferguson Sutherland interviews; Evelyn Pepper, in *Military Nurses of Canada*, 1: 56-57; Constance Bond Young, interview with Ella Beardmore, Omeemee, Ontario, 4 July 1989, MMA.
113 Mary Bray Hutton, in Joyce Hibbert, *Fragments of War: Stories from Survivors of World War II* (Toronto: Dundurn Press, 1985), 127.
114 Dempsey, "Canada's Blitz Sisters," 24.
115 Cynthia Enloe, *Maneuvers: The International Politics of Militarizing Women's Lives* (Berkeley and Los Angeles: University of California Press, 2000), 212.
116 Confidential DND personnel files, LAC.
117 Edna Rossiter, audiotaped interview with Nina Rumen, Vancouver, 27 October 1987, CRNBC; "Postwar Planning Activities: Opportunities in DVA Hospitals," *Canadian Nurse* 41, 9 (1945): 720; "Opportunities for Nurses with the DVA," *Canadian Nurse* 42, 3 (1946): 236-37; "Appointment Statistics," DHH.
118 Margery MacLean Root interview.
119 Margaret Allemang, audiotaped interview with author, Toronto, 26 April 2001.
120 Peter Neary and Shaun Brown, "The Veterans Charter and Canadian Women of World War II," in *The Good Fight: Canadians and World War II*, ed. J.L. Granatstein and Peter Neary (Toronto: Copp Clark, 1995), 388-89.
121 Ibid., 389, 410.
122 Carter, *Never Leave Your Head Uncovered*, 151.
123 Neary and Brown, "The Veterans Charter and Canadian Women," 391; "Postwar Planning Activities: Re-establishment Information," *Canadian Nurse* 41, 8 (1945): 636-38.
124 Tritt Aspler interview; Gertrude M. Hall, "Notes from National Office: Of Interest to Nursing Sisters," *Canadian Nurse* 41, 1 (1945): 53-54.
125 Beatrice Cole Hunter, audiotaped interview with author, Edmonton, Alberta, 13 October 2001.
126 Pauline Lamont Flynn, personal communication, 16 September 2002.
127 See Kathleen Canning, "Feminist History after the Linguistic Turn: Historicizing Discourse and Experience," *Signs* 19, 2 (1994): 368-404.
128 Eleanor MacGregor, "Defending the Empire," unpublished paper in possession of the author.
129 Wheeler Keays interview, CRNBC.
130 M. Dorothy Mawdsley, "The Position of Women in the Postwar World," *Canadian Nurse* 40, 8 (1944): 548-52.

Chapter 3: Shaping Nursing Sisters as "Officers" and "Ladies"
1 Kathleen (Rowntree) Bowman, in *The Military Nurses of Canada: Recollections of Canadian Military Nurses*, vol. 1, ed. E.A. Landells (White Rock, BC: Co-Publishing, 1995), 79; Jean Ellen (Wheeler) Keays, audiotaped interview with Sheila Zerr, White Rock, BC, 16 August 1994, Oral History Collection, College of Registered Nurses of British Columbia (hereafter CRNBC); Margaret Van Scoyoc, audiotaped interview with author, Ottawa, 13 June 2001.
2 Leisa D. Meyer, *Creating G.I. Jane: Sexuality and Power in the Women's Army Corps during World War II* (New York: Columbia University Press, 1996), 2-3.
3 Jean (MacBain) MacAulay, in *The Military Nurses of Canada: Recollections of Canadian Military Nurses*, vol. 2, ed. E.A. Landells (White Rock, BC: Co-Publishing, 1999), 111; See also Ruth Roach Pierson, "Wartime Jitters over Femininity," in *The Good Fight: Canadians and World War II*, ed. J.L. Granatstein and Peter Neary (Toronto: Copp Clark, 1995) and *"They're Still Women after All": The Second World War and Canadian Womanhood* (Toronto: McClelland and Stewart, 1986).
4 Kathleen (Dickey) Allan, in *Military Nurses of Canada*, 1: 358.
5 Kathryn McPherson, "'The Case of the Kissing Nurse': Femininity, Sexuality, and Canadian Nursing, 1900-1970," in *Gendered Pasts: Historical Essays in Femininity and Masculinity in Canada*, ed. Kathryn McPherson, Cecilia Morgan, and Nancy M. Forestell (Don Mills, ON: Oxford University Press, 1999), 180-81.
6 Paragraph 193, *King's Regulations and Orders for the Canadian Militia, 1939* (Ottawa: King's Printer, 1939; revised, 1947); W.R. Feasby, ed., *Official History of the Canadian Medical Services, 1939-1945*, vol. 1, *Organization and Campaigns* (Ottawa: Queen's Printer, 1956), 324.

7 Lotta Dempsey, "Canada's Blitz Sisters," *Maclean's Magazine*, 1 September 1943, 24.
8 Arthur Salusbury MacNalty and W. Franklin Mellor, eds., *Medical Services in War: The Principal Medical Lessons of the Second World War Based on the Official Medical Histories of the United Kingdom, Canada, Australia, New Zealand and India* (London: H.M.S.O., 1968), 77-78; Juliet Piggott, *Queen Alexandra's Royal Army Nursing Corps* (London: Leo Cooper, 1975), 73; Jan Bassett, *Guns and Brooches: Australian Army Nursing from the Boer War to the Gulf War* (New York: Oxford University Press, 1992), 3, 99, 142, 151, 165.
9 G.W.L. Nicholson, *Seventy Years of Service: A History of the R.C.A.M.C.* (Ottawa: Borealis Press, 1977), 141.
10 Harriet J.T. Sloan, in *We Were There: The Army, a Record for Canada*, vol. 5, ed. Jean E. Portugal (N.p.: Royal Canadian Military Institute Heritage Society, 1998), 2283-84.
11 Margery MacLean Root, audiotaped interview with author, Ottawa, 15 June 2001.
12 Margaret Fletcher to her family, 3 July 1943, Margaret Fletcher fonds, 1933-1945, SC042, University of Victoria Archives and Special Collections, BC Archives (hereafter Fletcher letters).
13 Helen K. Mussallem, audiotaped interview with author, Ottawa, 24 September 2001.
14 No. 1 CGH War Diary for 29 January 1941, RG 24, C-3, vol. 15666, serial 282, Library and Archives Canada (hereafter LAC).
15 Eva Wannop, audiotaped interview with author, Toronto, 25 April 2001.
16 Feasby, *Official History of the Canadian Medical Services*, 1: 439-42; G.W.L. Nicholson, *Canada's Nursing Sisters* (Toronto: Samuel Stevens Hakkert, 1975), 182-83.
17 Letter from #2 RCAF Training Command at Winnipeg to National Defence (Air), 16 March 1942, E-1-b, v. 3365, HQ400-1-1, LAC.
18 P. Wetzel, "Draft Narrative for the History of the RCAF (WDs) re. Women Medical Officers, Nursing Sisters, Physiotherapists, Orthopists, and Opthalmical Assistants," 181.003 (D1467), National Defence Department Directorate of History and Heritage (hereafter DHH); letters from H.A. Peacock to Commodore R.W. Ryan, 29 May 1942, RG 24, E-1-b, v. 3365, part 1, LAC; letter from Marion Lindeburgh to C.G. Power, 20 November 1942, RG24, series E-1-b, v. 3365, 400-2-1, part 1, LAC.
19 Letters, 29 September and 2 November 1940, from Major A.D. Kelly; letters, 27 May, 8 June, and 20 July 1942 between Matron-in-Chief Elizabeth Smellie and J.A. Sully; memo of 4, 17, and 20 August 1942; all from "Nursing Sisters, RCAF: Appointment of, policy governing," file 400-2-1, vol. 3365, series E-1-b, vol. 1, RG 24, LAC.
20 Feasby, *Official History of the Canadian Medical Services*, 1: 439-42.
21 Everett C. Hughes, Helen MacGill Hughes, and Irwin Deutscher, *Twenty Thousand Nurses Tell Their Story* (Philadelphia: J.B. Lippincott, 1958), 62.
22 Evelyn A. Pepper, Gaëtan (LaBonté) Kerr, Harriet J.T. Sloan, and Margaret D. McLean, "'Over There' in World War II," *Canadian Nurse* 62, 11 (1966): 32.
23 Frances Ferguson Sutherland, audiotaped interview with author, Edmonton, Alberta, 10 October 2001.
24 Marjorie (Cowan) Horton, in *Military Nurses of Canada*, 1: 553.
25 Betty Young Ramage Hamilton, audiotaped interview with author, Edmonton, Alberta, 12 October 2001.
26 Margaret H. Mills, audiotaped interview with Margaret Allemang, 5 April 1991, Oral History Collection, Margaret M. Allemang Centre for the History of Nursing (hereafter MMA).
27 Eleanor MacGregor, "Defending the Empire," unpublished paper in possession of author.
28 Ruth Littlejohn McIlrath, audiotaped interview with Nina Rumen, Vancouver and Burnaby, BC, 20 October 1987 and 23 November 1988, CRNBC; Ruth (Littlejohn) McIlrath, in *The Military Nurses of Canada: Recollections of Canadian Military Nurses*, vol. 3, ed. E.A. Landells (White Rock, BC: Co-Publishing, 1999), 18.
29 Florence Louise Jamieson, audiotaped interview with Margaret Allemang at Toronto, Ontario, 24 April and 3 May 1987, MMA.
30 Margaret Helena Kellough, audiotaped interview with Margaret Allemang, April and May 1987, MMA.
31 Margaret Van Scoyoc, interview with Lisa Weintraub, 4 June 1984, ISN 167825, LAC.
32 Margaret M. Allemang, audiotaped interview with author, Toronto, 26 April 2001.
33 Beatrice Cole Hunter, audiotaped interview with author, Edmonton, Alberta, 13 October 2001.
34 Constance Betty Nicolson Brown, audiotaped interview with author, Ottawa, 3 June 2001.
35 Doris Carter, *Never Leave Your Head Uncovered: A Canadian Nursing Sister in World War Two* (Waterdown, ON: Potlatch Publications, 1999), 4, 12.
36 Memo, 12 May 1941, Department of External Affairs, E-1-b, v. 3365, HQ400-1-1, LAC.
37 Evelyn Pepper, in *Military Nurses of Canada*, 1: 50.

38 Mary M. Bower White, audiotaped interview with author, Surrey, BC, 20 October 2001.
39 Mills interview, MMA.
40 Pauline Lamont Flynn, audiotaped interview with author, Ottawa, 3 April 2001.
41 McPherson, "The Case of the Kissing Nurse," 184.
42 Estelle Tritt Aspler, audiotaped interview with author, Westmount, Quebec, 13 August 2001.
43 Mary Bray Hutton, in *We Were There: The Navy, the Army, and the RCAF: A Record for Canada*, vol. 5, ed. Jean E. Portugal (Shelburne, ON: Battered Silicon Dispatch Box, 1998), 2243.
44 Kellough interview, MMA.
45 Doris Taylor Rasberry, audiotaped interview with author, Pointe Claire, Quebec, 19 June 2001.
46 Amy White, letter to her parents, 12 January 1944, M. Amy White fonds, MG 30 E508, LAC.
47 "Responsibilities of Members of Nursing Sister Service," Course in Aviation Nursing, Course No. 12, August 23rd-Septmber 14, 1944," Barbara R. Carr fonds, Royal Canadian Military Institute Library, Toronto.
48 "Army Nurses Are on the Go," *Canadian Nurse* 39, 7 (1943): 499.
49 "Navy Nurses Are Busier than Ever," *Canadian Nurse* 39, 9 (1943): 633.
50 "Unprecedented Times? Unprecedented Problems," *Canadian Nurse* 39, 8 (1943): 555.
51 "War Effort Speeded by New Success over Athlete's Foot," *Canadian Nurse* 40, 5 (1944): 349.
52 "Nursing Service, RCAMC, CASF," *Canadian Nurse* 36, 2 (1940): 87-88.
53 Carter, *Never Leave Your Head Uncovered*, 6-7.
54 "The RCAF Nursing Service," *Canadian Nurse* 40, 3 (1944): 164-66; "The Royal Canadian Naval Nursing Service," *Canadian Nurse* 40, 2 (1944): 96-98; Nicholson, *Canada's Nursing Sisters*, 183.
55 Elizabeth Dean Doe, audiotaped interview with author, Ottawa, 30 June 2001.
56 Doris V. Carter, audiotaped interview with author at Ottawa, Ontario, 22 June 2001.
57 Dorothy Surgenor Maddock, audiotaped interview with author, Ottawa, 26 June 2006.
58 John Murray Gibbon, "Our Canadian Nursing Sister," *Nursing Songs of Canada* (Toronto: Gordon V. Thompson, 1946), 8-9.
59 Kellough interview, MMA.
60 Pepper et al., "Over There," 26, 28.
61 Meyers, *Creating G.I. Jane*, 149-56.
62 Jean (MacBain) MacAulay, in *Military Nurses of Canada*, 2: 115.
63 Pauline Cox Walker, audiotaped interview with author, Kingston, Ontario, 13 June 2001; Margaret Moss, in *Military Nurses of Canada*, 1: 299.
64 Kay Christie, audiotaped interview with Joan Williams, 20 November 1975, ISN 196090, LAC; Kathleen G. Christie, audiotaped interview with Margaret Allemang, 5 April 1992 and 3 June 1992, MMA; Kay Christie, "Behind Japanese Barbed Wire: A Canadian Nursing Sister in Hong Kong," *Royal Canadian Military Institute Year Book* (Toronto: RCMI, 1979), 11-13.
65 Elizabeth M. Norman made a similar point regarding American nurses in *We Band of Angels: The Untold Story of American Nurses Trapped on Bataan by the Japanese* (New York: Random House, 1999), 39.
66 Irene (Stephenson) Mercier, in *Military Nurses of Canada*, 1: 224.
67 Mary T. Sarnecky, *A History of the U.S. Army Nurse Corps* (Philadelphia: University of Pennsylvania Press, 1999), 231, 273-75.
68 "Report of the Committee on Nursing and Nurse Education in Canadian Hospitals," Bulletin #36 (1941), 39, RNAO fonds, 96B-5-14, Archives of Ontario (hereafter AO).
69 Lamont Flynn interview.
70 Grace Patterson, audiotaped interview with Joan Williams, 18 November 1975, ISN 196088, LAC.
71 Pepper, in *Military Nurses of Canada*, 1: 57.
72 RCAF memo, 8 June 1944, HQ54-27-93-15 FD15 (Personnel 1B), RG24, E-1-b, vol. 3365, file 400-2-1, part II, LAC; Evelyn Pepper, Elizabeth L. (Burnham) Lowe, and Jessie Morrison, in *Military Nurses of Canada*, 1: 51, 57, 158, 241; Dorothy A. Macham, interview with Norma Fieldhouse, Toronto, 10 February 1988, MMA; Nicholson, *Canada's Nursing Sisters*, 124, 140-41.
73 Dorothy Macham, in *Military Nurses of Canada*, 1: 320.
74 Confidential personnel records, Department of National Defence, LAC.
75 Bray Hutton, in *We Were There*, ed. Portugal, 5: 2244.
76 Pepper, in *Military Nurses of Canada*, 1: 57.
77 Constance Bond Young, audiotaped interview with Ella Beardmore, 4 July 1989, MMA.
78 Dorothy Agnes Potts, audiotaped interview with Margaret M. Allemang, 30 September 1987, MMA.

79 MacGregor, "Defending the Empire."

80 Lenore Lancaster Menard, audiotaped interview with Terina Rindal, Lethbridge, Alberta, 14 March 1995, College and Association of Registered Nurses of Alberta Museum and Archives.

81 Anne Farries, "War Nurse Recalls Second World War Experiences," *Cranbrook Daily Townsman*, (Cranbrook, BC), 10 November 1992.

82 Irene Henderson Greenwood, in *Nursing Sisters' Association of Canada: Commemorative Issue and Membership Directory*, June 1994, 25.

83 M.J. Tuttle, "Analysis of Medial Repatriations: Canadian Army Overseas," *Journal of the Canadian Medical Services* 3, 3 (1946): 211.

84 Mary Beatrice (Nelson) Weir, in *Military Nurses of Canada*, 2: 237; Eleanor (Wallbridge) Lloyd, in *Military Nurses of Canada*, 3: 57; Lois Bayly Tewsley, audiotaped interview with author, Ottawa, 11 June 2001; Amy White, letters of 9 October 1944 and 19 February 1945, M. Amy White fonds, MG 30 E508, LAC.

85 Jean Mary Ciceri, audiotaped interview with Nina Rumen at Victoria, BC, 13 January 1987, CRNBC.

86 Confidential personnel records, Department of National Defence, LAC.

87 Anonymity requested.

88 McPherson, "The Case of the Kissing Nurse," 181-85.

89 Harriet J.T. Sloan, audiotaped interview with author, Ottawa, 14 March 2001.

90 Fletcher, letter to her father from No. 16 CGH, 13 November 1943, Fletcher letters.

91 Mary M. White, *Hello War, Goodbye Sanity* (N.p.: New Leaf, 1992), 34, 43-45, 72-73, 86-88, 91-95, 99-100, 105.

92 MacGregor, "Defending the Empire."

93 Fletcher, letter to her father from No. 16 CGH, 27 October 1942, Fletcher letters.

94 Dorothy A. Macham interview with Norma Fieldhouse at Toronto, 10 February 1988, MMA.

95 Fletcher, letters to her family, 17 February and 16 April 1945, Fletcher letters.

Chapter 4: Legitimating Military Nursing Work

1 J.L. Granatstein, *Canada's Army: Waging War and Keeping the Peace* (Toronto: University of Toronto Press, 2002), 230; Mark Zuehlke, *Ortona: Canada's Epic World War II Battle* (Toronto: Stoddart, 1999), 290-1; and Wallace Reyburn, "Medicine Goes to War," *Maclean's Magazine*, 1 September 1943, 18-19, 32, 34-35, 37.

2 F. Mills, "A Letter from a Field Surgical Unit, CMF (Overseas)," *Journal of the Canadian Medical Services* 1, 3 (1944): 187. ⁷

3 Margaret M. Allemang, audiotaped interview with author, Toronto, 26 April 2001; Cynthia Enloe, *Does Khaki Become You? The Militarization of Women's Lives* (Boston: South End Press, 1983), 108.

4 Gail Braybon and Penny Summerfield, *Out of the Cage: Women's Experiences in Two World Wars* (London: Pandora, 1987); Jan Bassett, *Guns and Brooches: Australian Army Nursing from the Boer War to the Gulf War* (New York: Oxford University Press, 1992), 2.

5 Wiebe E. Bijker and John Law, eds., *Shaping Technology/Building Society: Studies in Sociotechnical Change* (Cambridge, MA: MIT Press, 1992); Wiebe E. Bijker, Thomas P. Hughes, and Trevor J. Pinch, eds., *The Social Construction of Technological Systems: New Directions in the Social History of Technology* (Cambridge, MA: MIT Press, 1989); John Law and John Hassard, *Actor Network Theory and After* (Oxford: Blackwell, 1999).

6 Donald H. Avery, *The Science of War: Canadian Scientists and Allied Military Technology during the Second World War* (Toronto: University of Toronto Press, 1998), 4-8; Irvin Stewart, *Organizing Scientific Research for War: The Administrative History of the Office of Scientific Research and Development* (Boston: Little, Brown, 1948), 104-5.

7 William McNeill, *The Pursuit of Power: Technology, Armed Force, and Society since A.D. 1000* (Chicago: University of Chicago Press, 1982), 118 as cited in Alex Roland, "Technology and War: The Historiographical Revolution of the 1980s," *Technology and Culture* 34, 1 (1993): 126.

8 Ethel Johns, "The Time and Place of Meeting," *Canadian Nurse* 36, 8 (1940): 474; Marion Lindeburgh, "A New Year Message," *Canadian Nurse* 39, 1 (1943): 15-16.

9 Nathan Rosenberg, Annetine C. Gelijns, and Holly Dawkins, eds., *Sources of Medical Technology: Universities and Industry*, vol. 5 of *Medical Innovation at the Crossroads* (Washington, DC: National Academy Press, 1995); Susan E. Lederer, *Subjected to Science: Human Experimentation in America before the Second World War* (Baltimore: Johns Hopkins University Press, 1995); Stuart S. Blume, *Insight and Industry: On the Dynamics of Technological Change in Medicine* (Cambridge, MA: MIT Press, 1992), 72.

10 W.R. Feasby, ed., *Official History of the Canadian Medical Services, 1939-1945*, vol. 2, *Clinical Subjects* (Ottawa: Queen's Printer, 1956); G.W.L. Nicholson, *Seventy Years of Service: A History of the R.A.M.C.* (Ottawa: Borealis Press, 1977); Bill Rawling, *Death Their Enemy: Canadian Medical Practitioners and War* (Ottawa: author, 2001).

11 John C. Sheehan, *The Enchanted Ring: The Untold Story of Penicillin* (Cambridge, MA: MIT Press, 1982); Gladys L. Hobby, *Penicillin: Meeting the Challenge* (New Haven: Yale University Press, 1985).

12 Roy Porter, *The Greatest Benefit to Mankind: A Medical History of Humanity* (New York: W.W. Norton, 1997), 283, 245-303; Patricia D'Antonio, "Legacy of Domesticity," *Nursing History Review* 1 (1993): 229-46.

13 Kathryn McPherson, *Bedside Matters: The Transformation of Canadian Nursing, 1900-1990* (Toronto: Oxford University Press, 1996), 86-94; Margarete Sandelowski, *Devices and Desires: Gender, Technology, and American Nursing* (Chapel Hill: University of North Carolina Press, 2000), 72-78.

14 Isabel Hampton Robb, *Nursing: Its Principles and Practice for Hospital and Private Use*, 3rd ed. (Toronto: J.F. Hartz, 1914); Bertha Harmer and Virginia Henderson, *Textbook of the Principles and Practice of Nursing*, 4th ed. (New York: Macmillan, 1939).

15 Edna Rossiter, audiotaped interview with Nina Rumen, Vancouver, 28 October 1987, Oral History Collection of the College of Registered Nurses of British Columbia Library (hereafter CRNBC).

16 "Performance of Clinical Procedures by Graduate Nurses: A Special Study by Committee on Nursing and Nurse Education," in *Report of the Committee on Nursing and Nurse Education in Canadian Hospitals*, Bulletin # 36 (1941), 48, RNAO fonds, 96B-5-14, Archives of Ontario (hereafter AO).

17 "Report of the Executive Secretary of the CNA," *Canadian Nurse* 38, 9 (1942): 725.

18 Margaret Van Scoyoc, audiotaped interview with author, Kingston, Ontario, 13 June 2001.

19 Kathryn McPherson, "Science and Technique: Nurses' Work in a Canadian Hospital, 1920-1939," in *Caring and Curing: Historical Perspectives on Women and Healing in Canada*, ed. Dianne Dodd and Deborah Gorham (Ottawa: University of Ottawa Press, 1994), 71-101; Cynthia Toman, "Blood Work: Canadian Nursing and Blood Transfusion, 1942-1990," *Nursing History Review* 9 (2001): 51-78, and "Almonte's Great Train Disaster: Shaping Nurses' Roles and Civilian Use of Blood Transfusion," *Canadian Bulletin of Medical History* 21, 1 (2004): 145-59.

20 Fanny C. Munroe, "Military Nursing Service," *Canadian Nurse* 36, 8 (1940): 483.

21 Pauline Cox Walker, audiotaped interview with author, Kingston, Ontario, 13 June 2001. Marion C. (Story) McLeod Scrapbook, *Lady Nelson*, April 1943, College and Association of Registered Nurses of Alberta Museum and Archives (hereafter CARNA); Joan Doree, audiotaped interview with Nina Rumen, Vancouver, 11 February 1987, CRNBC; Ruth Littlejohn McIlrath, audiotaped interviews with Nina Rumen at Burnaby, BC, 20 October 1987 and Vancouver, 23 November 1988, CRNBC.

22 Harriet J.T. Sloan, audiotaped interview with author, Ottawa, 14 March 2001.

23 Elizabeth B. Pense Neil, interview with Norma Fieldhouse, Kingston, Ontario, March 1987, Oral History Collection, Margaret M. Allemang Centre for the History of Nursing, Toronto (hereafter as MMA); see also, Constance Bond Young, interview with Ella Beardmore, Omeemee, Ontario, 4 July 1989, MMA.

24 Letter, Margaret Fletcher to her family, 18 September 1943, Margaret Fletcher fonds, 1933-1945, SC042, University of Victoria Archives and Special Collections, BC Archives (hereafter Fletcher letters).

25 Pauline Lamont Flynn, audiotaped interview with author, Ottawa, 3 April 2001.

26 Eva Wannop, audiotaped interview with author, Toronto, 25 April 2001.

27 Constance Betty Nicolson Brown, audiotaped interview with author, Ottawa, 3 June 2001.

28 Lois Bayly Tewsley, audiotaped interview with author, Ottawa, 11 June 2001.

29 Beatrice Cole Hunter, audiotaped interview with author, Edmonton, Alberta, 13 October 2001.

30 Betty Young Ramage Hamilton, audiotaped interview with author, Edmonton, Alberta, 12 October 2001.

31 "RNAO Secretary-Treasurer Report for 1942-44," from the file "RNAO Secretary-Treasurer Report to the CNA Biennial Meetings, 1926-44," 3, 96B-6-06, AO.

32 "New Editions: For Wartime Teaching," *Canadian Nurse* 39, 7 (1943): 494-95; "New Books! New Editions and Revisions of Nursing Texts," *Canadian Nurse* 40, 11 (1944): 889.

33 Lily Clegg, in Jean E. Portugal, *We Were There: The Navy, the Army, and the RCAF: A Record for Canada*, vol. 5 (Shelburne, ON: Battered Silicon Dispatch Box, 1998), 2286.

34 Bond Young interview, MMA.

35 Rawling, *Death Their Enemy*, 197, 215, 220.

36 Feasby, "The Canadian Medical Services," 524-42, and *Official History of the Canadian Medical Services*, vol. 2: 277-95; Sheehan, *The Enchanted Ring*; Hobby, *Penicillin*.

37 Norman Miles Guiou, *Transfusion: A Canadian Surgeon's Story in War and in Peace* (Yarmouth, NS: Stoneycroft Publishers, 1985); Ted Allan and Sydney Gordon, *The Scalpel, the Sword: The Story of Dr. Norman Bethune* (Toronto: McClelland and Stewart, 1971); Richard Kapp, "Charles H. Best, the Canadian Red Cross Society, and Canada's First National Blood Donation Program," *Canadian Bulletin of Medical History* 12 (1995): 27-46.

38 "The Canadian Serum Project," *Journal of the Canadian Medical Services* 3, 4 (1946): 374; Feasby, *Official History of the Canadian Medical Services*, 2: 277-95; National Film Board, *Canadian Blood Saves Lives on All Fronts* (film, n.d.), ISN 82968; *Red Cross Blood Serves Canada*, ISN 23851; *Who Sheds His Blood* (film, 1939), ISN 160916; *Our Blood for Their Lives* (audiotape, 1941), ISN 82176; and *Miracle Fluid* (film, 1950), ISN 19404, Division of Documentary Art, Library and Archives Canada (hereafter LAC).

39 J.C. McC. Brown, "A Simple Method of Serum Transfusion in the Field," *Journal of the Canadian Medical Services* 3, 2 (1946): 144-46; T.S. Williams, "Resuscitation in Battle Casualties," *Journal of the Canadian Medical Services* 2, 5 (1945): 525-26; W.A. Scott, "Letter on Transfusion Service in Sicily and Italy," *Journal of the Canadian Medical Services* 1, 2 (1944): 108-9.

40 Teresa M. (Woolsey) Weir, in *The Military Nurses of Canada: Recollections of Canadian Military Nurses*, vol. 1, ed. E.A. Landells (White Rock, BC: Co-Publishing, 1995), 246.

41 Helen (Bright) Armstrong, in ibid., 183; Brenda McBryde, *A Nurse's War* (London: Chatto and Windus, 1979), 94.

42 "A Canadian F.T.U. – C.A. Overseas," *Journal of the Canadian Medical Services* 2, 2 (1945): 113-14.

43 Fletcher letters, 20 September and 30 October 1944.

44 Frances Ferguson Sutherland, audiotaped interview with author, Edmonton, Alberta, 10 October 2001.

45 E.J. Pampana, "Scientific Progress and the Victims of the War," *Canadian Nurse* 41, 1 (1945): 45-49; Katherine Inch, "The Bunyan Bag Treatment for Burns," *Canadian Nurse* 39, 3 (1943): 194.

46 Alice Whiteside Gray, "Penicillin," *Canadian Nurse* 40, 1 (1944): 21; and Rawling, *Death Their Enemy*, 132-33.

47 "Life-Saving Drugs for the Wounded," *Canadian Nurse* 36, 7 (1940): 450; Pampana, "Scientific Progress," 46; Hobby, *Penicillin*, 31.

48 Perrin H. Long and Eleanor A. Bliss, *The Clinical and Experimental Use of Sulfanilamide, Sulfapyridine and Allied Compounds* (New York: Macmillan, 1939): 11; Hobby, *Penicillin*, 31.

49 Sheehan, *The Enchanted Ring*, xiii; "Memorandum on Penicillin," *Journal of the Canadian Medical Services* 2, 1 (1944): 62-68.

50 Hobby, *Penicillin*, 145, 172, 208-9; "Squibb Had Penicillin Ready," *Canadian Nurse* 40, 10 (1944): 801.

51 Fletcher letters, 28 October 1943; and in *Military Nurses of Canada*, 1: 87.

52 Estelle Tritt Aspler, audiotaped interview with author, Westmount, Quebec, 13 August 2001; David P. Adams, *"The Greatest Good to the Greatest Number": Penicillin Rationing on the American Home Front, 1940-1945* (New York: Peter Lang, 1991), 10-11; G.W.L. Nicholson, *Seventy Years of Service*, 185-87.

53 Gwladys M. Rees Aikens, *Nurses in Battledress: The World War II Story of a Member of the QA Reserves* (Halifax: Cymru Press, 1998), 101.

54 Helen K. Mussallem, audiotaped interview with author, Ottawa, 24 September 2001.

55 No. 1 FSU War Diary, 17 February 1944, RG 24, C-3, vol. 15940, LAC; "Notes on Penicillin," 20 January 1944, from scrapbook compiled by Frances Ferguson Sutherland, CARNA.

56 Gaëtane Labonté Kerr, audiotaped interview with Lisa Weintraub, 11 April 1985, Oral History Collection, Concordia University, ISN 167796, LAC.

57 Claudia Tennant, in *Nursing Sisters of Canada Commemorative Directory* (Edmonton: Nursing Sisters' Association of Canada, 1994), 38-39.

58 Evelyn Pepper, in *Military Nurses of Canada*, 1: 53 and 56.

59 Jessie (Smith) Jamieson, in *The Military Nurses of Canada: Recollections of Canadian Military Nurses*, vol. 2, ed. E.A. Landells (White Rock, BC: Co-Publishing, 1999): 157; Margaret H. Mills, interview with Margaret M. Allemang, 5 April 1991, MMA; Susan Isabel Rowland, interview with Ella Beardmore, 15 May 1988, MMA; Rita (Murphy) Morin, in *Military Nurses of Canada*, 2: 179; Berna Tuckwell Thompson, interview with Ella Beardmore, Scarborough, Ontario, 10 June 1988, MMA; Mary Bray, in Jean Portugal, *We Were There*, 5: 2238; Doree interview, CRNBC; Kellough interview, MMA.

60 Anselm Strauss, Shizuko Fagerhaugh, Barbara Suczek and Carolyn Wiener, eds., *Social Organization of Medical Work* (Chicago: University of Chicago Press, 1985), 246-51 and 268-72; Jocalyn Lawler, *Behind the Screens: Nursing, Somology, and the Problem of the Body*, North American ed. (Don Mills, ON: Benjamin/Cummings Publishing, 1993), 44-50; Sandelowski, *Devices and Desires*, 10-11.

61 Weir, in *Military Nurses of Canada*, 1: 245; Rawling, *Death Their Enemy*, 150-52.
62 Feasby, *Official History of the Canadian Medical Services*, 1: 146; 139-42, 146-48, 155, 198, and 313; Dean Swift, "The Laboratory Diagnosis of Malaria," *Journal of the Canadian Medical Services* 1, 5 (1944): 573-78; Rawling, *Death Their Enemy*, 177-78; Nicholson, *Seventy Years of Service*, 164.
63 Doris V. Carter, *Never Leave Your Head Uncovered: A Canadian Nursing Sister in World War Two* (Waterdown, ON: Potlatch Publications, 1999), 68-69.
64 Doris V. Carter, audiotaped interview with author, Ottawa, 22 June 2001.
65 Bertha Harmer and Virginia Henderson, *Textbook of the Principles and Practice of Nursing*, 4th ed. (New York: Macmillan, 1939), 763-72.
66 Margaret Roe Dewart, audiotaped interview with author, Edmonton, Alberta, 15 October 2001.
67 J.A. MacFarland, "Trends in Military Surgery," *Canadian Nurse* 37, 2 (1941): 97-99; E.A. MacNaughton, "Early Wound Closure and Treatment in Plaster of Ten Compound Fractures of the Femur from the Normandy Front," *Journal of the Canadian Medical Services* 2, 3 (1945): 237-47.
68 Mary Bray, in *We Were There*, ed. Portugal, 5: 2238-39.
69 Barbara Ross, in ibid., 2252.
70 Fletcher letters, 25 June and 20 September 1944.
71 Feasby, *Official History of the Canadian Medical Services*, 2: 200, 207, and 203-4.
72 E. Gertrude Ferguson, "Continuous Gastric Drainage," *Canadian Nurse* 36, 6 (1940): 341-44.
73 "A Salute to Our Nursing Sisters," *Canadian Nurse* 39, 12 (1943): 796.
74 Grace Paterson, audiotaped interview with Joan Williams, 18 November 1975, ISN 196088, LAC.
75 Patricia Moll, audiotaped interview with Lisa Weintraub, 5 July 1985, ISN 167813, LAC.
76 Van Scoyoc, audiotaped interview with Lisa Weintraub, 4 June 1984, ISN 167825, LAC.
77 Adams, "The Greatest Good," 10.
78 David A. Gordon, *The Stretcher Bearers* (Stroud, ON: Pacesetter Press, 1995), 68.
79 MacNalty and Mellor, *Medical Services in War*, 140.
80 R.I. Harris, "Treatment of War Fractures," *Journal of the Canadian Medical Services* 2, 1 (1944): 10.
81 No. 4 CGH war diary for 30 June 1944, as cited in Nicholson, *Seventy Years*, 209.
82 Dorothy Surgenor Maddock, audiotaped interview with author, Ottawa, 26 June 2001; Rawling, *Death Their Enemy*, 152-53.
83 Sloan, in *We Were There*, ed. Portugal, 5: 2282.
84 See, for example, Patricia D'Antonio and Julie Fairman, "Organizing Practice: Nursing, the Medical Model, and Two Case Studies in Historical Time," *Canadian Bulletin of Medical History*, 21, 2 (2004): 411-29; Julie Fairman and Joan Lynaugh, *Critical Care Nursing: A History* (Philadelphia: University of Pennsylvania Press, 1998); and Sandelowski, *Devices and Desires: Gender, Technology, and American Nursing*.
85 D.A. Macham, "The Nursing Care of Burns," *Canadian Nurse* 39, 2 (1943): 110-12; Kathleen H. Clifford and Katherine Miller, "Nursing Aspects of Pressure Emulsion Dressings for Burns," *Canadian Nurse* 39, 1 (1943): 26.
86 Rita Donovan, *As for the Canadians: The Remarkable Story of the RCAF's "Guinea Pigs" of World War II* (Ottawa: Buschek Books, 2000), 38-43; Alfreda F. Dearden, "An Operating Room Set-up for Plastic Surgery," *Canadian Nurse* 29, 2 (1943): 109-12.
87 Joan Doree, in *Military Nurses of Canada*, 2: 97.
88 "History of the RCAF Plastic Surgery and Jaw Injury Unit," *Journal of the Canadian Medical Services* 4, 1 (1946): 91.
89 Donovan, *As for the Canadians*, 20 and 128.
90 Frances Oakes, audiotaped interview with author, Guelph, Ontario, 15 May 2001.
91 Amy White, letter of 2 April 1944 to her parents from HMCS *Niobe*, M. Amy White fonds, MG 30-E508, LAC (hereafter White letters).
92 Andrew MacPhail, *The Medical Services: Official History of the Canadian Forces in the Great War, 1914-1919* (Ottawa: King's Printer, 1925), 276-79.
93 A.M. Doyle, "Psychiatry with the Canadian Army in Action in the C.M.F.," *Journal of the Canadian Medical Services* 3, 2 (1946): 100; Terry Copp and Bill McAndrew, *Battle Exhaustion: Soldiers and Psychiatrists in the Canadian Army, 1939-1945* (Montreal and Kingston: McGill-Queen's University Press, 1990), 43; Bill McAndrew, "The Soldier and the Battle," in *The Good Fight: Canadians and the Second World War*, ed. J.L. Granatstein and Peter Neary (Toronto: Copp Clark, 1995), 128; Joanna Bourke, "The Emotions in War: Fear and the British and American Military, 1914-45,"*Historical Research* 74, 185

(2001): 314-30.

94 Copp and McAndrew, *Battle Exhaustion*, 8-9 and 39-40; Jonathan C. Meakins, "'PULHEMS' Profiles for Army Medical Officers," *Journal of the Canadian Medical Services* 1, 3 (1944): 236-41.

95 W.O. Glidden, "Psychiatry and Post-Discharge Problems," *Journal of the Canadian Medical Services* 1, 1 (1943): 52-56; McAndrew, "The Soldier and the Battle," 130-34.

96 W.R. Feasby, in MacNalty and Mellor, *Medical Services in War*, 526-27.

97 Doree, in *Military Nurses of Canada*, 2: 95-98; Copp and McAndrew, *Battle Exhaustion*, 25.

98 Copp and McAndrew, *Battle Exhaustion*, 16-17; Feasby, *Official History of the Canadian Medical Services*, 2: 64

99 Copp and McAndrew, *Battle Exhaustion*, 69.

100 Doyle, "Psychiatry with the Canadian Army," 93; A.M. Doyle, "Report of the Neuropsychiatrist on the Sicilian Campaign," *Journal of the Canadian Medical Services* 1, 2 (1944): 106-7.

101 Verna L. White Lister, personal communication with author, Vancouver, 18 October 2001 and in *Military Nurses of Canada*, 1: 254-56.

102 Marjorie MacLean Root, audiotaped interview with author, Ottawa, 15 June 2001.

103 Copp and McAndrew, *Battle Exhaustion*, 32, 71.

104 Doyle, "Psychiatry with the Canadian Army," 95-100; Feasby, *Official History of the Canadian Medical Services*, 2: 64.

105 G.S. Burton, "Report on No. 1 Canadian Neuropsychiatric Wing," *Journal of the Canadian Medical Services* 2, 5 (1945): 531-32; Feasby, *Official History of the Canadian Medical Services*, 2: 76; Doyle, "Psychiatry with the Canadian Army," 97.

106 Veryl Margaret Tipliski, "Parting at the Crossroads: The Emergence of Education for Psychiatric Nursing in Three Canadian Provinces, 1909-1955," *Canadian Bulletin of Medical History* 21, 2 (2004): 253-79; Chris Dooley, "'They Gave Their Care, but We Gave Loving Care': Defining and Defending Boundaries of Skill and Craft in the Nursing Service of a Manitoba Mental Hospital during the Great Depression," *Canadian Bulletin of Medical History* 21, 2 (2004): 229-51.

107 C.M. Crawford, "What about Psychiatric Nursing?" *Canadian Nurse* 40, 11 (1944): 834; John Murray Gibbon and Mary S. Mathewson, *Three Centuries of Canadian Nursing* (Toronto: Macmillan, 1947), 388-89 and 416-17.

108 H.E. MacDermot, *History of the School of Nursing of the Montreal General Hospital* (Montreal: Alumnae Association, 1940), 75; Valerie Knowles, *Leaving with a Red Rose: A History of the Ottawa Civic Hospital School of Nursing* (Ottawa: Ottawa Civic Hospital School of Nursing Alumnae Association, 1981), 57.

109 Jean Mary Ciceri, audiotaped interview with Nina Rumen, 13 January 1987, CRNBC; Copp and McAndrew, *Battle Exhaustion*, 14, 24; Aikens, *Nurses in Battledress*, 59.

110 Anne Farries, "War Nurse Recalls Second World War Experiences," *Cranbrook Daily Townsman*, 10 November 1992.

111 Florence Louise Jamieson, interview with Margaret M. Allemang, Toronto, 24 April and 3 May 1987, MMA; Florence Jamieson in *The Military Nurses of Canada: Recollections of Canadian Military Nurses*, vol. 3, ed. E.A. Landells (White Rock, BC: Co-Publishing, 1999), 108-10.

112 Rae Fellowes, "Nursing Care of 'Immersion Foot,'" *Canadian Nurse* 39, 9 (1943): 581-82.

113 Kay Christie, audiotaped interview with Joan Williams, 20 November 1975, ISN 196090, LAC; Kay Christie, "Behind Japanese Barbed Wire: A Canadian Nursing Sister in Hong Kong," *Royal Canadian Military Institute Year Book* (Toronto: RCMI, 1979), 11-13; Kathleen G. Christie, "M. & V. for Christmas Dinner," *Canadian Nurse* 63, 12 (1967): 28-30; Bill McNeil, *Voices of a War Remembered: An Oral History of Canadians in the Second World War* (Toronto: Doubleday, 1991), 96-104.

114 Christie, "M. & V. for Christmas Dinner," 29.

115 Ibid.

116 Christie interview, HCM 28-82.

117 Ibid.

118 Christie interview, LAC.

119 Dorothy M. (Grainger) Anderson, in *Military Nurses of Canada*, 1: 415.

120 Bonnie Bullough, "The Lasting Impact of World War II on Nursing," *American Journal of Nursing* 76, 1 (1976): 118-20; Mary T. Sarnecky, *A History of the U.S. Army Nurse Corps* (Philadelphia: University of Pennsylvania Press, 1999), 398-99.

121 McPherson, *Bedside Matters*, 187-92, 203-4.

122 Ethel Johns, "The Shape of Things to Come," *Canadian Nurse* 37, 2 (1941): 83-84.

123 RNAO Placement Service Advisory Committee Minutes and Reports (1945-46), 96C-1-08 and RNAO Postwar Planning Committee – Minutes, Reports, and Correspondence (1944-46), 96C-1-09, AO; Ethel Johns, "Background for Postwar Planning," *Canadian Nurse* 40, 3 (1944): 161-62.

124 Lyle M. Creelman, "With UNRRA in Germany," *Canadian Nurse* 43, 7 (1947): 532, 552-56; "With UNRRA in Germany," *Canadian Nurse* 43, 8 (1947): 605-10; and "With UNRRA in Germany," *Canadian Nurse* 43, 9 (1947): 710-12.

125 Personal communication with Jan Robertson of Surrey, BC, November 2005.

126 Barbara Logan Tunis, *In Caps and Gowns: The Story of the School for Graduate Nurses, McGill University, 1920-1964* (Montreal: McGill University Press, 1966), 81-83, 126-27.

127 C.B. Parker to J.W. Tice, letters of 7 July 1945 and 10 July, 1945, HQ file 400-1-1, vol. 3365, E-1-b, RG 24, LAC.

128 "Postwar Planning Activities," *Canadian Nurse* 41, 4 (1945): 301-2.

129 Laura Holland, "How Can Nurses Fight for Peace?" *Canadian Nurse* 41, 7 (1945): 549-51.

130 H. Evelyn Mallory, "The Time for Action Is Now," *Canadian Nurse* 42, 3 (1946): 201-3.

131 "Opportunities in Nursing in Canada," *Canadian Nurse* 42, 6 (1946): 494-95.

132 Report, 1 March 1946, "RNAO Placement Service Advisory Committee Minutes and Reports (1945-46)," 96C-1-08, AO.

133 Report, 13 September 1946, "RNAO Placement Service Advisory Committee Minutes and Reports (1945-46)," p. 3, 96C-1-08, AO.

134 Holland, "How Can Nurses Fight for Peace?" 550.

135 Marion Lindeburgh, "Postwar Planning Committee," *Canadian Nurse* 42, 9 (1946): 791-92; Tunis, *In Caps and Gowns,* 83; "Extension of Time Limit for Candidates for University Courses in Nursing," *Canadian Nurse* 42, 3 (1946): 233-34.

136 Ethel Johns, "The Home Front," *Canadian Nurse* 37, 9 (1941): 604-5.

137 "Building for the Future," *Canadian Nurse* 36, 7 (1940): 415-16; "Activities of the School for Graduate Nurses, McGill University," *Canadian Nurse* 39, 5 (1943): 327-28; "A Timely and Generous Gift," *Canadian Nurse* 38, 8 (1942): 546-48; Fanny Munroe, "Government Grant Committee," *Canadian Nurse* 42, 9 (1946): 782-83; Marion Lindeburgh, "The Grant from the Federal Government," *Canadian Nurse* 38, 9 (1942): 607.

138 Ellen Jean Wheeler Keays, audiotaped interview with Sheila Zerr, White Rock, BC, 16 August 1994, CRNBC.

139 See editorials in the *Ottawa Citizen,* 28 February and 4 March 1949 for public complaints, as well as "Judicial Inquiry, v. I-III," City of Ottawa Archives, MG 38, vol. 36 and the final report as "Civic Hospital," Minutes of the City Council, 2 August 1949, pp. 662-76, City of Ottawa Archives.

140 MacDermot, *History of the School of Nursing,* 77.

141 McPherson, *Bedside Matters,* 222; Weir, *Survey of Nursing,* 306-7.

142 Dorothy G. Riddell, "Training Nursing Assistants," *Canadian Nurse* 43, 11 (1947): 851-54; MacDermot, *History of the School of Nursing,* 77-78.

143 Ruby G. Hull, "Recovery," *Canadian Nurse* 41, 9 (1945), 700-2; Florence E. Dunn and Miriam G. Shupp, "The Recovery Room: A Wartime Economy," *American Journal of Nursing* 43, 3 (1943): 279; Agnes Leon, "Postanesthetic and Postoperative Recovery Units," *American Journal of Nursing* 52, 4 (1952): 430.

144 M. Décary, "Hospital Penicillin Treatment Centre," *Canadian Nurse* 43, 11 (1947): 847-50.

145 "What You Want to Know about Nursing" (Montreal: Canadian Nurses Association, n.d.), 18, from "RNAO Background/Supplemental Material for CNA Nurse Recruitment, 1944-45," RNAO fonds, 96B-5-20, AO.

146 A.E. Archer, "Health Insurance," *Journal of the Canadian Medical Services* 1, 2 (1944): 162; Jacalyn Duffin, "The Guru and the Godfather: Henry Sigerist, Hugh MacLean, and the Politics of Health Care Reform in 1940s Canada," *Canadian Bulletin of Medical History* 9 (1992): 191-218; C. David Naylor, *Private Practice, Public Payment: Canadian Medicine and the Politics of Health Insurance, 1911-1966* (Montreal and Kingston: McGill-Queen's University Press, 1986).

147 Bullough, "The Lasting Impact of World War II on Nursing," 120.

148 McPherson, *Bedside Matters,* 211; Agnes Calliste, "Women of 'Exceptional Merit': Immigration of Caribbean Nurses to Canada," *Canadian Journal of Women and the Law* 6, 1 (1993): 85-102; Tania Das Gupta, "Anti-Black Racism in Nursing in Ontario," *Studies in Political Economy* 51 (Fall 1996): 97-116; Karen Flynn, "Proletarianization, Professionalization, and Caribbean Immigrant Nurses," *Canadian Woman Studies/Cahiers de la femme* 18, 1 (1998): 57-60.

149 Marion Myers, "Sub-committee on Male Nurses," *Canadian Nurse* 44, 6 (1948): 470-71.

Chapter 5: "The Strain of Peace"

1 "Prayer on Hearing V-E Day Proclamation," Marguerite McLimont, NS, at Bologna, Italy, in May 1945, read by Florence Louise Jamieson in audiotaped interview with Margaret M. Allemang, Toronto, 24 May and 3 June 1987, Oral History Collection, Margaret M. Allemang Centre for the History of Nursing at Toronto (hereafter MMA).
2 Constance Betty Nicolson Brown, audiotaped interview with author, Ottawa, 3 June 2001.
3 A.P. Cohen, *The Symbolic Construction of Community* (New York: Tavistock Publications, 1985), 9, 12-13, 16.
4 Benedict Anderson, *Imagined Communities: Reflections on the Origin and Spread of Nationalism*, rev. ed. (New York: Verso, 1991), 6-7.
5 Charles Wetherell, Andrejs Plakans, and Barry Wellman, "Social Networks, Kinship, and Community in Eastern Europe," *Journal of Interdisciplinary History* 24, 4 (1994): 646.
6 John C Walsh and Steven High, "Rethinking the Concept of Community," *Histoire sociale/Social History* 32, 64 (1999): 256, 261-62.
7 Brenda McBryde, *Quiet Heroines: Nurses of the Second World War* (Saffron Walden, Essex: Cakebreads Publications, 1989), 230.
8 Jenéa Tallentire, "Strategies of Memory: History, Social Memory, and the Community," *Histoire sociale/ Social History* 34, 67 (2001): 198.
9 Cynthia Enloe, *Maneuvers: The International Politics of Militarizing Women's Lives* (Berkeley and Los Angeles: University of California Press, 2000), 218.
10 Tallentire, "Strategies of Memory," 202-3, 206.
11 Joan I. Roberts and Thetis M. Group, *Feminism and Nursing: An Historical Perspective on Power, Status, and Political Activism in the Nursing Profession* (Westport, CT: Praeger, 1995), 133-40, 147; Cynthia Enloe, *Does Khaki Become You? The Militarization of Women's Lives* (Boston: South End Press, 1983), 100.
12 Nina Rumen, personal communication; E. June Parker, audiotaped interview with author, Ottawa, 23 November 2001.
13 Joseph R. Llobera, "The Role of Historical Memory in Catalan National Identity," *Social Anthropology* 6, 3 (1998): 333.
14 Walsh and High, "Rethinking the Concept of Community," 256, 261-62; Tallentire, "Strategies of Memory," 197, 199.
15 Pauline Cox Walker, audiotaped interview with author, Kingston, Ontario, 13 June 2001.
16 "Nursing Sisters' Association of Canada: Membership Directory, 1958" in possession of Lt. Colonel/NS (retired) Harriet J.T. Sloan of Ottawa.
17 Margaret Van Scoyoc, audiotaped interview with author, Kingston, Ontario, 13 June 2001.
18 Karen D. Davis, "Women Join the Navy, 1942-1946 and 1951-1954: Social/Historical Processes and Their Decision to Join," Second Inter-University Colloquium of Sociology Students, McGill University, 26-28 March 1993, 83-92. See examples such as anecdotes posted on the Veterans Affairs Canada/Anciens Combattants Canada website: www.vac-acc.gc.ca.
19 Jan Bassett, *Guns and Brooches: Australian Army Nursing from the Boer War to the Gulf War* (New York: Oxford University Press, 1992), 95; McBryde, *Quiet Heroines*, 231; Diane Burke Fessler, *No Time for Fear: Voices of American Military Nurses in World War II* (East Lansing: Michigan State University Press, 1996), 3.
20 Kathryn McPherson, *Bedside Matters: The Transformation of Canadian Nursing, 1900-1990* (Toronto: Oxford University Press, 1996), 25-47; Barbara Melosh, *"The Physician's Hand": Work, Culture and Conflict in American Nursing* (Philadelphia: Temple University Press, 1982); Susan M. Reverby, *Ordered to Care: The Dilemma of American Nursing, 1850-1945* (New York: Cambridge University Press, 1987).
21 McPherson, *Bedside Matters*, 64-66, 147-50.
22 Lois Bayly Tewsley, audiotaped interview with author, Ottawa, 11 June 2001.
23 Jean MacBain MacAulay, in *The Military Nurses of Canada: Recollections of Canadian Military Nurses*, vol. 2, ed. E.A. Landells (White Rock, BC: Co-publishing, 1999), 112.
24 Norma Fieldhouse, interview with Margaret M. Allemang, Toronto, 16 February 1988, MMA.
25 Isabel Morrison Fraser, audiotaped interview with author, Ottawa, 27 November 2001.
26 Lettie Turner, in *Nurses on the Battlefield*, TV documentary, producers Lori Kuffner and Barbara Campbell (Cooper Rock Pictures, 2001).
27 Doris V. Carter, *Never Leave Your Head Uncovered: A Canadian Nursing Sister in World War Two* (Waterdown, ON: Potlatch Publications, 1999), 53-54.
28 Elizabeth Dean Doe, audiotaped interview with author, Ottawa, 30 June 2001.

29 Margaret Van Scoyoc, audiotaped interview with Lisa Weintraub, 4 June 1984, ISN 167825, and Gaëtane LaBonté Kerr, interview with Lisa Weintraub, 11 April 1985, ISN 167796, Concordia University fond, Oral History Project, Library and Archives Canada (hereafter LAC).

30 Patricia Moll, audiotaped interview with Lisa Weintraub, 5 July 1985, ISN 167813, Concordia University fond, Oral History Project, LAC.

31 Frances Oakes, audiotaped interview with author, Guelph, Ontario, 15 May 2001.

32 Harriet J.T. Sloan, audiotaped interview with author, Ottawa, 14 March 2001.

33 Doris V. Carter, audiotaped interview with author, Ottawa, 22 June 2001.

34 Beatrice Cole Hunter, audiotaped interview with author, Edmonton, Alberta, 13 October 2001.

35 Kathleen G. Christie, "Experiences as a Prisoner-of-War, World War 2," transcribed interview with Charles G. Roland on 8 December 1982, HCM 28-82, Oral History Archives, Hannah Chair for the History of Medicine, McMaster University, Hamilton, Ontario (hereafter HCM 28-82).

36 Christie interview, LAC.

37 Christie interview, HCM 28-82.

38 Kathleen G. Christie, "M. & V. for Christmas Dinner," *Canadian Nurse* 63, 12 (1967): 30.

39 Kay Christie, audio-interview with Margaret M. Allemang, Toronto, Ontario, 5 April 1992, MMA.

40 Christie interview, HCM 28-82.

41 Cohen, *Symbolic Construction of Community*, 13, 28, 33, and 36.

42 Carter, *Never Leave Your Head Uncovered*; Mary M. White, *Hello War, Goodbye Sanity* (N.p.: New Leaf, 1992).

43 Carter interview; and Mary M. Bower White, audiotaped interview with author, Surrey, BC, 20 October 2001.

44 Penny Starns, *Nurses at War: Women on the Frontline, 1939-45* (Stroud, Gloucestershire: Sutton Publishing, 2000), xii-xvii, 12-15; Juliet Piggott, *Queen Alexandra's Royal Army Nursing Corps* (London: Leo Cooper, 1975), 73.

45 Kay Christie, "Behind Japanese Barbed Wire: A Canadian Nursing Sister in Hong Kong," *Royal Canadian Military Institute Year Book* (Toronto: RCMI, 1979), 13; Kay Christie, interview with Margaret M. Allemang, Toronto, 5 April 1992, MMA; Christie interview, HCM 28-82.

46 Claire (Murray) Bowman, in *The Military Nurses of Canada: Recollections of Canadian Military Nurses*, vol. 1, ed. E.A. Landells (White Rock, BC: Co-publishing, 1995), 319.

47 Constance Bond Young, interview with Ella Beardmore, Omeemee, Ontario, 4 July 1989, MMA.

48 C.P. Stacey, *Official History of the Canadian Army in the Second World War*, vol. 1, *Six Years of War: The Army in Canada, Britain and the Pacific* (Ottawa: Queen's Printer, 1955), 44-45; G.W.L. Nicholson, *Canada's Nursing Sisters* (Toronto: Samuel Stevens Hakkert, 1975), 130-31.

49 Estell Tritt Aspler, audiotaped interview with author, Westmount, Quebec, 13 August 2001.

50 Helen K. Mussallem, audiotaped interview with author, Ottawa, 24 September 2001.

51 Margaret Fletcher, letters of 10 September and 28 October 1943 to her family, Margaret Fletcher fonds, 1933-1945, SC042, University of Victoria Archives and Special Collections, BC Archives (hereafter Fletcher letters).

52 Dorothy A. Macham, in *Military Nurses of Canada*, 1: 311.

53 Margaret Roe Dewart, audiotaped interview with author, Edmonton, Alberta, 15 October 2001.

54 Suzanne Giroux, "Overseas Mail," *Canadian Nurse* 39, 5 (1943): 344.

55 Carter, *Never Leave Your Head Uncovered*, 7, 41.

56 Ibid., 149-51.

57 McPherson, *Bedside Matters*, 12, 15-18, and 30; Knowles, *Leaving with a Red Rose*, 22; John Murray Gibbon and Mary S. Mathewson, *Three Centuries of Canadian Nursing* (Toronto: Macmillan, 1947), 156.

58 Fletcher letters, 12 January 1944.

59 Ibid., 7 September 1943.

60 Ruby Heap, "From the Science of Housekeeping to the Science of Nutrition: Pioneers in Canadian Nutrition and Dietetics at the University of Toronto's Faculty of Household Science, 1900-1950," in *Challenging Professions: Historical and Contemporary Perspectives on Women's Professional Work*, ed. Elizabeth Smyth, Sandra Acker, Paula Bourne, and Alison Prentice (Toronto: University of Toronto Press, 1999), 141-70 and Heap, "Training Women for a New 'Women's Profession': Physiotherapy Education at the University of Toronto, 1917-40," *History of Education Quarterly* 35, 2 (1995): 135-58; Nicholson, *Canada's Nursing Sisters*, 199-205.

61 C.P. Stacey, *Official History of the Canadian Army in the Second World War*, 1: 432.

62 W.R. Feasby, ed., *Official History of the Canadian Medical Services, 1939-1945*, vol. 1, *Organization and Campaigns* (Ottawa: Queen's Printer, 1956), 302-3.
63 Carter, *Never Leave Your Head Uncovered*, 142.
64 Mabel (Glew) Tweddell, in *Military Nurses of Canada*, 1: 194-95.
65 Van Scoyoc interview, LAC.
66 Anne A. (Gair) Evans, in *Military Nurses of Canada*, 1: 348.
67 Margaret H. Mills, interview with Margaret M. Allemang, Toronto, 5 April 1991, MMA.
68 Ruth Littlejohn McIlrath, audiotaped interview with Nina Rumen, 20 October 1987 and 23 November 1988, Oral History Collection, College of Registered Nurses of British Columbia Library (hereafter CRNBC).
69 Jamieson interview, MMA.
70 Fletcher letter, 21 January 1945.
71 Van Scoyoc interview, LAC.
72 Dorothy Agnes Potts, interview with Margaret M. Allemang, Toronto, Ontario, 30 September 1987, MMA.
73 Bond Young interview, MMA.
74 Van Scoyoc interview, LAC.
75 Elizabeth B. Pense Neil, interview with Norma Fieldhouse, Kingston, March 1987, MMA.
76 Eleanor (Jones) MacGregor, "Defending the Empire," unpublished paper in possession of author.
77 Margaret M. Allemang, audiotaped interview with author, Toronto, 26 April 2001.
78 Fletcher letter, 29 April 1945.
79 Margaret Dewart and Jessie Morrison, "Formation of the First Unit: Edmonton, 1920," *Nursing Sisters' Association of Canada: Commemorative Issue and National Directory* (Edmonton: Nursing Sisters' Association of Canada, 1990), 81.
80 Jessie Morrison, "Address to Royal Alexandra Hospital Nurses Alumnae – Edmonton, December 9, 1974," Jessie Morrison fonds, 87.4, 91.30 and 92.10, College and Association of Registered Nurses of Alberta Museum and Archives (hereafter as CARNA); Dewart and Morrison, "Formation of the First Unit," 81-82, CARNA; Nicholson, *Canada's Nursing Sisters*, 106-12.
81 Nicholson, *Canada's Nursing Sisters*, 109, 224.
82 "Nursing Sisters' Association of Canada," *Canadian Nurse* 43, 1 (1947): 71.
83 Morrison, "Address to Royal Alexandra Hospital Nurses Alumnae."
84 Lotta Dempsey, "Canadian Nurses Will Recall War Years," *Globe and Mail*, 21 June 1975.
85 Kay Poulton in Bill McNeil, *Voices of a War Remembered: An Oral History of Canadians in World War Two* (Toronto: Doubleday, 1991), 91.
86 "Nursing Sisters' Association of Canada," *Canadian Nurse* 42, 3 (1946): 246.
87 "Nursing Sisters' Association of Canada: Membership Directory, 1958" in possession of Lt. Colonel/NS (retired) Harriet J.T. Sloan, Ottawa.
88 Cohen, *Symbolic Construction of Community*, 50.
89 Jay Winter, *Sites of Memory, Sites of Mourning: The Great War in European Cultural History* (New York: Cambridge University Press, 1995), 34, 224; Jonathan Vance, *Death So Noble: Memory, Meaning, and the First World War* (Vancouver: UBC Press, 1997), 260.
90 Winter, *Sites of Memory*, 9.
91 Janéa Tallentire, "Strategies of Memory," 211.
92 Kathryn McPherson, "Carving Out a Past: The Canadian Nurses' Association War Memorial," *Histoire sociale/Social History* 29, 58 (1996): 418-19.
93 The Jean Matheson Memorial Pavilion of the Shaughnessy Military Hospital, Vancouver, the Rena McLean Memorial Hospital on Prince Edward Island, and Mount Wake, British Columbia (named for NS Gladys Maude Wake) commemorate First World War nursing sisters. Three memorial windows are located in British Columbia – one in Victoria and two in Vancouver; a fourth window is in Kingston, Ontario.
94 Woodlawn Cemetery, Memorial Boulevard, information, http://www.city.saskatoon.sk.ca/org/parks.
95 "Why Buy Victory Bonds?" *Canadian Nurse* 40, 4 (1944): 258. Emphasis in original.
96 John Murray Gibbon, "Our Canadian Nursing Sister," arranged by Harold Eustace Key (Toronto: Gordon V. Thompson, 1946). Gibbon is better known for John Murray Gibbon and Mary S. Mathewson, *Three Centuries of Canadian Nursing* (Toronto: Macmillan, 1947).
97 Nicholson, *Canada's Nursing Sisters*, 223-24.
98 Minutes of the NSAC, Ottawa unit, 11 May 2001; Sarah Staples, "Nurse Returns to Dieppe to Mark 60th Anniversary," *Ottawa Citizen*, 10 August 2002.

99 *Angels of Mercy: The Story of Nursing Sisters from World Wars I and II* (Sound Venture Productions, 1994); *Nurses on the Battlefield* (Cooper Rock Pictures, 2001); CBC, "Remembrance Day Town Hall," with Peter Mansbridge at Vimy House, Ottawa, 11 November 2000; and *The English Patient* (Miramax Films, Tiger Moth Productions, 1996).

100 Ethel Cryderman, "War Memorial Committee," *Canadian Nurse* 42, 9 (1946): 792; Margaret E. Kerr, "War Memorial Committee," *Canadian Nurse* 44, 6 (1948): 480.

101 Kerr, "War Memorial Committee," 481.

102 "The Nursing Sisters Association of Canada, 1920-1966," CARNA.

103 Anne Marie Rafferty with Geertje Boschma, "The Essential Idea," in *Nurses of All Nations: A History of the International Council of Nurses, 1899-1999*, ed. Barbara L. Brush and Joan E. Lynaugh (Philadelphia: Lippincott, 1999), 44.

104 Ibid.

105 Joan E. Lynaugh, "From Chaos to Transformation," in Brush and Lynaugh, *Nurses of All Nations*, 113-14 and 120.

106 Nicholson, *Canada's Nursing Sisters*, 224-26; Morrison, "Address to Royal Alexandra Hospital Nurses Alumnae."

107 Veterans' Affairs Canada, Orders and Decorations, Royal Red Cross class 2, www.vac-acc.gc.ca.

108 Nicholson, *Canada's Nursing Sisters*, 203.

109 Macham interview, MMA and in *Military Nurses of Canada*, 1: 309.

110 Concordia University Oral History Project, Concordia University fonds, LAC; Kathryn McPherson, "Nurses and Their Work," Oral History Collection, Provincial Archives of Manitoba.

111 The British Columbia History of Nursing Professional Practice Group in Vancouver and the Margaret M. Allemang Centre for the History of Nursing in Toronto led projects to collect Nursing Sisters' oral histories. Edith Landells solicited and collected accounts from military nurses across Canada, independently publishing them as a three-volume anthology between 1995 and 1999.

112 Morrison, "Address to Royal Alexandra Hospital Nurses Alumnae."

Conclusion

1 Kathryn McPherson, *Bedside Matters: The Transformation of Canadian Nursing, 1900-1990* (Toronto: Oxford University Press, 1996), 207-8, 210-15, 257-59.

2 George M. Weir, *Survey of Nursing Education in Canada* (Toronto: University of Toronto Press, 1932), 50-65.

3 "RCAMC Nursing Sisters on Duty in Hong Kong," *Canadian Nurse* 38, 1 (1942): 32.

4 Norah (Mallandaine) Noiles, in *The Military Nurses of Canada: Recollections of Canadian Military Nurses*, vol. 1, ed. E.A. Landells (White Rock, BC: Co-Publishing, 1995, 147.

Selected Bibliography

Canadian Nursing Sister Oral History Collections

Library and Archives Canada
Ella Beardmore, audiotaped interview with Joan Williams, 26 November 1975, ISN 196092
Kay Christie, audiotaped interview with Joan Williams, 20 November 1975, ISN 196090
Gaëtane LaBonté Kerr, audiotaped interview with Lisa Weintraub, 11 April 1985, ISN 167796
Patricia Moll, audiotaped interview with Lisa Weintraub, 5 July 1985, ISN 167813
Grace Patterson, audiotaped interview with Joan Williams, 18 November 1975, ISN 196088
Margaret Van Scoyoc, audiotaped interview with Lisa Weintraub, 4 June 1984, ISN 167825

Margaret M. Allemang Centre for the History of Nursing
Kathleen G. Christie, audiotaped interview with Margaret Allemang, 5 April 1992 and 3 June 1992
Norma Fieldhouse, audiotaped interview with Margaret Allemang, 16 February 1988
Florence Louise Jamieson, audiotaped interview with Margaret Allemang, 24 April and 3 May 1987
Margaret Helena Kellough, audiotaped interview with Margaret Allemang, April and May 1987
Dorothy A. Macham, audiotaped interview with Norma Fieldhouse, 10 February 1988
Margaret H. Mills, audiotaped interview with Margaret Allemang, 5 April 1991
Elizabeth Pense Neil, audiotaped interview with Norma Fieldhouse, March 1987
Elizabeth Harpham Orford, audiotaped interview with Margaret Allemang, 9 October 1991 and 26 January 1993
Dorothy Agnes Potts, audiotaped interview with Margaret Allemang, 30 September 1987
Helen Morton Rendall, audiotaped interview with Margaret Allemang, 14 and 21 March 1986
Susan Isabel Rowland, audiotaped interview with Ella Beardmore, 15 May 1988
Berna Thompson Tuckwell, audiotaped interview with Ella Beardmore, 10 June 1988
Eva R. Wannop, audiotaped interview with Margaret Allemang, 28 August 1991
Constance Bond Young audiotaped interview with Ella Beardmore, 4 July 1989

McMaster University Hannah Chair for History of Medicine, Oral History Archives
Kathleen G. Christie, "Experiences as a Prisoner-of-War, World War 2," interview with Charles G. Roland, 8 December 1982, HCM 28-82.

College and Association of Registered Nurses of Alberta Museum and Archives
Kay Christie, audiotaped interview with Bill McNeil, "Voice of the Pioneer," January 1992, Kay Christie fonds, 94.41
Joan Suzanne Verral (Maynard) Ferguson, audiotaped interview with Kristi Rigaux, Lethbridge, Alberta, 7 March 1995
Lenore Lancaster Menard, audiotaped interview with Terina Rindal, Lethbridge, Alberta, 14 March 1995

College of Registered Nurses of British Columbia Oral History Collection
Jean Mary Ciceri, audiotaped interview with Nina Rumen, Victoria, 13 January 1987

Joan Doree, audiotaped interview with Nina Rumen, Vancouver, 11 February 1987
Ellen Jean (Wheeler) Keays, audiotaped interview with Sheila Zerr, White Rock, BC, 16 August 1994
Eleanor Kunderman, audiotaped interview with Audrey Stegen, Gibson's, British Columbia, 26 October 1987
Enid Matheson, audiotaped interview with Elizabeth Kirkwood, Hawaii, 22 February 1989
Ruth Littlejohn McIlrath, audiotaped interview with Nina Rumen, Vancouver, on 23 November 1988
    and at Burnaby, BC, 20 October 1987
Edna Rossiter, audiotaped interview with Nina Rumen, Vancouver, 27 October 1987.

Archival Collections

Library and Archives Canada
Nursing Sisters' Association of Canada fonds
Canadian Nurses Association fonds
Department of National Defence (RG 24)
Department of External Affairs (RG 25)
M. Amy White fonds, MG30-E508

Department of National Defence Directorate of History and Heritage
Royal Canadian Army Medical Corps fonds
Royal Canadian Air Force Nursing Service fonds
Royal Canadian Navy Nursing Services fonds
South African Military Nursing Service, 1939-1947 fonds

Archives of Ontario
"Performance of Clinical Procedures by Graduate Nurses: A Special Study by Committee on Nursing
    and Nurse Education," Canadian Hospital Council and Canadian Nurses Association, 1940-1941,
    Registered Nurses Association of Ontario fonds, 96B-5-14.
Report of the Committee on Nursing and Nurse Education in Canadian Hospitals, Canadian Hospital
    Council (1941), Registered Nurses Association of Ontario fonds, 96B-5-14.
Report of the Committee on Nursing and Nurse Education in Canadian Hospitals, Canadian Hospital
    Council (1943), Registered Nurses Association of Ontario fonds, 96B-5-14.

College and Association of Registered Nurses of Alberta Museum and Archives
Oral History Collection: Nursing Sisters
Agnes McLeod Scrapbook Collection
Frances Ferguson Sutherland Scrapbook Collection

Winnipeg General Hospital Health Sciences Centre Nurses Alumnae Archives
Nursing Sisters Collection

University of Victoria, Archives and Special Collections
Margaret Fletcher fonds

Other Sources

Abel-Smith, Brian. *A History of the Nursing Profession.* London: Heinemann, 1966.
Abella, Irving, and Harold Troper. *None Is too Many: Canada and the Jews of Europe, 1933-1948.* Toronto:
    Lester and Orpen Dennys, 1982.
Adami, J. George. *War Story of the Canadian Army Medical Corps.* Vol. 1, *The First Contingent to the
    Autumn of 1915.* Toronto: Canadian War Records Office, 1918. Canadian Institute of Historical
    Microfilms, #73232.
Adams, David P. *"The Greatest Good to the Greatest Number": Penicillin Rationing on the American
    Home Front, 1940-1945.* New York: Peter Lang, 1991.
Agnew, G. Harvey. *Canadian Hospitals, 1920-1970: A Dramatic Half Century.* Toronto: University of

Toronto Press, 1974.

Aikens, Gwladys M. Rees. *Before and after the Battles: From Wales to Canada via Two World Wars.* Halifax, NS: Cymru Press, 2001.

—. *Nurses in Battledress: The World War II Story of a Member of the Q.A. Reserves.* Halifax, NS: Cymru Press, 1998.

Allard, Geneviève. "Des anges blanc sur le front: L'expérience de guerre des infirmières militaires Canadiennes pendant la première guerre mondiale." *Bulletin d'histoire politique* 8, 2-3 (2000): 119-33.

Anderson, Benedict. *Imagined Communities: Reflections on the Origin and Spread of Nationalism.* Rev. ed. New York: Verso, 1991.

Angels of Mercy: The Story of Nursing Sisters from World Wars I and II. Sound Venture Productions, 1994.

Archard, Theresa. *G.I. Nightingale: The Story of an American Army Nurse.* New York: W.W. Norton, 1945.

Avery, Donald H. *The Science of War: Canadian Scientists and Allied Military Technology during the Second World War.* Toronto: University of Toronto Press, 1998.

Axelrod, Paul. *Making a Middle Class: Student Life in English Canada during the Thirties.* Montreal and Kingston: McGill-Queen's University Press, 1990.

Ayerst, McKenna, and Harrison. *Penicillin.* Montreal: Ayerst, McKenna, and Harrison, 1963.

Bassett, Jan. *Guns and Brooches: Australian Army Nursing from the Boer War to the Gulf War.* New York: Oxford University Press, 1992.

Beamish, Rahno M. *Fifty Years a Canadian Nurse: Devotion, Opportunities and Duty.* New York: Vantage Press, 1970.

Bijker, Wiebe E., Thomas P. Hughes, and Trevor J. Pinch. *The Social Construction of Technological Systems: New Directions in the Social History of Technology.* Cambridge, MA: MIT Press, 1989.

Blume, Stuart S. *Insight and Industry: On the Dynamics of Technological Change in Medicine.* Cambridge, MA: MIT Press, 1992.

Bothwell, Robert, Ian Drummond, and John English. *Canada since 1945: Power, Politics, and Provincialism.* Rev. ed. Toronto: University of Toronto Press, 1996.

Bourke, Joanna. "The Emotions in War: Fear and the British and American Military, 1914-45." *Historical Research* 74, 185 (2001): 314-30.

Brand, Dionne. "'We weren't allowed to go into factory work until Hitler started the war': The 1920s to the 1940s." In *We're Rooted Here and They Can't Pull Us Up,* ed. Peggy Bristow, Dionne Brand, Linda Carty, Afua P. Cooper, Sylvia Hamilton, and Adrienne Shadd, 171-91. Toronto: University of Toronto Press, 1994.

Braybon, Gail, and Penny Summerfield. *Out of the Cage: Women's Experiences in Two World Wars.* London: Pandora, 1987.

Brittain, Vera. *Chronicle of Youth: War Diary, 1913-1917,* ed. Alan Bishop with Terry Smart. London: Gollancz, 1981.

—. *Testament of Youth.* New York: Seaview Books, 1980.

Brown, Robert Craig, and Ramsay Cook. *Canada, 1896-1921: A Nation Transformed.* Toronto: McClelland and Stewart, 1974.

Bruce, Herbert A. *Politics and the Canadian Army Medical Corps: A History of Intrigue, Containing Many Facts Omitted from the Official Records, Showing How Efforts at Rehabilitation Were Baulked.* Toronto: William Briggs, 1919.

Bruce, Jean. *Back the Attack: Canadian Women during the Second World War – at Home and Abroad.* Toronto: Macmillan, 1985.

Bullough, Bonnie. "The Lasting Impact of World War II on Nursing." *American Journal of Nursing* 76, 1 (1976): 118-20.

Burns, E.L.M. *Manpower in the Canadian Army, 1939-45.* Toronto: Clarke, Irwin, 1956.

Callon, Michel. "The Sociology of an Actor-Network: The Case of the Electric Vehicle." In *Mapping the Dynamics of Science and Technology: Sociology of Science in the Real World,* ed. Michel Callon, John Law, and Arie Rip, 19-34. Basingstoke: Macmillan, 1986.

Canada. *Report of the National Health Survey.* Part 8, *Nurses.* Ottawa: King's Printer, 1945.

Canadian Broadcasting Corporation. "Remembrance Day Town Hall," with Peter Mansbridge at Vimy House, Ottawa on 11 November 2000.

Canadian Nurses Association. *The Leaf and the Lamp: The Canadian Nurses' Association and the Influences Which Shaped Its Origins and Outlook during Its First Sixty Years.* Ottawa: Canadian Nurses' Association, 1968.

Care, Dean, David Gregory, John English, and Peri Venkatesh. "A Struggle for Equality: Resistance to

Commissioning of Male Nurses in the Canadian Military, 1952-1967." *Canadian Journal of Nursing Research* 28, 1 (1996): 103-17.

Carter, Doris V. *Never Leave Your Head Uncovered: A Canadian Nursing Sister in World War Two.* Waterdown, ON: Potlatch Publications, 1999.

Christie, Kathleen G. "M. & V. for Christmas Dinner." *Canadian Nurse* 63, 12 (1967): 28-30.

—. "Report by Miss Kathleen G. Christie, Nurse with the Canadian Forces at Hong Kong, as Given on Board the SS *Gripsholm*, November 1943." *Canadian Military History* 10, 4 (2001): 27-34.

Christie, Kay. "Behind Japanese Barbed Wire: A Canadian Nursing Sister in Hong Kong." *Royal Canadian Military Institute Year Book* (Toronto: RCMI, 1979): 11-13.

—. "Kay Christie, Toronto, Ontario." In *Voices of a War Remembered: An Oral History of Canadians in World War II*, ed. Bill McNeil, 96-104. Toronto: Doubleday, 1991.

Coburn, Judi. "'I see and am silent': A Short History of Nursing in Ontario." In *Health and Canadian Society: Sociological Perspectives*, ed. David Coburn, Carl D'Arcy, Peter New, and George Torrance, 182-201. Toronto: Fitzhenry and Whiteside, 1981.

Cohen, A.P. *The Symbolic Construction of Community.* New York: Tavistock Publications, 1985.

Cook, Tim. "Clio's Soldiers: Charles Stacey and the Army Historical Section in the Second World War." *Canadian Historical Review* 83, 1 (2002): 29-57.

Cooter, Roger. *Surgery and Society in Peace and War: Orthopaedics and the Organization of Modern Medicine, 1880-1948.* Houndmills, Basingstoke: Macmillan, 1993.

Cooter, Roger, Mark Harrison, and Steve Sturdy, eds. *Medicine and Modern Warfare.* Amsterdam and Atlanta: Rodopi, 1999.

Copp, Terry, and Bill McAndrew, *Battle Exhaustion: Soldiers and Psychiatrists in the Canadian Army, 1939-1945.* Montreal and Kingston: McGill-Queen's University Press, 1990.

D'Antonio, Patricia. "Legacy of Domesticity." *Nursing History Review* 1 (1993): 229-46.

Day, Frances Martin, Phyllis Spence, and Barbara Ladouceur, eds. *Women Overseas: Memoirs of the Canadian Red Cross Corps.* Vancouver: Ronsdale Press, 1998.

Dempsey, Lotta. "Canada's Blitz Sisters." *Maclean's Magazine*, 1 September 1943, 24.

Dombrowski, Nicole Ann, ed. *Women and War in the Twentieth Century: Enlisted with or without Consent.* New York: Garland, 1999.

Donahue, M. Patricia. "Reflections on the Changing Image of Nurses in Wartime." *Caduceus: A Humanities Journal for Medicine and the Health Sciences* 11, 1 (1995): 53-58.

Donovan, Rita. *As for the Canadians: The Remarkable Story of the RCAF's "Guinea Pigs" of World War II.* Ottawa: Buschek Books, 2000.

Dooley, Chris. "'They Gave Their Care, but We Gave Loving Care': Defining and Defending Boundaries of Skill and Craft in the Nursing Service of a Manitoba Mental Hospital during the Great Depression." *Canadian Bulletin of Medical History*, 21, 2 (2004): 229-51.

Elshtain, Jean Bethke. *Women and War.* New York: Basic Books, 1987.

The English Patient. Miramax Films, Tiger Moth Productions, 1996.

Enloe, Cynthia. *Does Khaki Become You? The Militarisation of Women's Lives.* Boston: South End Press, 1983.

—. *Maneuvers: The International Politics of Militarizing Women's Lives.* Berkeley and Los Angeles: University of California Press, 2000.

Feasby, W.R. "The Canadian Medical Services." In *Medical Services in War: The Principal Medical Lessons of the Second World War Based on the Official Medical Histories of the United Kingdom, Canada, Australia, New Zealand and India*, ed. Arthur Salusbury MacNalty and W. Franklin Mellor, 469-559. London: H.M.S.O., 1968.

—, ed. *Official History of the Canadian Medical Services, 1939-1945.* Volume 1. *Organization and Campaigns.* Ottawa: Queen's Printer, 1956.

—, ed. *Official History of the Canadian Medical Services, 1939-1945.* Volume 2. *Clinical Subjects.* Ottawa: Queen's Printer, 1953.

Fessler, Diane Burke. *No Time for Fear: Voices of American Military Nurses in World War II.* East Lansing: Michigan State University Press, 1996.

Flynn, Karen. "Proletarianization, Professionalization, and Caribbean Immigrant Nurses." *Canadian Woman Studies/Cahiers de la femme* 18, 1 (1998): 57-60.

Galambos, Louis, and Jeffrey L. Sturchio. "The Pharmaceutical Industry in the Twentieth Century: A Reappraisal of the Sources of Innovation." *History and Technology* 13 (1996): 83-100.

Gibbon, John Murray. "Our Canadian Nursing Sister." In *Nursing Songs of Canada*, 8-9. Toronto:

Gordon V. Thompson, 1946.

Gibbon, John Murray, and Mary S. Mathewson. *Three Centuries of Canadian Nursing.* Toronto: Macmillan, 1947.

Glassford, Larry A. *Reaction and Reform: The Politics of the Conservative Party under R.B. Bennett, 1927-1938.* Toronto: University of Toronto Press, 1992.

Goldie, Sue M., ed. *Florence Nightingale: Letters from the Crimea, 1854-1856.* Manchester: Mandolin, 1997.

Goostray, Stella. *Memoirs: Half a Century in Nursing.* Boston: Boston University Mugar Memorial Library, 1969.

Gordon, David A. *The Stretcher Bearers.* Stroud, ON: Pacesetter Press, 1995.

Gossage, Carolyn. *Greatcoats and Glamour Boots: Canadian Women at War, 1939-1945.* Toronto: Dundurn Press, 1991.

Granatstein, J.L. *Canada's Army: Waging War and Keeping the Peace.* Toronto: University of Toronto Press, 2002.

—. *Canada's War: The Politics of the Mackenzie King Government, 1939-1945.* Toronto: Oxford University Press, 1975.

Granatstein, J.L., and J.M. Hitsman. *Broken Promises: A History of Conscription in Canada.* Toronto: Oxford University Press, 1977.

Granatstein, J.L., and Peter Neary, eds. *The Good Fight: Canadians and World War II.* Toronto: Copp Clark, 1995.

Grayzel, Susan R. *Women's Identities at War: Gender, Motherhood, and Politics in Britain and France during the First World War.* Chapel Hill: University of North Carolina Press, 1999.

Greenhous, Brereton. *Official History of the Royal Canadian Air Force: Crucible of War, 1939-1945.* Volume 3. Toronto: University of Toronto Press, 1986.

Guest, Dennis. *The Emergence of Social Security in Canada.* 2nd ed. Vancouver: University of British Columbia Press, 1985.

Guiou, Norman Miles. *Transfusion: A Canadian Surgeon's Story in War and in Peace.* Yarmouth, NS: Stoneycroft Publishers, 1985.

Hacker, Carletta. "The Bluebirds Who Went Over." *Canadian Nurse* 65, 11 (1969): 31-34.

Harmer, Bertha, and Virginia Henderson. *Textbook of the Principles and Practice of Nursing.* 4th ed. New York: Macmillan, 1939.

Headrick, Daniel. *The Tools of Empire: Technology and European Imperialism in the Nineteenth Century.* New York: Oxford University Press, 1981.

Heap, Ruby. "From the Science of Housekeeping to the Science of Nutrition: Pioneers in Canadian Nutrition and Dietetics at the University of Toronto's Faculty of Household Science, 1900-1950." In *Challenging Professions: Historical and Contemporary Perspectives on Women's Professional Work,* ed. Elizabeth Smith, Sandra Acker, Paula Bourne, and Alison Prentice, 141-70. Toronto: University of Toronto Press, 1999.

—. "'Salvaging War's Waste': The University of Toronto and the 'Physical Reconstruction' of Disabled Soldiers during the First World War." In *Ontario since Confederation: A Reader,* ed. Edgar-André Montigny and Lori Chambers, 214-34. Toronto: University of Toronto Press, 2000.

—. "Training Women for a New 'Women's Profession': Physiotherapy Education at the University of Toronto, 1917-1940." *History of Education Quarterly* 35, 2 (1995): 135-58.

Heap, Ruby, and Meryn Stuart. "Nurses and Physiotherapists: Issues in the Professionalization of Health Care Occupations during and after World War I." *Health and Canadian Society/Santé et société canadienne* 3, 1-2 (1995): 179-93.

Heaton, Leonard D. *Internal Medicine in World War II.* Volume 1. *Activities of Medical Consultants.* Washington, DC: Office of the Surgeon General (Army), 1961.

Hegarty, Marilyn E. "Patriot or Prostitute? Sexual Discourses, Print Media, and American Women during World War II." *Journal of Women's History* 10, 2 (1998): 112-36.

Herbert, Melissa S. *Camouflage Isn't Only for Combat: Gender, Sexuality, and Women in the Military.* New York: New York University Press, 1998.

Hershberger, Ann Graber, "Mennonite Nurses in World War II: Maintaining the Thread of Pacifism in Nursing." *Nursing History Review* 11 (2003): 147-66.

Hibbert, Joyce. *Fragments of War: Stories from Survivors of World War II.* Toronto: Dundurn Press, 1985.

Higonnet, Margaret R. "Not So Quiet in No-Woman's Land." In *Gendering War Talk,* ed. Miriam Cooke and Angela Woollacott. Princeton: Princeton University Press, 1993.

—. *Nurses at the Front: Writing the Wounds of the Great War.* Boston: Northeastern University Press, 2001.

Higonnet, Margaret Randolph, Jane Jenson, Sonya Michel, and Margaret Collins Weitz, eds. *Behind the Lines: Gender and the Two World Wars.* New Haven: Yale University Press, 1987.

Higonnet, Margaret, and L.-R. Patrice. "The Double Helix." In *Behind the Lines: Gender and the Two World Wars,* ed. Margaret Randolph Higonnet, Jane Jenson, Sonya Michel, and Margaret Collins Weitz, 31-47. New Haven: Yale University Press, 1987.

Hillmer, Norman, Bohdan Kordan, and Lubomyr Luciuk. *On Guard for Thee: War, Ethnicity, and the Canadian State, 1939-1945.* Ottawa: Canadian Committee for the History of the Second World War, 1988.

Hine, Darlene Clark. *Black Women in White: Racial Conflict and Cooperation in the Nursing Profession, 1890-1950.* Bloomington and Indianapolis: Indiana University Press, 1989.

Hobby, Gladys L. *Penicillin: Meeting the Challenge.* New Haven: Yale University Press, 1985.

Howell, Joel D. *Technology in the Hospital: Transforming Patient Care in the Early Twentieth Century.* Baltimore: Johns Hopkins University Press, 1995.

Hughes, Everett C. *Twenty Thousand Nurses Tell Their Story.* Philadelphia: J.B. Lippincott, 1958.

Hughes, Thomas P. "The Evolution of Large Technological Systems." In *The Social Construction of Technological Systems,* ed. Wiebe E. Bijker, Thomas P. Hughes, and Trevor J. Pinch. Cambridge, MA: MIT Press, 1989.

Hume, Edgar Erskine. *Victories of Army Medicine: Scientific Accomplishments of the Medical Department of the United States Army.* London: J.B. Lippincott, 1943.

Hutchinson, John F. *Champions of Charity: War and the Rise of the Red Cross.* Boulder, CO: Westview Press, 1996.

—. "Rethinking the Origins of the Red Cross." *Bulletin of the History of Medicine* 63 (1989): 557-78.

International Committee of the Red Cross. *Rights and Duties of Nurses, Military and Civilian Medical Personnel under the Geneva Conventions of August 12, 1949: Red Cross Principles.* Geneva: International Committee of the Red Cross, 1970.

Jackson, Kathi. *They Called Them Angels: American Military Nurses of World War II.* Westport, CT: Praeger, 2000.

James, Paul. *Nation Formation: Towards a Theory of Abstract Community.* London: Sage Publications, 1996.

Jarrell, Richard A., and James P. Hull. *Science, Technology and Medicine in Canada's Past: Selections from Scientia Canadensis.* Thornhill, ON: Scientia Press, 1991.

Kalisch, Phillip A.. "How Army Nurses Became Officers." *Nursing Research* 25, 3 (1976): 164-77.

Kalisch, Phillip A., and Beatrice J. Kalisch. "The Cadet Nurse Corps in World War II." *American Journal of Nursing* 76 (1976): 240-42.

—. "Nurses under Fire: World War II Experiences of Nurses in Bataan." *Nursing Research* 25 (1976): 409-29.

—. "The Women's Draft: An Analysis of the Controversy over the Nurses' Selective Service Bill of 1945." *Nursing Research* 22, 5 (1973): 402-13.

Kalisch, Philip A., and Margaret Scobey. "Female Nurses in American Wars: Helplessness Suspended for the Duration." *Armed Forces and Society* 9, 2 (1983): 215-44.

Kapp, Richard. "Charles H. Best, the Canadian Red Cross Society, and Canada's First National Blood Donation Program." *Canadian Bulletin of Medical History* 12 (1995): 27-46.

Keddy, Barbara A. "Private Duty Nursing: Days of the 1920s and 1930s in Canada." *Canadian Woman Studies* (Fall 1986): 99-102.

Keshen, Jeff. "Revisiting Canada's Civilian Women during World War II." *Histoire sociale/Social History* 30, 60 (1997): 239-66.

Keshen, Jeffrey A. *Propaganda and Censorship during Canada's Great War.* Edmonton: University of Alberta Press, 1996.

—. *Saints, Sinners, and Soldiers: Canada's Second World War.* Vancouver: UBC Press, 2004.

Knowles, Valerie. *Leaving with a Red Rose: A History of the Ottawa Civic Hospital School of Nursing.* Ottawa: Ottawa Civic Hospital School of Nursing Alumnae Association, 1981.

Landells, E.A., ed. *The Military Nurses of Canada: Recollections of Canadian Military Nurses.* Volumes 1-3. White Rock, BC: Co-Publishing, 1995-99.

Latour, Bruno. *Science in Action: How to Follow Scientists and Engineers through Society.* Cambridge, MA: Harvard University Press, 1987.

Law, John, and John Hassard, eds. *Actor Network Theory and After.* Oxford: Blackwell Publishers, 1999.

Lawler, Jocalyn. *Behind the Screens: Nursing, Somology, and the Problem of the Body.* North American ed. Don Mills, ON: Benjamin/Cummings Publishing, 1993.

—. *The Body in Nursing.* Melbourne: Churchill Livingstone, 1997.

Leef, C.D. Stewart. *The Fifteenth Canadian Field Ambulance, RCAMC: A Short History.* 2nd ed. Montreal: Data Resolutions, 1998.

Leon, Agnes. "Postanesthetic and Postoperative Recovery Units." *American Journal of Nursing* 52, 4 (1952): 430-32.

"Lesson Plan: Medical Assistants (Course B & SA)." Borden, ON: Royal Canadian Army Medical Corps Training School, n.d.

Lockeberg, Liv-Ellen. "The Colonel Is a Lady – and a Nurse." *Canadian Nurse* 67, 11 (1971): 23-25.

Lorentzen, Lois Ann, and Jennifer Turpin, eds. *The Women and War Reader.* New York: New York University Press, 1998.

MacDermot, H.E. *History of the School of Nursing of the Montreal General Hospital.* Montreal: Alumnae Association, 1940 (re-issued 1961).

MacNalty, Arthur Salusbury, and W. Franklin Mellor, eds. *Medical Services in War: The Principal Medical Lessons of the Second World War Based on the Official Medical Histories of the United Kingdom, Canada, Australia, New Zealand and India.* London: H.M.S.O., 1968.

Mann, Susan. *Margaret Macdonald: Imperial Daughter.* Montreal and Kingston: McGill-Queen's Press, 2005.

—, ed. *The War Diary of Clare Gass, 1915-1918.* Montreal and Kingston: McGill-Queen's Press, 2000.

—. "Where Have all the Bluebirds Gone? On the Trail of Canada's Military Nurses 1914-1918." *Atlantis* 26, 1 (2001): 35-43.

Manual of Instruction for the Royal Naval Sick Berth Staff. Ottawa: King's Printer, n.d.

McBryde, Brenda. *A Nurse's War.* London: Chatto and Windus, 1979.

—. *Quiet Heroines: Nurses of the Second World War.* Saffron Walden, Essex: Cakebreads Publications, 1989.

McGann, Susan. *The Battle of the Nurses: A Study of Eight Women Who Influenced the Development of Professional Nursing, 1880-1930.* London: Scutari Press, 1992.

McGee, Molly. "Report on Canadian Red Cross Corps, World War II, Italy, and the role of the Nursing Sister." Canadian Broadcasting Corporation, ISN 249814, LAC.

McNeil, Bill, ed. *Voices of a War Remembered: An Oral History of Canadians in World War Two.* Toronto: Doubleday, 1991.

McPherson, Kathryn. *Bedside Matters: The Transformation of Canadian Nursing, 1900-1990.* Toronto: Oxford University Press, 1996.

—. "'The Case of the Kissing Nurse': Femininity, Sexuality, and Canadian Nursing, 1900-1970." In *Gendered Pasts: Historical Essays in Femininity and Masculinity in Canada,* ed. Kathryn McPherson, Cecelia Morgan, and Nancy M. Forestell, 179-98. Toronto: Oxford University Press, 1999.

—. "Carving Out a Past: The Canadian Nurses' Association War Memorial." *Histoire sociale/Social History* 29, 58 (1996): 417-29.

—. "Science and Technique: Nurses' Work in a Canadian Hospital, 1920-1939." In *Caring and Curing: Historical Perspectives on Women and Healing in Canada,* ed. Dianne Dodd and Deborah Gorham, 71-101. Ottawa: University of Ottawa Press, 1994.

—. "Women's Studies and Women's History." *Atlantis* 25, 1 (2000): 144-47.

Mecca, Jo-Anne. "'Neither Fish, Flesh, nor Fowl': The World War I Army Nurse." *Minerva: Quarterly Report on Women and the Military* 13, 2 (1995): 1-19.

Melosh, Barbara. *"The Physician's Hand": Work, Culture and Conflict in American Nursing.* Philadelphia: Temple University Press, 1982.

Meyer, Leisa D. *Creating G.I. Jane: Sexuality and Power in the Women's Army Corps during World War II.* New York: Columbia University Press, 1996.

Morton, Desmond. *A Military History of Canada.* 3rd ed. Toronto: McClelland and Stewart, 1992.

—. *A Peculiar Kind of Politics: Canada's Overseas Ministry in the First World War.* Toronto: University of Toronto Press, 1982.

Morton, Desmond, and Glenn Wright. *Winning the Second Battle: Canadian Veterans and the Return to Civilian Life, 1915-1930.* Toronto: University of Toronto Press 1987.

Neary, Peter, and J.L. Granatstein, eds. *The Veteran's Charter and Post-World War II Canada.* Montreal and Kingston: McGill-Queen's University Press, 1998.

Newell, M. Leslie. "'Led by the Spirit of Humanity': Canadian Military Nursing, 1914-1929." MA thesis, University of Ottawa, 1996.

Nicholls, T.B. *Organization, Strategy and Tactics of the Army Medical Services in War.* London: Baillière, Tindall and Cox, 1945.

Nicholson, G.W.L. *Canada's Nursing Sisters.* Toronto: Samuel Stevens Hakkert, 1975.

—. *Official History of the Canadian Army in the Second World War*. Volume 2. *The Canadians in Italy, 1943-1945*. Ottawa: Queen's Printer, 1957.

—. *Seventy Years of Service: A History of the R.C.A.M.C.*. Ottawa: Borealis Press, 1977.

Norman, Elizabeth M. "How Did They All Survive? An Analysis of American Nurses' Experiences in Japanese Prisoner-of-War Camps." *Nursing History Review* 3 (1995): 105-27.

—. *We Band of Angels: The Untold Story of American Nurses Trapped on Bataan by the Japanese*. New York: Random House, 1999.

—. *Women at War: The Story of Fifty Military Nurses Who Served in Vietnam*. Philadelphia: University of Philadelphia Press, 1990.

Norman, Elizabeth M., and Sharon Elfried. "The Angels of Bataan." *Image: The Journal of Nursing Scholarship* 25, 2 (1993): 121-26.

Nurses on the Battlefield. Lori Kuffner and Barbara Campbell, Cooper Rock Pictures, 2001.

Nursing Sisters' Association of Canada. *Nursing Sisters' Association of Canada: Commemorative Issue and Membership Directory*. Edmonton: Nursing Sisters' Association of Canada, June 1994.

Royal Canadian Army Medical Corps. *Pay and Allowance Regulations for the Canadian Army, 1946*. Ottawa: King's Printer, 1946.

Penfield, Wilder. *Canadian Army Manual of Military Neurosurgery*. Ottawa: Department of National Defence, 1941.

Pickstone, John V., ed. *Medical Innovations in Historical Perspective*. Manchester: Macmillan, 1992.

Pierson, Ruth Roach. "Beautiful Soul or Just Warrior: Gender and War." *Gender and History* 1, 1 (1989): 77-86.

—. *Canadian Women and the Second World War*. Historical monograph no. 37. Ottawa: Canadian Historical Association, 1983.

—. *"They're Still Women after All": The Second World War and Canadian Womanhood*. Toronto: McClelland and Stewart, 1986.

—. "Women's Emancipation and the Recruitment of Women into the Labour Force in World War II." In *The Neglected Majority: Essays in Canadian Women's History*, ed. Susan Mann Trofimenkoff and Alison Prentice, 125-45. Toronto: McClelland and Stewart, 1977.

Piggott, Juliet. *Queen Alexandra's Royal Army Nursing Corps*. London: Leo Cooper, 1975.

Porter, Roy. "Before the Fringe: 'Quackery' and the Eighteenth-Century Medical Market." In *Studies in the History of Alternative Medicine*, ed. Roger Cooter, 1-27. Basingstoke: Macmillan in association with St Antony's College Oxford, 1988.

—. *The Greatest Benefit to Mankind: A Medical History of Humanity*. New York: W.W. Norton, 1997.

Portugal, Jean E., ed. *We Were There: The Navy, the Army, and the RCAF: A Record for Canada*. 7 vols. Shelburne, ON: Battered Silicon Dispatch Box, 1998.

Quiney, Linda J. "Assistant Angels: Canadian Voluntary Aid Detachment Nurses in the Great War." *Canadian Bulletin of Medical History* 15, 1 (1998): 189-206.

—. "'Sharing the Halo': Social and Professional Tensions in the Work of World War I, Canadian Volunteer Nurses." *Journal of the Canadian Historical Association*, 8 (1998): 105-24.

—. "'Tradition and Transformation': Recent Scholarship in Canadian Nursing History." *Journal of Canadian Studies* 34, 3 (1999): 282-91.

Rawling, Bill. *Death Their Enemy: Canadian Medical Practitioners and War*. Ottawa: author, 2001.

—. "Providing the Gift of Life: Canadian Medical Practitioners and the Treatment of Shock on the Battlefield." *Canadian Military History* 10, 1 (2001): 7-20.

Reverby, Susan M. *Ordered to Care: The Dilemma of American Nursing, 1850-1945*. New York: Cambridge University Press, 1987.

Richards, Stanley T. *Operation Sick Bay*. West Vancouver, BC: Cantaur Publishing, 1994.

Robb, Isabel Hampton. *Nursing: Its Principles and Practice for Hospital and Private Use*. 3rd ed. Toronto: J.F. Hartz, 1914.

Roberts, Julia. "British Nurses at War, 1914-1918: Ancillary Personnel and the Battle for Registration." *Nursing Research* 45, 3 (1996): 167-72.

Roberts, Leslie. *There Shall be Wings: A History of the Royal Canadian Air Force*. Toronto: Clarke, Irwin, 1959.

Roland, Alex. "Technology and War: The Historiographical Revolution of the 1980s." *Technology and Culture* 34, 1 (1993): 117-35.

Roland, Charles G. *Long Night's Journey into Day: Prisoners of War in Hong Kong and Japan, 1941-1945*. Waterloo, ON: Wilfrid Laurier University Press, 2001.

—. "Massacre and Rape in Hong Kong: Two Case Studies Involving Medical Personnel and Patients."

Journal of Contemporary History 32, 1 (1997): 43-61.

Rose, Sonya O. "Race, Empire and British Wartime National Identity, 1939-1945." *Historical Research* 74, 184 (2001): 220-37.

Rosenberg, Charles E. *The Care of Strangers: The Rise of America's Hospital System.* New York: Basic Books, 1987.

Rosenberg, Nathan, Annetine C. Gelijns, and Holly Dawkins, eds. *Sources of Medical Technology: Universities and Industry.* Washington, DC: National Academy Press, 1995.

Royal Army Medical Corps. *Training Pamphlet No. 3.* Canada: King's Printer, 1944.

Royal Canadian Army Medical Corps. *Field Service Pocket Book, Part II.* Pamphlet No. 6 Administration. Canada: King's Printer, 1944.

—. *King's Regulations and Orders for the Canadian Militia, 1939.* Ottawa: King's Printer, 1939.

—. *Notes for Nursing Instructors and Nursing Procedures for Use in Military Hospitals R.C.A.M.C. 1943 (Provisional)* HQ 54-27-35-30, vol. 2.

Sage, W.D.M. *Battlefield Nurse: Letters and Memories of a Canadian Army Overseas Nursing Sister in World War II.* Vancouver: Sage Family Publications, 1994.

Sandelowski, Margarete. *Devices and Desires: Gender, Technology, and American Nursing.* Chapel Hill: University of North Carolina Press, 2000.

Sarnecky, Mary T. *A History of the U.S. Army Nurse Corps.* Philadelphia: University of Pennsylvania Press, 1999.

—. "Nurses at Pearl Harbor: The Real Story ..." *Reflections on Nursing Leadership,* Fourth Quarter (2001): 16-20.

—. "Nursing in the American Army from the Revolution to the Spanish-American War." *Nursing History Review* 5 (1997): 49-69.

Schneider, William H. "Blood Transfusion in Peace and War, 1900-1918." *Social History of Medicine* 10, 1 (1997): 105-26.

Sheehan, John C. *The Enchanted Ring: The Untold Story of Penicillin.* Cambridge, MA: MIT Press, 1982.

Sheffield, R. Scott. "'Of Pure European Descent and of the White Race': Recruitment Policy and Aboriginal Canadians, 1939-1945." *Canadian Military History* 5, 1 (1996): 8-15.

Smith, Angela K. *The Second Battlefield: Women, Modernism and the First World War.* Manchester: Manchester University Press, 2000.

Snell, James G. *The Citizen's Wage: The State and the Elderly in Canada, 1900-1951.* Toronto: University of Toronto, 1996.

Stacey, C.P. *Official History of the Canadian Army in the Second World War.* Volume 1. *Six Years of War: The Army in Canada, Britain and the Pacific.* Ottawa: Queen's Printer, 1955.

—. *Official History of the Canadian Army in the Second World War.* Volume 3. *The Victory Campaign: The Operations in North-West Europe, 1944-1945.* Ottawa: Queen's Printer, 1960.

Starns, Penny. *March of the Matrons: Military Influence on the British Civilian Nursing Profession, 1939-1969.* Peterborough, UK: DSM, 2000.

—. *Nurses at War: Women on the Frontline, 1939-45.* Stroud, Gloucestershire: Sutton Publishing, 2000.

Stevens, Susan Y. "Sale of the Century: Images of Nursing in the Movietonews during World War II." *Advances in Nursing Science* 12, 4 (1990): 44-52.

Stewart, Irvin. *Organizing Scientific Research for War: The Administrative History of the Office of Scientific Research and Development.* Boston: Little, Brown, 1948.

Strauss, Anselm, Shizuko Fagerhaugh, Barbara Suczek, and Carolyn Wiener, eds. *Social Organization of Medical Work.* Chicago: University of Chicago Press, 1985.

Strong-Boag, Veronica. *The New Day Recalled: Lives of Girls and Women in English Canada, 1919-1939.* Toronto: Copp Clark Pitman, 1988.

Struthers, James. *The Limits of Affluence: Welfare in Ontario, 1920-1970.* Toronto: University of Toronto Press, 1994.

—. *No Fault of Their Own: Unemployment and the Canadian Welfare State, 1914-1941.* Toronto: University of Toronto Press, 1983.

—. "Welfare to Workfare: Poverty and the 'Dependency Debate' in Post-Second World War Ontario." In *Ontario since Confederation: A Reader,* ed. Edgar-André Montigny and Lori Chambers, 429-53. Toronto: University of Toronto Press, 2000.

Stuart, Meryn. "Seeking Stability in the Midst of Change." In *Nurses of All Nations: A History of the International Council of Nurses, 1899-1999,* ed. Barbara L. Brush and Joan E. Lynaugh, 71-110.

Philadelphia: Lippincott, 1999.

—. "Ideology and Experience: Public Health Nursing and the Ontario Rural Child Welfare Project, 1920-1925." *Canadian Bulletin of Medical History* 6 (1989): 111-31.

—. "Shifting Professional Boundaries: Gender Conflict in Public Health, 1920-1925." In *Caring and Curing: Historical Perspectives on Women and Healing in Canada*, ed. Dianne Dodd and Deborah Gorham. Ottawa: University of Ottawa Press, 1994.

—. "War and Peace: Professional Identities and Nurses' Training, 1914-1930." In *Challenging Professions: Historical and Contemporary Perspectives on Women's Professional Work*, ed. Elizabeth Smyth, Sandra Acker, Paula Bourne, and Alison Prentice, 171-93. Toronto: University of Toronto Press, 1999.

Summers, Anne. *Angels and Citizens: British Women as Military Nurses, 1854-1914*. London and New York: Routledge, 1988.

Tallentire, Jenéa. "Strategies of Memory: History, Social Memory, and the Community." *Histoire sociale/ Social History* 34, 67 (Spring 2001): 197-212.

Taylor, Eric. *Front-line Nurse: British Nurses in World War II*. London: R. Hale, 1997.

Thompson, E.P. *The Making of the English Working Class*. New York: Pantheon Books, 1963.

Thompson, John Herd, with Allen Seager. *Canada, 1922-1939: Decades of Discord*. Toronto: McClelland and Stewart, 1985.

Thompson, Paul. *The Voices of the Past: Oral History*. Oxford: Oxford University Press, 1978.

Tice, J.W. "Medical Problems in the RCAF." *Aviation Medicine* (February 1943): 4-9.

Tice, J.W., and J.A. Jones. "The RCAF 35 Bed Hospital." *Canadian Hospital* 20, 12 (1943): 20-22.

Tidy, Henry Letheby, and J.M. Browne Kutschback, eds. *Inter-allied Conferences on War Medicine, 1942-1945: Convened by the Royal Society of Medicine*. London: Staples Press, 1947.

Tipliski, Veryl Margaret. "Parting at the Crossroads: The Emergence of Education for Psychiatric Nursing in Three Canadian Provinces, 1909-1955." *Canadian Bulletin of Medical History*, 21, 2 (2004): 253-79.

Toman, Cynthia. "Blood Work: Canadian Nursing and Blood Transfusion, 1942-1990." *Nursing History Review* 9 (2001): 51-78.

—. "'Body Work': Nurses and the Delegation of Medical Technology at the Ottawa Civic Hospital, 1947-1972." *Scientia Canadensis*, 29, 2 (2006): 155-75.

—. "Frontlines and Frontiers: War as Legitimate Work for Nurses, 1939-1945." *Histoire sociale/Social History*, 40, 79 (May 2007): 45-75.

—. "'An Officer and a Lady': Shaping the Canadian Military Nurse, 1939-1945." In *Out of the Ivory Tower: Feminist Research for Social Change*, ed. Andrea Martinez and Meryn Stuart, 89-115. Toronto: Sumach Press, 2003

—. "'Trained brains are better than trained muscles': Scientific Management and Canadian Nursing, 1910-1939." *Nursing History Review* 11 (2003): 89-108.

Tomblin, Barbara Brooks. *G.I. Nightingales: The Army Nurse Corps in World War II*. Lexington: University Press of Kentucky, 1996.

Tunis, Barbara Logan. *In Caps and Gowns: The Story of the School for Graduate Nurses, McGill University, 1920-1964*. Montreal: McGill University Press, 1966.

Vance, Jonathan F. *Death So Noble: Memory, Meaning, and the First World War*. Vancouver: UBC Press, 1997.

Vickers, Jeanne. *Women and War*. Atlantic Highlands, NJ: Zed Books, 1993.

Walsh, John C., and Steven High. "Rethinking the Concept of Community." *Histoire sociale/Social History* 32, 64 (1999): 255-73.

Waters, Anna May. "Report by Miss Anna May Waters: Nurse with the Canadian Forces at Hong Kong, as Given on Board the SS *Gripsholm*, November 1943." *Canadian Military History* 10, 4 (2001): 51-58.

Watson, E.H.A. *History Ontario Red Cross, 1914-1946: The Story of Red Cross Activities in Ontario in World War I, in the Peacetime Period from 1919 to 1939 and of the Work of the Ontario Division in World War II*. Toronto: Ontario Division Red Cross, n.d.

Weir, George M. *Survey of Nursing Education in Canada*. Toronto: University of Toronto Press, 1932.

Wellman, Barry, and Barry Leighton. "Networks, Neighborhoods, and Communities: Approaches to the Study of the Community Question." *Urban Affairs Quarterly* 14, 3 (1979): 363-90.

Wetherell, Charles, Andrejs Plakans, and Barry Wellman. "Social Networks, Kinship, and Community in Eastern Europe." *Journal of Interdisciplinary History* 24, 4 (1994): 639-63.

White, Mary M. *Hello War, Goodbye Sanity*. N.p.: New Leaf, 1992.

Winter, Jay. *Sites of Memory, Sites of Mourning: The Great War in European Cultural History*. New York:

Cambridge University Press, 1995.

Wright, Harold M. *Salute to the Air Force Medical Branch on the 75th Anniversary, Royal Canadian Air Force.* Ottawa: author, 1999.

Ziegler, Mary. *We Serve That Men May Fly: The Story of the Women's Division Royal Canadian Air Force.* Hamilton, ON: R.C.A.F. (W.D.) Association, 1973.

Index

Fund, 195-96; nurses' private memories
and accounts, 198; nurses' war memorials
and tributes, 191-92, 195-98; nursing sisters'
memorials, First vs Second World War, 191-92;
nursing sisters' participation with men's
commemorations, 194-95; portrayals of nursing
sisters in 1940s, 192-93; purpose, 190; social
memory, relationship with, 190-91; symbolic
community, relationship with, 190-91. *See also*
collective social memory; symbolic community
community, 169, 176-78. *See also*
symbolic community
comportment of nurses: as both officers and
ladies, 92-94, 99-100, 116; fraternization with
enlisted men to be avoided, 102, 115; gender-
and class-based regulations and policies, 12,
93; lady-like behaviour, expectation of, 100-3,
101(p), 114-16; marriage as career-limiting
move, 113; nurses' required presence at social
events, 102-3; pregnancy, 113-14; sexuality
issues, 114-16; wearing of trousers, 107-8
Concordia University Oral History Project, 198
Connaught Laboratories, 127
conscription, 5, 20-21
Cook, Tim, 9
Cooper, Frances, NS, 76(t)
Cowan, Marjorie, NS, 97
Cox, Pauline, NS: on adjusting to postwar life,
159, 171; on adverse conditions in military
nursing, 80-81; on availability of female
clothing, 109; biographical profile, 208;
on improvisation by nurses, 138; learning
from other nurses, 122; on military nurse
community postwar, 175; sinking of ship and
rescue, 77-78, 77(p); on triage and evacuation,
141; on Trueta method of wound care, 136

dangers of military nursing: adverse weather,
80; bombing, strafing, and accidents,
79-80; deaths on active duty, 75-76, 76(t);
on hospital ships, 80; mental and physical
toll, 84-86; military precautions regarding
nurses' safety, 83-84; military's control
of public perception, 11, 72-75, 200-1;
occupational hazards, 80-81; prisoners of
war, 81-83; silence regarding dangers, 72-75,
79-80, 87, 192, 204; travel during wartime,
76-78; Victory Bond poster portrayal, 192-93;
women "supposed to be protected," 79, 200
DDT use, 81
Dean, Elizabeth, NS/Dietician: biographical
profile, 208; on military nurse community,
174; on nurses' uniform, 104; on-call
experience for nursing emergencies,
36; on relationships with nurses, 183
Defence Scheme No. 3 (1938), 29, 55

demobilization: careers and activities after war,
12, 156-60; civilian nursing not appealing,
156-59, 163-64, 166, 202; demobilization of
nurses, 12, 183-84; education allowances
postwar, 88-89, 158, 163; lack of welcome
home, 186-87; military nurses remaining
in nursing postwar, 161-64; military's lack
of concern over nurses' future careers,
87-91; nurses as expendable workforce,
52, 87-91; official discharge orders, 89-90;
postwar quota for military nurses, 88, 156;
re-establishment credits, 88-89; stereotypical
assumptions regarding nurses' future role,
87-91, 157-58; veterans' benefits, men vs
women, 87, 88-90; war service gratuity, 88-89
demographic profile of military nurses: age,
38-39, 110-12, 204; class, 47-50; comparison
with nurses of other countries, 50-51;
economic status, 39; education, 38-39, 40-41,
121; experience when enlisting, 40, 204;
female profession, 41-42; language, 46-47;
marriage bar, 42-44; province where enlisted,
40; race and ethnicity, 44-46; religion, 47
Dempsey, Lotta, 74, 87, 94, 188
Department of Veterans Affairs: on
ambition of military nurses postwar,
161-62; stereotypical assumptions regarding
nurses' future role, 87-88, 90-91, 157-58
Depression: attraction of military nursing, 11,
13-14, 18, 39, 92, 200; civilian nursing during,
13-16, 39; male-focused assistance, 14
DeVere, M.N., NS, 54(p)
Dick, Edith, Matron, 75
Dickey, Kathleen, NS, 93
Donnacona (RCN medical unit), 61
Donovan, Rita, NS, 147
Doree, Joan, NS, 70-71, 122, 145-46
Dorgan, Jean, NS, 65
dressings for wounds, 134-36, 145(p)
duration of service: marriage as career-limiting
move, 113; nurses' service, 5, 11, 166-67, 200,
201; recall of older nurses near war's end, 111-12

education: area of contention among military
nurses, 183; demographic profile of military
nurses, 38-39, 40-41, 121; education allowances
postwar, 88-89, 158, 163; education for military
nurses postwar, 158, 162-63, 203; enlistment
requirements and First Nations abilities, 45;
postgraduate courses after nurses' training, 41
education allowances, 88-89, 158, 162-63
Ellis, Kathleen, 26, 28, 35
Elshtain, Jean, 8
enlistment: applications, 27-28, 30(t);
appointments, 32(t); attraction of military
nursing, 11, 13-14, 18, 39, 92; availability of

Canadian nurses, 29(t); changing needs over course of war, 29, 31-33; concerns over civilian nursing shortage, 11, 18, 22-23, 25, 26, 28-29; eligibility requirements, 21-22, 38; impact on civilian hospitals, 53-54; lists of available nurses circumvented, 22-24; oversubscription, 4-5, 19, 20, 23, 27-28, 30(t); proportional representation, 23, 55; race and ethnicity issues, 3, 21; selection of "right" kind of nurse, 20-25, 200. *See also* demographic profile of military nurses
Enloe, Cynthia, 7, 18
ethnicity, 21, 44-46
evacuation and triage, 63-64, 139-42

Farries, Anne, NS, 113, 152
Feasby, W.R., 64-65, 137
Fellowes, Rae, Matron, 153
femininity: "femaleness" allegedly main contribution of nurses, 64, 100-2; gendered construction of, 21, 92-94, 107-8, 113, 201; gendered officer rank of nurses, 94-96; intersecting masculine and feminine identities of nurses, 92-94; military's control of public perception of nurses' femininity, 11, 57, 72-75, 103-5, 200-1; nurses' required presence at social events, 102-3; nursing as ideal postwar profession, 90-91; saluting issue, 96-97; sexuality issues, 114-16; stereotypical view of nurses, 5, 8, 41-42, 80, 87, 170, 192-93; uniforms of nursing sisters, 94, 103-10, 111(p); wartime service as threat to, 12; wearing of trousers, 107-8; while climbing rope ladders, 80
Ferguson, Frances, NS: biographical profile, 208-9; care of burn patients, 147-48; military service highlight of life, 184; on need for medical assistants postwar, 164; on saluting as masculine behaviour, 97; on use of technology, 129; on work of medical orderlies, 70; on workload at casualty clearing stations, 69-70
field ambulances, 63
field dressing stations, 63, 64
field surgical units, 10, 57, 63-65
field transfusion units, 64, 127
Fieldhouse, Norma, NS, 173
First Nations peoples, 21, 44-45
First World War: commemoration of nursing sisters, 191-92; conscription, 20; literature on women's contribution to war effort, 6-7; loss of civilian medical personnel to military, 22-23, 53-54. *See also* military nurses (First World War)
Fitzgerald, Gladys, NS, 76(t)
Fleming, Alexander, 130
Fletcher, Margaret, NS: on abdominal wound care, 136-37; on blood transfusions, 129; on

civilian patients, 68; on east-west rivalries of nurses, 180; on loss of male friendships postwar, 116; on nurse exchanges, 123; on official silence re dangers, 74; on penicillin, 131; on rank and relationship with patients, 94; resentment regarding postings, 182-83; on returning to civilian life, 185, 187; on sexuality issues, 114-15; on treatment of POWs, 86-87
Florey, Howard, 131
French-Canadian nurses, 21, 46

Gair, Anne, NS, 185
Gannon, Frances, NS, 76(t)
gender: all women in forces listed as nurses (pre-1941), 35; ambivalence regarding nurses as soldiers, 5, 74, 100, 201, 202; assignment of duties and, 125-33, 200; comportment of nurses (*see* comportment of nurses); danger to nurses (*see* dangers of military nursing); Depression assistance male focused, 14; female military nurses only, 21, 42; "gender bending," 106-8, 126, 201; gendered officer rank of nurses, 94-96; marriage as career-limiting move, 113; masculine environment of military, 4, 5, 21, 52; nurses' rank and relationship with physicians, 99; nursing as almost exclusively female profession, 41-42, 93; pregnancy and termination of military career, 113-14; role in shaping social memory, 170; sexuality issues, 114-16; social expectations regarding masculinity and femininity, 92-94, 107-8, 113, 201; war as "gendering activity," 7-8. *See also* femininity; masculinity; military nurses as soldiers
Geneva Convention, 5, 82, 204
Gibbon, John Murray, 193
Gilday, Lorne, 164
Giroux, Suzanne, Matron, 26, 181
Glew, Mabel, NS, 184
Gordon, Molly, NS, 81
grafts, pedicle, 146(p), 147
Grainger, Dorothy, NS, 15, 156
Grayzel, Susan, 7

Hall, G.R., 61(p)
Harmer, Bertha, 135
Henderson, Irene, NS, 113
Hendricks, "Freddie," NS, 173(p)
Herringer, Betty, NS, 85
Higonnet, Margaret, 7, 8
Hillman, Muriel, NS, 86(p)
Hine, Darlene Clark, 44
HMCS *Conestoga*, 61
HMCS *Naden*, 61
HMCS *Niobe*, 33, 36, 61, 148
HMCS *Stadacona*, 61

Studies in Canadian Military History

John Griffith Armstrong, *The Halifax Explosion and the Royal Canadian Navy: Inquiry and Intrigue*

Andrew Richter, *Avoiding Armageddon: Canadian Military Strategy and Nuclear Weapons, 1950-63*

William Johnston, *A War of Patrols: Canadian Army Operations in Korea*

Julian Gwyn, *Frigates and Foremasts: The North American Squadron in Nova Scotia Waters, 1745-1815*

Jeffrey A. Keshen, *Saints, Sinners, and Soldiers: Canada's Second World War*

Desmond Morton, *Fight or Pay: Soldiers' Families in the Great War*

Douglas E. Delaney, *The Soldiers' General: Bert Hoffmeister at War*

Michael Whitby, ed., *Commanding Canadians: The Second World War Diaries of A.F.C. Layard*

Martin Auger, *Prisoners of the Home Front: German POWs and "Enemy Aliens" in Southern Quebec, 1940-46*

Tim Cook, *Clio's Warriors: Canadian Historians and the Writing of the World Wars*

Serge Marc Durflinger, *Fighting from Home: The Second World War in Verdun, Quebec*

Richard O. Mayne, *Betrayed: Scandal, Politics, and Canadian Naval Leadership*

P. Whitney Lackenbauer, *Battle Grounds: The Canadian Military and Aboriginal Lands*

Cynthia Toman, *An Officer and a Lady: Canadian Military Nursing and the Second World War*